Mental Wellness
in **Adults** with
Down Syndrome

Mental Wellness in **Adults** with **Down Syndrome**

A Guide to Emotional and Behavioral Strengths and Challenges

Dennis McGuire, Ph.D. & Brian Chicoine, M.D.

Woodbine House ◆ 2006

Front cover photo courtesy of Jackie Dodson.
Back cover photo courtesy of Lynn Hoffman-Brouse.

All rights reserved under International and Pan American Copyright Conventions. Published in the United States of America by Woodbine House, Inc., 6510 Bells Mill Rd., Bethesda, MD 20817. 800-843-7323. www.woodbinehouse.com

Publisher's note: The information contained in this book is not intended as a substitute for consultation with your child's healthcare providers. Although the authors, editor, and publisher made every attempt to ensure that the information in this book was up to date and accurate at the time of publication, recommended treatments and drug therapies may change as new medical or scientific information becomes available. Additionally, the authors, editor, and publisher are not responsible for errors or omissions or for consequences from application of this book. Any practice described in this book should be applied by the reader in close consultation with a qualified physician.

Library of Congress Cataloging-in-Publication Data

McGuire, Dennis Eugene.
  Mental wellness in adults with Down syndrome : a guide to emotional and behavioral strengths and challenges / Dennis McGuire and Brian Chicoine. -- 1st ed.
      p. cm.
  Includes bibliographical references and index.
  ISBN-13: 978-1-890627-65-2
  ISBN-10: 1-890627-65-8
  1. Down syndrome. I. Chicoine, Brian. II. Title.
  RC571.M354 2006
  616.85'8842--dc22

                                                                          2006009504

Printed in the United States of America

First edition

10   9   8   7   6   5   4   3   2

Table of Contents

Acknowledgements vii

Introduction xi

SECTION 1: ASSESSMENT

Chapter 1   Mental Health Assessment.. 1

Chapter 2   Assessing the Physical/Mental Health Connection.......................... 9

SECTION 2: ISSUES IN PROMOTING AND ADDRESSING MENTAL HEALTH IN ADULTS WITH DOWN SYNDROME

Chapter 3   Family and Community Support 29

Chapter 4   What is Normal?: Understanding "Normal," "Usual," and "Common" Behavior in People with Down Syndrome 45

Chapter 5   Memory...65

Chapter 6   Communication Skills 85

Chapter 7   Self-esteem and Self-image..105

Chapter 8   Self-talk, Imaginary Friends, and Fantasy Life 137

Chapter 9   The Groove and Flexibility... 147

Chapter 10 Life Span Issues: "Teenage Behavior," Isolation, Withdrawal, Retirement 169

Section 3: Mental Illness

Chapter 11   Mental Illness and Its Precipitants 187

Chapter 12   Assessment of Mental Illness 205

Chapter 13   Treatment Approaches for Mental Illness 211

Chapter 14   Mood Disorders 255

Chapter 15   Anxiety Disorders 277

Chapter 16   Obsessive-Compulsive Disorder 291

Chapter 17   Psychotic Disorders 309

Chapter 18   Eating Refusal 315

Chapter 19   Challenging Behavior 323

Chapter 20   Self-injurious Behavior 349

Chaper 21   Tic Disorders and Repetitive Movements 357

Chapter 22   Autism 373

Chapter 23   Alzheimer Disease 385

Addendum 1   Medication Table 401

Addendum 2   Consent Form 414

References.. 415

Index... 421

Acknowledgements

We want to thank our patients with Down syndrome who have graciously let us into their world, and what an interesting world it is (as we will explain in this book). When you see people who are as genuine and caring as people with Down syndrome, you cannot help but be affected by them. We also give a very special thanks to their families. They are the true experts on Down syndrome and they have been extremely open and supportive of our efforts to learn more about the issues and challenges facing people with Down syndrome.

We cannot understate the importance of the support we receive from our parent organization, Advocate Health Care, James H. Skogsbergh, MD, President and CEO; Advocate Lutheran General Hospital, Bruce C. Campbell, Dr.P.H, President; our practice group, Advocate Medical Group, Debra Geisler, CEO; by Ron Ferguson, MD, Chairman of Family Medicine, and by Vice Presidents John Perrone and Nancy Christie, who are Directors of our program.

We have also benefited greatly from the support of the Advocate Charitable Foundation staff and of our own advisory group made up of leaders and concerned individuals from the community at large and the Down syndrome community.

We also want to acknowledge our exceptional colleagues and staff at the Center. They have shared the dream and passion to serve and learn more about our patients and they have been there to make our job so much easier. Present colleagues and staff include Janet Bilodeau, CNP, Nurse Practitioner; Laura Iatropoulos, Practice Manager; Fernando Serrano, Certified Medical Assistant; Jenny Howard-Lobough and Nancy Geary, Support and Advocacy; Shirley Lange, Patient Representative; Carol Jacobsen, Transcriptionist; and Eileen Walsh, RD, Nutritionist. *We would also like to acknowledge colleagues and staff who have worked with us in the past, including Steffi Gratigny, MD, Julie Shapiro, MD, Donna Mirro, Nancy Halligan, Karen Cornell, Mary Sue Minkus, and Sharon Giannone.* We also thank our dedicated volunteers who give their time and talent to the Center, including Catherine Chicoine, Pat Brandt, Pat Lasch, and Audrey

Kupsco. Thanks also to Judith Gravdal, who is the Family Medicine Residency Director, for editing assistance.

We have been extremely fortunate to be able to refer to specialists in the Advocate Medical Group and the Hospital who have treated our patients with great respect and dignity. We have also been fortunate to have met many skilled professionals from around the country and the world at national conferences and at the Down Syndrome Medical Interest Group meetings. These people have encouraged and stimulated us, and the meetings have been fertile ground for the discussion of problems and issues encountered in our clinical work.

Finally, there would not be a Center and this book would not exist without the vision, determination, and support of our partner, The National Association for Down Syndrome (NADS). We would like to especially thank Sheila Hebein, the Executive Director of this group, who has been the driving force behind the Center. Not only is she a superb advocate for people with Down syndrome, but she has also been a wonderful mentor to us. May we continue to be blessed by people like her and by the people with Down syndrome, their families, by our administration, staff and volunteers, colleagues, and families from around the country and so many others who have supported our work at the Center.

We also need to acknowledge several people who have been instrumental in the development of this book.

Our sincere thanks goes to our editor, Sue Stokes, at Woodbine House. She has been superb at guiding, editing, questioning, challenging, and encouraging us throughout the entire process. She has helped us to think and to clarify our writing. As a result, the book is so much more than we would have ever hoped.

We would also like to thank Joan Medlen, RD, the founder and editor of the excellent newsletter, *Disability Solutions,* and of the popular book, *The Down Syndrome Nutrition Handbook* (2004). She has published our material and has been very supportive of our work and the Center. We value her opinion, and her encouragement was helpful in our decision to write this book.

Dennis's personal acknowledgement:

I would like to thank my wife, Dr. Elina Manghi, and my son, Martin, for their enormous patience and tolerance through the many hours I have spent on weeknights and weekends absorbed in writing the book. I am proud to say that despite the time spent on the book, my son has been very encouraging of my work. He has also shown a level of maturity, compassion, and understanding in how he relates to people with Down syndrome which makes me very proud.

My wife, Elina, has also been very patient with me during this period, but in addition I need to acknowledge the benefit that I have gained from the depth and breadth of her knowledge and expertise as a psychologist in the field. She generously took time from her own work to read and to help with ideas and suggestions. She has been particularly helpful in sections of the book dealing with memory, testing, AD/HD, autism, and counseling, in which she has considerable experience and expertise. I am very fortunate that she not only encourages me but she also shares my passion for discovering more about people with Down syndrome.

Brian's personal acknowledgement:

I would like to thank the Family Medicine faculty who support and share patient-care responsibilities with me and who are truly colleague-friends: Ron Ferguson, Judith Gravdal, Stuart Goldman, Greg Kirschner, Don Novey, Bruce Perlow, Tamar Perlow, Bill Briner, Mayank Shah, and Robin O'Meara.

I would also like to thank my family, who teach me valuable lessons that guide me in serving people with Down syndrome:

- ◆ My father, who taught me about duty and honesty, two important ideals that live on in his children;
- ◆ My mother, who continues to teach about compassion and caring;
- ◆ My siblings, Mary Jo, David, Mark, Beth Ann, Mike, and Julie, with whom I continue to learn respect and appreciation for the many valuable ways we can share the gifts we are given and the lessons we have learned;
- ◆ My daughters, Emily, Caitlin, and Laura, who teach me about and share with me what is important in my life;
- ◆ My wife, Kathy, for her understanding and acceptance of me and others that opened my eyes to the possibility of caring for adults with Down syndrome long before it was even a consideration. Her love and encouragement are reflected in any positive contribution I am able to make.

Introduction

As you hold this rather large volume in your hands, you probably have a number of questions. Perhaps the most natural one
is, why is there so much to say about the subject? Is the mental health of adolescents
and adults with Down syndrome really such a complex matter that we need an ency-
clopedic guide? You might also wonder: Are mental health problems inevitable in all
people with Down syndrome? Will it be worth my while to read this book, even if the
individual(s) with Down syndrome I know seem to be perfectly healthy?

We would like to reassure you at the outset that mental health problems are *not*
inevitable in people with Down syndrome. That is one reason we wrote this book—
to point out ways that parents, adult siblings, teachers, paid caregivers, and others
can effectively promote and maintain mental wellness in adolescents and adults with
Down syndrome. But we also wrote this book because there are some biological differences as well as common environmental stresses that can make people with Down
syndrome more susceptible to mood, emotional, and other mental health problems.
We hoped to make it easier for other practitioners to recognize these problems and
pursue treatments that will help the person regain his normal abilities and outlook
on life. We also hoped to clarify that there are some common characteristics of Down
syndrome that can be mistaken for evidence of mental illness, but are nothing more
than harmless quirks or useful coping strategies.

Our goal is not just to educate parents and support people about these issues,
however. We would also like to help adults with Down syndrome actively participate
in the process of achieving good health. Health is more than the absence of disease.
It is a sense of physical, mental, and spiritual well being. It is a process that involves
health promotion, health screening, and early intervention for health problems. It is
reasonable for adults with Down syndrome and their families to assume that they can
(and should) be part of this process that leads to improved health. While there are
clearly physical and psychological problems that limit the health of some individuals

with Down syndrome, good health for most and improved health for all are reasonable expectations.

Many families have described how health problems of people with Down syndrome were ignored because the problem was assumed to be (or "written off" as being) "just part of the Down syndrome." In fact, people with Down syndrome are susceptible to many of the "usual" health problems that occur in people without Down syndrome. In addition, there are illnesses and conditions that are more common in people with Down syndrome. These problems may alter health and, therefore, cause a change in the status of the person. These changes are often not directly linked to the syndrome but to one of these conditions. While there is no proven treatment for Down syndrome itself, most often the additional health issues are diagnosable and treatable. Therefore, changes that are just assumed to be a manifestation of Down syndrome can lead to unnecessary impairment because of under-diagnosis or under-treatment of other conditions.

These ideas are true for both physical and mental health issues. The focus of this book will be on mental health issues. Physical health issues will be addressed as they relate to or affect mental health.

WHAT IS MENTAL HEALTH?

By "mental health," we mean having the emotional wellbeing that allows us to cope with the activities and stresses of everyday life. Mental health is more than just diagnosing and treating mental illness. It is part of each person's life: seeking to optimize our enjoyment, our sense of purpose, and our ability to participate in the activities of daily life. Mental health is a process. It can be optimized through mental health promotion strategies. These strategies are ideally part of daily living, as well as part of regular healthcare promotion with your healthcare provider.

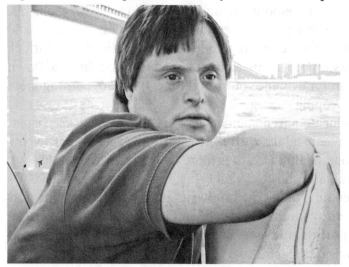

To promote mental health, it is imperative to understand the continuum of normal behavior and mental health issues. A behavior may be healthy and serve a useful purpose, but if it becomes excessive or impairs function, it may move along the continuum into the "abnormal range." While there are clear diagnostic guidelines for mental illness, there is certainly some degree of subjective interpretation of the symptoms. In addition, the environment in which the person lives, if supportive enough, may help prevent the behavior from becoming or from being labeled as maladaptive. Mental health promotion strategies can help emphasize the positive aspects of behavior and keep the behavior on the healthy side of the continuum.

As mentioned previously, it is important to understand that a change in behavior is often not "just the Down syndrome." Conversely, it is also critical to understand that there are typical strengths and weaknesses and common characteristics of people with Down syndrome. To optimally promote mental health in a person with Down syndrome, it is necessary to understand and appreciate both of these opposing concepts.

WHO WE ARE
◆ ◆ ◆ ◆ ◆ ◆ ◆ ◆ ◆ ◆ ◆ ◆ ◆ ◆ ◆ ◆

We, the authors, are the directors of the Adult Down Syndrome Center of Lutheran General Hospital in Park Ridge, Illinois. A little history of how we came to work at the Center should help you understand our perspective on mental health issues in adolescents and adults with Down syndrome.

In the late 1980s, parents in the Chicago metropolitan area were becoming increasingly frustrated by the lack of good quality medical and psychosocial care for their adult children with Down syndrome. Too often, these parents found that when their children with Down syndrome developed changes in behavior, healthcare professionals would tell them it was "just the Down syndrome" and there was no treatment. Another common concern was that any time a person with Down syndrome experienced a decline in cognitive function, a limited evaluation always seemed to lead to a diagnosis of Alzheimer disease. Families often felt that their son or daughter was not receiving a thorough evaluation. They wanted to be able to bring the person with Down syndrome to a place where he or she would get a thorough evaluation from practitioners who understood the medical and psychosocial issues of people with Down syndrome.

Many of these concerned parents belonged to The National Association for Down Syndrome (NADS), the oldest parent group serving people with Down syndrome in the United States. In 1991, the staff and parents of the group went to the administration of Lutheran General Hospital. They requested that a clinic for adults with Down syndrome be developed. It opened in 1992. Initially, patients were served two mornings a month. The original staff included a physician (the second author), Ph.D.-trained social worker (the first author), and a certified medical assistant. Dr. McGuire had been working with NADS through a fellowship they provided to the University of Illinois-Chicago where Dr. McGuire was employed. The clinic was a natural extension of his work because he realized that medical conditions often were part of the cause for the psychosocial problems he was addressing. Dr. Chicoine had recently joined the faculty in the Lutheran General Department of Family Medicine residency program. He had previous experience in working with adults with intellectual disabilities and eagerly helped develop the clinic. A nutritionist and an audiologist were also available to see the patients.

Today the Center has grown and is now open full-time. It is the result of a unique collaborative effort between The National Association for Down Syndrome, Advocate Medical Group, and Advocate Lutheran General Hospital. The staff includes a physician, nurse practitioner, Ph.D.-trained social worker, two certified medical assistants, clerical staff, outreach specialist, advocate, and research assistant. Nutrition and audiology services are also provided.

To date, the Adult Down Syndrome Center has served over 3000 patients, aged 12 to 83. The patients use the center in one of three ways: as their primary healthcare center; for an annual complete evaluation and regular follow-up for specific problems (most commonly for psychosocial issues); or for annual evaluations only. The patients who live furthest away are most commonly in the last group. They use the extensive report (that is completed for each patient after an annual evaluation) with their practitioners closer to home, with whom they follow up for their other healthcare needs. In all, between the physician, nurse practitioner, and social worker, we have over 5500 visits per year. We work as a team in treating patients, particularly when there are mental health concerns. This approach allows us to address all the issues that promote health (mental and physical) as well as contribute to mental or physical health problems.

This book is a compilation of the information we have gathered through serving adolescents and adults with Down syndrome and their families and care providers. We view the Adult Down Syndrome Center as a repository of knowledge. Through listening to people with Down syndrome and their families and care providers, we have learned much of what is written on these pages. When we heard something from one person, we asked others whether that was true for them as well. Through this process, we have developed a greater understanding of mental health and mental illness in people with Down syndrome.

"TWO SYNDROMES"

A word on the concept of "Two Syndromes" is important. Some families that include children or young adults with Down syndrome have heard us speak or have read a piece of material from us and have commented that it doesn't seem to fit with their life experience. Certainly some of this interpretation may be from the variance in people with Down syndrome and the variance in families. Some of it, however, may be because it sometimes seems as if there are "Two Syndromes." The childhood experience of families with older sons and daughters was often very different from that experienced by families now. In the past, based on the information provided by healthcare and education professionals, families often had very low expectations for their son or daughter. Good health care was often unavailable to children with Down syndrome. School, social, recreational, and work opportunities were often limited or nonexistent.

We now know that early intervention is very beneficial for children with Down syndrome (Anderson et al., 2003; Guralnick, 1998). The benefits of early intervention, as well as more inclusive and academically challenging school experiences, are being appreciated and enjoyed in childhood and early adulthood. As this generation of young people ages, it will be very interesting to see what the long-term benefits will be. Studies in the general population suggest that improved learning and educational opportunities may reduce cognitive decline and reduce the risk of Alzheimer disease (Snowdon, 2001; Levenson, 1978). What will be the effect on people with Down syndrome? Historically, impaired verbal and communication skills have had a great impact on both the physical and mental health of people with Down syndrome. Presumably, the improved skills being seen in many young people who have received speech therapy from a young age will affect their health in adulthood. The improved ability to report and discuss their concerns and to participate in treatment should reduce illness as well as lessen the severity of problems.

The concept of "Two Syndromes" is theoretical at this point. However, it will be very interesting to watch the differences in adults with Down syndrome who have had very different life experiences. It is also important to understand that we are also seeing the beneficial effect of these positive experiences for our older patients. In other words, it is not too late even if these opportunities were not available at a younger age. Good health care, work opportunities, and social opportunities have been very positive experiences for our older patients as well.

A WORD ABOUT THE CASE STORIES

Throughout this book you will find many case stories about adolescents or adults with Down syndrome we have seen. We have changed the names, and, in some cases, other identifying information to protect their identities, but their problems and solutions are real.

In addition, note that we sometimes refer to adolescents and adults with Down syndrome simply as "people" or "adults" for simplicity's sake, and will make it clear when we are using the word "people" to refer to individuals who do *not* have Down syndrome. In addition, at times for simplicity's sake, we will abbreviate Down syndrome as DS.

IN CONCLUSION

As you proceed through this book, we recommend keeping "Joe" in mind. Joe is both an example and a compilation of our healthy patients. Joe is 29 years old and is healthy, physically and mentally. What has helped Joe be healthy? What are the experiences that Joe has had that contributed to health?

- Joe is accepted as an individual.
- He is given choices.
- Expectations are placed on him that are neither too low or too high.
- Joe regularly exercises.
- His need for routine is supported, but flexibility is encouraged.
- Joe gets annual health evaluations and good health care at other times when needed.
- Communication skills were emphasized from a young age.
- Vocational training was part of his schooling.
- He has an enjoyable, stimulating job that allows him to use his strengths.
- He is part of a supportive community.
- He has opportunities to help others.
- He participates in his religious community.
- He has opportunities to be integrated in society (with people without disabilities) but also has opportunities to congregate with other people with disabilities.
- And Joe is heard. When he expresses concerns, people listen.

Joe has taken these opportunities and works very well in his job and has an enjoyable social and family life. In short, Joe is healthy. Our hope is that by sharing the information in this book, we can help all adults with Down syndrome be healthy, like Joe.

Chapter **1**

Mental Health

. . . .

Assessment

. . . .

The evaluation of a person with Down syndrome (DS) for mental health issues should not begin when there is a problem. Where physical health is concerned, it is well recognized that health promotion, disease prevention, and early assessment of disease are essential to optimize health and limit illness. Similarly, mental health promotion, prevention of mental illness, and early assessment of mental illness are essential parts of mental health care. Educating people with DS, their families, and care providers about ways to optimize mental health is an important part of the process.

Even if an adolescent or adult with Down syndrome does not seem to have any mental health problems, it is very useful to assess the aspects of his life that can promote mental health, or, conversely, increase the likelihood of mental illness. Understanding a person's support system, his connection to friends, the activities available to him, his community involvement, and other aspects of his life help develop a picture of the person and can help provide guidance in ways to optimize mental health.

We recommend that our patients at the Adult Down Syndrome Center see us annually for a comprehensive mental health assessment starting in adolescence and throughout the adult years.

Of course, if the adult with Down syndrome experiences changes in mental health or behavior, he should have a thorough assessment as soon as possible. A complete evaluation of his physical health status will also often provide a great deal of insight into the cause of the problem.

In *To Kill a Mockingbird,* Atticus Finch stated, "You never really understand a man until you stand in his shoes and walk around in them." At the Adult Down Syndrome Center, our assessment is designed to do this as best as we can. While we will never be able to understand all that it means to be a person with Down syndrome, our assessment is designed to maximize our understanding. The goals of the assessment include:

- understanding a person's strengths and weaknesses;
- appreciating the positive and negative aspects of the environment where he lives;
- assessing the contribution of physical health challenges; and
- discerning how the person deals with stresses in life.

If an adult with Down syndrome has experienced a change in his mental health status or there is a behavioral concern, the assessment is similar. It is important to understand his strengths and the supportive aspects of the environment. Those will be important issues to emphasize in developing a health-promoting treatment plan. In addition, we focus particularly on the areas that may be contributing to the problem so that these can be understood and addressed.

In the course of assessing these issues, we typically evaluate:

- the relationship between social health and mental health;
- expressive language skills;
- self-esteem;
- self-talk;
- cognitive issues, including the need for repetition, processing speed, understanding of time, and abstract thinking abilities;
- range of emotions;
- the presence of factors that could precipitate mental illness;
- symptoms of mental illness (if any); and
- physical health.

These areas are discussed in detail below.

WHERE TO GET AN EVALUATION

Of course, it is not practical or possible for all adults with Down syndrome to be evaluated at our Center (or another center serving adults with Down syndrome). In fact, the demand is so great, we generally have to restrict our practice to residents of Illinois. If you are seeking a mental health assessment elsewhere, it may be up to you to ensure that all of the above areas are evaluated as described in this chapter. Ideally, you will be able to take the person with DS to a comprehensive Down syndrome clinic where the staff understand these issues, and where professionals with different specialty areas work together to evaluate individuals with Down syndrome. Dr. Len Leshin has a web page that lists clinics for people with Down syndrome (www.ds-health.com).

If you are not able to visit a Down syndrome clinic, you may need to seek a series of assessments from a variety of professionals. You can then ask one of them to be the case manager and help you interpret what all the separate assessments mean. We have found that the combined efforts of the following professionals work very well:

- ◆ A medical doctor (family physician or internist), to rule out medical problems and to prescribe medications, if needed;
- ◆ A psychologist, social worker, or other professional qualified to assess social skill and support issues, as well as emotional/behavioral disturbances;
- ◆ A teacher, job coach, or counselor at a job site who can provide valuable information about the work or school environment, the person's behavior before the problem arose, and the problems the person may be experiencing outside the home.

In addition, a psychiatrist or a neurologist may be consulted, depending on the need.

AREAS ASSESSED

THE RELATIONSHIP BETWEEN SOCIAL HEALTH AND MENTAL HEALTH

> *"For anyone to receive unbidden words of encouragement, this is the material a true gift is made of."*
> —Christopher deVinck, ***The Power of the Powerless***

No one is generally able to achieve mental health completely independently. A sense of wellbeing usually requires a sense of connection to others. For instance, most of us need to feel that we are loved and accepted by others to feel really good about ourselves. This is just as true for people with Down syndrome. Because adolescents and adults with Down syndrome usually have a greater degree of dependence on others in most areas of life, their reliance on others to achieve mental health is not surprising.

However, the important contribution that friends and family provide is often overlooked as an important aspect of health for people with DS.

A number of years ago, a large state facility closed in Illinois. The adults with intellectual disabilities were moved to new, smaller residenc-

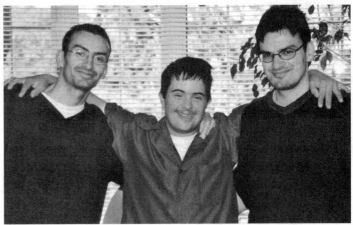

es. Some of the residents had very significant communication challenges. There was little obvious social interaction between these residents. To the observer's eye, they did not seem to rely on each other for social stimulation. When the residents were tracked over time, however, it was found that those who moved to a residence together with other people from the old facility did better than those who moved to separate facilities. This was true even for those who had very significant communication challenges. Even the survival rate was better for those who moved with their peers. Social interaction is part of our life-sustaining activity, even when it is not obvious to others (Heller, 1982).

People with Down syndrome need interaction with family, friends, peers, and others, just as other people do. The absence of any of these groups can be a significant problem. This can be true even if there never was any perceived interaction with the group, as discussed in the preceding paragraph.

Also important for mental health is meaningful participation in community life. Participating in activities, hobbies, and community events promotes a sense of wellbeing, boosts self-esteem, and helps a person develop and improve social skills. Physical activity, social events, travel, learning new ideas, and opportunities to interact with other people while doing these activities can all be beneficial. So too is employment in a job that the *person with Down syndrome* finds interesting and fulfilling. Chapter 3 describes in more detail why social connections are essential to the mental wellbeing of adults with Down syndrome.

In our Center, the social worker assesses the individual's social health. Information is gathered via a checklist of questions addressing family support, friendships, recreational opportunities, other support systems, the work or school environment, and other issues of daily life. Both the person with DS and his family answer the questions. If appropriate, staff of a residential facility or day program, teachers, and other important people in the person's life are also questioned.

In addition, each staff person in the Center is aware of his or her role in assessing a patient's social health. Often the person will reveal an important piece of information during a less formal part of the assessment. For example, as part of the "warming up" part of the interview, the physician asks, "What do you do for fun?" This part of the interview is less threatening, gives the person with DS an opportunity to "warm up" to the interview, and often reveals important information. The person with Down syndrome may also reveal important information pertaining to his social health to the receptionist, nurse, or others. This information is shared with other staff in the Center to optimize data gathering.

EXPRESSIVE LANGUAGE SKILLS

Another area to assess is the person's expressive language skills—that is, his or her ability to communicate a message to others using spoken language, gestures, or an augmentative or alternative method. The ability or inability to express oneself has a significant impact on promotion of mental health and prevention of mental illness.

At the Center, we do a basic, informal assessment of communication skills. We focus on articulation, intelligibility, and overall communication abilities. If additional assessment or treatment is needed, we refer the adult to a speech-language pathologist. We have found that 75 percent of our patients are understood by familiar others most of the time. Only 28 percent are understood by unfamiliar others most of the time. Clearly, intelligibility is important to assess.

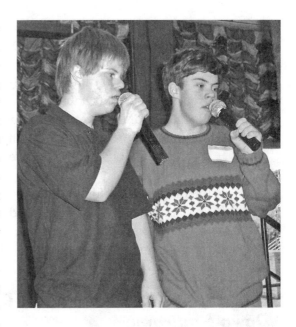

In addition to understanding verbal skills, it is essential to do a basic assessment of the adult's ability to express feelings. We also question the family about the adult's ability to express feelings. In our experience, most people with Down syndrome are open and honest in expressing feelings nonverbally, even though many have difficulty expressing feelings verbally. Unfortunately, we find that many caregivers have difficulty interpreting the cause or source of the person's nonverbal expressions.

When the family or caregivers of a person with Down syndrome have difficulty understanding his nonverbal expressions, the person is more likely to have a mental illness diagnosis. For our patients *without* mental illness diagnoses, 78 percent of them had caregivers who reported that they could understand the nonverbal expressions of the person with Down syndrome most of the time. For those with a mental illness diagnosis, only 26 percent had caregivers who stated they could understand the person's nonverbal expression of feelings most of the time.

The cause and effect are not clear from these data. In other words, the data do not prove that the caregiver's inability to understand nonverbal expressions leads to a higher incidence of mental illness. However, we believe that this is the case. Therefore, knowing how well a person with Down syndrome can express his feelings is essential to understanding mental health and assessing for mental illness risk. Chapter 6 provides further discussion of how this information is used to promote mental health.

ADDITIONAL AREAS OF ASSESSMENT

The mental health assessment also includes evaluations of several other important areas related to social and emotional functioning. These areas are assessed through questions in the medical exam and the semi-structured psychosocial evaluation, and more informally by talking with the adult with Down syndrome and his parents or caregivers. These areas include:

◆ memory (discussed in Chapter 5),

◆ issues of self-esteem (Chapter 7),

◆ self-talk (Chapter 8),

◆ the tendency toward repetition (Chapter 9),

◆ processing speed (Chapter 4),

◆ the understanding of time (Chapter 4),

◆ the ability to use abstract thinking (Chapter 4),

◆ the difference or similarity between chronological and developmental age (Chapter 4),

◆ the range of emotions (Chapter 4),

◆ lifespan issues, such as issues of adolescence and geriatrics (Chapter 10),

◆ factors that may precipitate mental illness (Chapter 11), and

◆ the assessment of mental health disorders (Section 3).

Diagnosis of Mental Health Disorders in Adults with Down Syndrome

For the assessment of mental health symptoms and disorders in adolescents and adults with Down syndrome, we use *The Diagnostic and Statistical Manual of Mental Disorders*, fourth edition, text revision (DSM-IV-TR). However, like other mental health professionals in the field of intellectual disabilities, we have found that the DSM-IV-TR criteria need to be adapted for use with people with Down syndrome and other intellectual disabilities (Sovner, 1986). This is because of the verbal expressive language and conceptual difficulties that may limit the person's ability to report his symptoms.

Emphasis in our adapted criteria is on the observed changes in behavior rather than self-report. For example, the DSM-IV-TR criteria for major depression include such observable behavioral changes as withdrawal, a loss of interest in things previously enjoyed, change in sleeping and eating habits, loss of energy and fatigue, etc. Parents or other caregivers have no difficulty observing and reporting on these symptoms.

However, the original DSM-IV-TR criteria also include such self-reported symptoms as verbal expressions of sadness and feelings of guilt and worthlessness, which are rarely expressed by persons with DS. Although feelings of guilt and worthlessness have no behavioral corollary, we have found that most caregivers readily observe evidence of sadness in facial expressions and body language (slumping shoulders, etc.), as well as in our criteria of a "loss of spark, life, and vitality." What also helps in this process is that family members are often very astute observers of someone with DS in their care. We feel confident that even without self-report, the observed changes in behavior do allow an accurate diagnosis of mental health disorders.

See Chapter 12 for further discussion of assessment of mental illness.

PHYSICAL HEALTH

The assessment of mental health is incomplete if physical health is not also assessed. For all people, there is a great deal of interaction between physical and mental health. For people with Down syndrome, there appears to be more interaction and, thus, a greater need to assess and understand physical health problems.

Physical health problems can directly affect mental health. Some physical problems can have mental illness symptoms as a part of the disease. For example, depression can be a manifestation of hypothyroidism. Physical problems can also indirectly contribute to mental illness. For example, prolonged pain or chronic illness can lead to depression. These are aspects of physical health that are well recognized in people with or without Down syndrome.

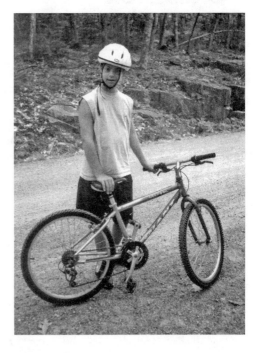

Another reason it is important to understand the interaction between physical health and mental health is that people with Down syndrome often have expressive language difficulties. People who have difficulty expressing their physical discomfort are more likely to have mental health or behavioral problems.

A thorough history and physical exam is part of the mental health assessment. In addition, if there are mental health or behavioral problems, additional testing is often necessary. This may include blood tests, x-rays, EEGs, and others. Often more testing is required for a person with Down syndrome than for someone without Down syndrome. If he is unable to provide an accurate history or tell us if he is having symptoms of physical disease, additional testing can help us rule out a physical cause for the behavioral change. Further information on the interaction between physical and mental health is provided in Chapter 2.

ASSESSMENT RESULTS

For many adults with Down syndrome, this will be the end of the assessment. They are doing well. We recommend that parents or whoever requested the assessment receive a written report of the results and an opportunity to discuss them. Areas of strength should be emphasized and other ways that mental health can be optimized discussed. Many times parents or other caregivers are relieved to learn that the particular behavior being discussed is common in people with Down syndrome and should be viewed as a characteristic rather than a mental illness. Treatment recommendations, if any, should be thoroughly explained and implemented or appropriate referral(s) should be made. If it appears that the adult with Down syndrome may have a mental illness, further assessment may be recommended, as discussed in Section 3.

Conclusion

The assessment of the mental health of a person with Down syndrome ideally begins before there is a problem. It is important to understand the individual's strengths and weaknesses; to assess the environment, including the social contacts and support of family and friends; and to evaluate the link between physical and mental health. This information can be used to promote mental health as well as to better understand mental illness and the appropriate treatment. Additional issues to consider in evaluating a person with Down syndrome are addressed throughout the rest of the book.

Chapter 2

Assessing the
Physical Health/
Mental Health
Connection

As discussed in the previous chapter, every thorough mental health assessment should also include an assessment of physical health to ensure that physical health problems are not affecting mental wellbeing in any way. This is true whether or not the adult with Down syndrome is suspected of having any kind of mental illness. Discovering physical health problems early in their course may prevent them from causing mental health problems.

When evaluating an adult with Down syndrome for changes in mental health or behavioral problems, it is important to do more than put on your "psychiatry hat." We often find that there is an underlying physical condition that is causing or contributing to the mental illness or the behavioral change. Furthermore, treating the mental illness or the behavioral symptoms without attention to the physical health issues will generally contribute to at least partial failure of the treatment of the mental illness or the behavioral symptoms.

It may be advisable to have the physical exam *before* the mental health assessment. This may be especially true if there are no experts in mental health of adults with DS in your community.

We sometimes find that a physical problem is or was the direct cause of a mental health problem and sometimes it is a contributing factor. However, in either case, as time goes by, the problem often develops other "layers," and treatment of the physical problem alone is not adequate. It is necessary to address the problem from all aspects: physical, psychological, and social. For example, consider an adult with DS who develops a medical problem that includes the symptom of depressed mood. A common scenario in these situations is that the person withdraws and is less interested in participating in activities, work, etc. In addition, her mood change may lead to interpersonal conflicts. Therefore, when treating the problem, it is not enough to focus on any one of these areas and neglect the others. It is important to evaluate and treat for the underlying physical problem. However, it is also generally necessary to address the psychological and social aspects of the problem as well as the physical problem. (This is addressed in detail in the chapters in Section 3.)

> *Sandy is a young woman with Down syndrome who had a birth trauma to her left shoulder that resulted in reduced use of her arm. Through therapy, however, the function of her arm had greatly improved. On her first visit to the Adult Clinic, Sandy had a depressed mood, did not want to go to work, and was significantly limiting her social interaction with people other than her immediate family. In reviewing her history, we found that shortly before these symptoms began, she had slipped on the ice and fallen on her left shoulder, resulting in further impairment of her arm's function. In Sandy's case, physical therapy for her shoulder was a major part of the treatment for her presenting complaint of depressed mood. She was able to recover with physical therapy, emotional support of her family, and a gentle reintroduction into her previously active social life.*

Some patients will require greater intervention for the psychological and social issues. Some will require medications for the psychological problem, in addition to therapy and other interventions. However, we have repeatedly found that providing that care without addressing the underlying or contributing medical problems will limit the overall success of treatment.

AREAS TO BE ASSESSED

◆ ◆ ◆ ◆ ◆ ◆ ◆ ◆ ◆ ◆ ◆ ◆ ◆ ◆ ◆ ◆ ◆ ◆ ◆

Table 1 shows the tests and procedures that should be completed to identify the physical problems that most commonly contribute to mental health problems in adolescents and adults with Down syndrome. The next sections explain in more detail why these problems are important to rule out. While the table suggests guidelines for assessing physical conditions, it is important to understand that *any* medical problem can contribute to making any psychological problem more significant. Any physical problem that makes a person feel physically worse will likely increase the symptoms of the psychological condition.

Table 1: Important Physical Conditions to Assess

Condition/Problem	Possible Impact on Mental Health	Test or Procedure*
Pain	Depression, behavior change, aggression, anxiety	Interview adult w/DS and family/caregiver; thorough physical exam; additional procedures as indicated based on history and physical exam.
Hearing impairment	Anxiety, apparent loss of cognitive skills, depression, agitation, aggression	Hearing test from audiologist at least every 2 years, or more frequently if indicated by possible change in hearing
Vision impairment	Anxiety, depression, apparent loss of cognitive skills, depression, agitation	Complete vision exam at least every 2 years or more frequently if indicated by possible change in vision
Seizures	Aggression, depression, apparent loss of cognitive skills	EEG and imaging of brain (CT scan or MRI)
Cervical subluxation	Loss of skills (particularly reduction in ambulation skills; loss of muscle function; incontinence), anxiety, agitation, depression	Thorough neurological exam (as part of physical exam); lateral cervical spine x-rays in flexion, extension, and neutral; CT scan and/or MRI of cervical spine
Urinary tract problems (includes urinary tract infections and difficulty/inability to empty the urinary bladder)	Development of incontinence, agitation, anxiety	Urinalysis (urine test) and possibly urine culture; ultrasound of the bladder and kidneys (a pre- and post-void ultrasound is helpful to assess for problems with emptying the bladder)

(continued on next page)

Condition/Problem	Possible Impact on Mental Health	Test or Procedure*
Arthritis	Agitation; depression; apparent loss of skills	Physical exam; x-rays
Diabetes	Apparent loss of skills; urinary incontinence; agitation; depression	Blood sugar (further testing indicated if blood sugar suggests diabetes)
Dental concerns	Agitation, poor eating, depression, aggressive behavior	Thorough dental exam; dental x-rays as indicated
Hypothyroidism (underactive thyroid)	Depression; loss of cognitive skills; appetite change	Blood test for TSH, T3, and T4 (we screen all of our patients every year with a TSH and then T3 and T4 if the TSH is abnormal)
Hyperthyroidism	Anxiety; hyperactivity; depression; loss of cognitive skills	Blood test for TSH, T3, and T4.
Sleep apnea and other sleep difficulties	Depression, loss of cognitive skills, agitation, psychoses	Observe sleep and keep a sleep log; formal sleep study in a sleep lab may be indicated
Gastrointestinal problems	Loss of appetite, depression, agitation, anxiety	Stool test for blood; blood tests for anemia (CBC), celiac disease, liver disease, gall bladder disease; x-rays, ultrasounds, CT scans, and endoscopy as indicated by history, physical, and other tests
Medication side effects	Can contribute to essentially any behavioral or psychological change	Careful history to look for potential link to medication; possible trial off the medication

It is assumed that a complete history and thorough physical exam is performed for each of the presenting problems. Although areas of focus for the history and physical are specified here, additional testing may be indicated.

PAIN

Pain is one aspect of physical conditions that can affect mental health. Many illnesses and injuries can cause pain. Common causes of pain in people with Down syndrome include: dental problems, gastroesophageal reflux, bladder problems (especially the inability to empty the bladder), ear infections, gastrointestinal discomfort secondary to celiac disease or constipation, and arthritis or subluxation of the joints (especially in the cervical spine). Pain can also be caused by emotional distress, but this section focuses on pain caused by physical health problems or injuries.

We are often asked, "Does a person with Down syndrome have a reduced ability to perceive pain (an increased pain tolerance) or does she have a reduced ability to communicate the pain so we only think she is not experiencing the pain?" The answer appears to be "both." Families often tell us that their son or daughter (sister, brother) has an increased pain tolerance. "He never complains. Even when he had the broken arm, he complained of very little pain."

A study of mice provides supporting evidence of these observations. There is a "mouse model" for Down syndrome. Mice with trisomy 16 (an extra sixteenth chromosome) have many similar health characteristics to people with trisomy 21 (Down syndrome). One study compared the response to pain of mice with trisomy 16 to mice with the normal number of chromosomes (for a mouse). The mice with trisomy 16 showed a significantly reduced response to painful stimuli. The authors concluded that the mice with trisomy 16 had a reduced ability to perceive pain (an increased pain tolerance) (Martinez-Cue et al., 1999).

While you might assume that a reduced ability to perceive pain would have some good points, there can also be some important negative aspects. An increased pain tolerance reduces a person's drive to remove herself from a painful situation and to avoid further contact with the painful stimuli. It also reduces the drive to seek help or treatment for the pain. We have had patients whose sole complaint was that they were "passing out" and found them to have a hemoglobin (blood count) of 4 or 5 (1/3 of normal) due to a bleeding ulcer of the stomach. The situation became life threatening because their increased pain tolerance allowed them to avoid seeking help for the condition earlier.

Sometimes it is clear that people with Down syndrome perceive pain but have a reduced ability or desire to communicate the pain. Some patients avoid communicating a painful condition because they know from previous experience that if they report it, they may have to have tests or an evaluation that they find uncomfortable or unpleasant. Other patients communicate their discomfort, but in a way that we have difficulty understanding. Particularly when someone has limited communication skills, she may communicate pain through behavior. For example:

> When we first began evaluating Patrick for depression, one of his
> symptoms was striking his head repeatedly. A CT scan of his head showed
> a chronic sinus infection in the area where he was striking his head. The
> depressive symptoms were improving with antidepressant medications but

the head-striking symptoms did not improve until the sinus infection was treated. The pain he was experiencing was contributing to his symptoms, and treatment of both the mental health and physical health issues was important to achieve the goal of improving his condition.

Pain can also have an effect if it persists and the person is unable to communicate the problem. Chronic pain can lead to depression and agitated behavior and exacerbate other mental health problems. There can be a great deal of interplay between chronic pain and depression, with each one contributing to or worsening the other. Therefore, addressing both is an important part of treating either.

Keys to Recognizing Painful Episodes

➤ **Watch for subtle signs.**
A grimace, pointing, a different spoken phrase, sweating for no apparent reason, change in appetite, and holding a limb differently can all be signs to note. There are probably many more that you have noticed as well.

➤ **Watch for behavioral changes.**
Pain can often be expressed by a behavioral change, especially if a person with Down syndrome has very limited verbal or nonverbal communication skills. Behavioral changes could include: less activity, more activity, seeking more attention, seeking less attention, a sad appearance, anger, emotional lability (sudden and frequent changes of emotions), reduced emotion, and many others. It is important to consider any behavioral change as a means of communication for a potential underlying physical problem.

➤ **Consider the possibility of increased pain tolerance.**
Remember that people with Down syndrome may have a reduced ability to perceive pain. Keep an eye on someone who has what appears to be a minor complaint. If the pain persists longer than expected or there are other symptoms that suggest something more serious (despite the person having little complaint), it could be time for further evaluation.

VISION

Impaired vision also affects mental health. Declining vision can be a scary problem for anyone. Having a reduced ability to understand the decline can make it even more frightening. In addition, most people with worsening vision will try to compensate by using their intellect and by increasing the use of their other senses. However, with an intellectual disability, there is "less to fall back on." Also, as noted below, hearing problems are more common in people with Down syndrome. Furthermore, as noted above, pain sensation appears to be reduced, so there is less ability to compensate with other senses. Therefore, vision loss can be even more traumatic for a person with Down syndrome.

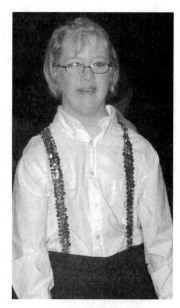

Adults with Down syndrome have the usual vision problems, including near-sightedness, far-sightedness, astigmatism, and glaucoma. There are also some problems that are more common. For example, cataracts occur at a younger age in adults with DS. In addition, many adults with DS have had strabismus (crossing of the eyes) from a young age. This can be a particular problem for depth perception. Furthermore, many people with Down syndrome appear to have depth perception problems even if they don't have strabismus. Depth perception impairment plays a role in mental health issues. People with poor depth perception may have more concerns about crossing from one surface to another or walking in places where there are different levels. For example, we have frequently heard that when people with DS are depressed and more fearful, they are afraid to go on escalators or to walk on the second level of a mall where there is a glass wall that overlooks the opening to the lower level.

Clearly, possible changes in vision are important to consider when assessing a change in mood, anxiety, an apparent loss of cognitive skills, and other changes. The loss of vision can be frightening and confusing.

> Sara, a woman in her mid-30s, developed a progressive, uncorrectable loss of vision. She became aggressive and developed repetitive behavior consistent with obsessive-compulsive disorder (OCD). She also developed an increased tactile defensiveness (she was very frightened when touched). Treatment included prescribing medications to help with her aggressiveness and compulsive symptoms and enlisting the help of experts on the care of people with blindness to help her negotiate her environment and reduce the fear she was experiencing. She also received "desensitization therapy" from an occupational therapist to reduce her tactile defensiveness. In addition, the staff where she lived developed a system of giving her advance warning before touching her or before asking her to move on to another task or activity. Reducing sudden, unexpected transitions to new activities made life less frightening for her.

HEARING

A decline in hearing can also be an emotionally difficult situation. Impaired hearing has a profound impact on our ability to communicate with others. In addition, if our hearing is impaired, we are deprived of a wonderful warning system that lets us know that someone or something is approaching or is nearby. If we don't hear people coming, their sudden, unexpected arrival can be anxiety provoking. Interaction with the world can be more frightening under these circumstances. Furthermore, daily joyful occurrences can be missed because good hearing helps let us know that those opportunities are there. In addition, as described with impaired vision, the person with Down syndrome probably has a reduced ability to compensate for this loss.

High frequency hearing loss (hearing of high-pitched sounds) is more common in people with Down syndrome. It can occur even in individuals who previously had normal hearing. One aspect of this loss is the reduced ability to distinguish different consonant sounds, making it harder to discriminate what is being said. An adult may sometimes seem to hear what is said but do something different than asked. He is hearing the sounds but not understanding the words. Therefore, what may appear to be defiance, oppositional behavior, or a decline in intellectual skills may actually be impaired hearing. Hearing assessment and hearing aids may be a significant part of the treatment of some mental health and behavioral problems.

Many children with Down syndrome experience recurrent middle ear infections and temporary loss of hearing related to fluid buildup in the middle ear. This can also occur in adults, but is much less common than in children. However, when it does occur, it can cause temporary hearing loss and be a significant problem.

Cerumen impaction (earwax blocking the ear canal) is more common in people with Down syndrome. Irrigating wax out of someone's ears may not ordinarily be considered a part of treating psychological or behavior problems, but if earwax is contributing to reduced communication, it may be an important piece of the treatment. Sometimes this relatively simple cause for hearing loss can lead to misunderstandings and frustration on the part of the person with Down syndrome. We have seen this situation escalate into more significant behavioral problems. As in other areas discussed, miscommunication can lead to significant psychosocial problems.

SEIZURES

Seizure disorders are more common in people with Down syndrome. The new onset of seizures has two peaks in people with Down syndrome. The first peak occurs in the first two years of life, and the second in adulthood. As discussed in the chapter on Alzheimer disease, sometimes seizures that start in adulthood are associated with Alzheimer disease.

Particularly if seizures are poorly controlled, they can lead to a sense of poor health, episodes of confusion, recurrent injuries, and a sense of fear and frustration. The fear may become emotionally paralyzing and cause the person to limit her activities. For some people, the unpredictability and randomness of the occurrences of seizures can be significant psychological stressors.

In addition, undiagnosed seizures can sometimes be mistaken for behavioral problems. Looking for other symptoms or clues during a "behavioral episode" can direct the assessment. Abnormal movements of the extremities or eyes, temporary loss of body control or consciousness, a period of fatigue or confusion after the episode, and other symptoms may suggest seizures. Some families have provided very helpful information by videotaping an episode. A careful neurological exam during the physical exam is recommended if seizures are suspected. An EEG, imaging studies (CT scan or MRI of the brain), and a referral to a neurologist may also be indicated.

CERVICAL SUBLUXATION

Atlanto-axial instability, the slipping of the first vertebrae in the neck on the second vertebrae, is more common in people with Down syndrome. There are seven vertebrae in the neck, and slippage (cervical subluxation) can occur at any of these other vertebrae, as well. This can cause discomfort. When the slippage is great enough, the vertebrae can put pressure on the spinal cord and cause neurological changes, weakness of the arms and/or legs, bowel and/or bladder incontinence, and impaired gait (walking). The physician will also find increased reflexes (a more brisk movement) in response to the reflex hammer. In addition, there is often a significant emotional component to this problem since the fear of the discomfort and of the changes occurring in the person's nervous system can be quite disturbing.

A person with Down syndrome can develop cervical subluxation at any time in her life. We have seen a number of patients who did not have the problem earlier in life develop it as they reached adolescence or adulthood. Significant trauma to the neck, such as a fracture, could cause this problem. Most of the time, however, it seems to be related to aging and the degeneration of joints. Osteoarthritis does seem to occur at a younger age in people with Down syndrome and one area where this can be a particular problem is in the cervical spine. It is important for the practitioner to regularly ask about symptoms that could be related to cervical subluxation and also perform a neurological exam for muscle strength and reflexes.

A young man came to the Adult Down Syndrome Center with a global decline in his cognitive skills, as well as bowel and bladder incontinence and unsteady gait. As discussed in Chapter 23, these are some of the symptoms seen in Alzheimer disease, and his family was concerned that he was developing Alzheimer disease. Our evaluation revealed that he was depressed and that he had increased reflexes. X-rays showed subluxation (slippage) of the third cervical vertebrae on the fourth. Antidepressants markedly improved his mood and enabled him to regain his former cognitive abilities. He also underwent surgery to stabilize his neck and to eliminate the pressure of the vertebrae on his spinal cord. With the assistance of physical therapy, supportive counseling, and the antidepressant medication, he resumed his previous level of function and daily activities.

ARTHRITIS

One of the medical conditions seen more frequently and at a younger age in people with Down syndrome is osteoarthritis (the arthritis generally associated with aging). The joints degenerate, cause discomfort, and eventually become less mobile and less functional. This can cause "slowing down physically." Pain-related issues are similar to those discussed above. Asking questions about joint discomfort or changes in mobility is part of the assessment for arthritis. The physical exam should include assessing joint structure, signs of inflammation, and joint mobility. X-rays of the joints may also be needed.

Jean's story provides a good illustration of the issues of aging and osteoarthritis. When she was 46, she was brought to us for an evaluation because of "behavior problems." The problem started when she would walk into the center of her workshop, stop, and urinate all over the floor. Workshop staff claimed, "She is being defiant because she doesn't like to work." We discovered that Jean was actually doing a good job at work most of the time. She would sit at her station and had a good production level. However, she was "frequently absent from her station for prolonged periods of time."

Our assessment found that, with age, Jean had developed a reduced bladder capacity and the need to urinate more frequently. In addition, she had progressive arthritis and she was walking more slowly and cautiously. Unfortunately, the workshop was in a building about the size of half a football field and her workstation was on the opposite end of the building from the bathrooms. Her frequent absences from her workstation were due to urinary frequency and her "defiant" behavior was caused by an inability to get to the toilet in time. Her reduced rate of walking secondary to her arthritis, the distance to the bathroom, and her reduced bladder capacity all made it impossible for her to make it to the bathroom in time. Jean's treatment included moving her work station closer to the bathroom, using medications to reduce the discomfort and immobility caused by her arthritis, assessing and treating her bladder condition, and providing emotional support for the physical changes she was experiencing. No psychiatric medications or other behavioral treatment were necessary.

URINARY TRACT AND BLADDER PROBLEMS

Bladder problems can cause emotional issues, as well. Decreased muscle tone in the bladder, which appears to be more common in people with Down syndrome, can cause retention of urine and difficulty voiding. The large, distended bladder, can, in turn, cause discomfort and overflow, leading to incontinence. A number of our patients have developed agitated behavior in response to this discomfort. Often, agitated behavior is treated with antidepressant or antipsychotic medications, many of which have the unintentional side effect of relaxing the bladder muscle even more and even further reducing the ability to empty the bladder. This can lead to even more agitation.

Incomplete emptying of the bladder can also lead to increased urinary tract infections, which can be uncomfortable and result in behavioral changes. If there is a change in behavior, particularly if it is accompanied by any change in urination, we recommend performing a urinalysis. An ultrasound of the bladder pre- and post-void may also be indicated to assess whether the person is emptying her bladder normally.

DIABETES MELLITUS

Type 2 diabetes mellitus (DM) is more common in people with Down syndrome. Type 2 DM was previously called adult onset DM or non-insulin DM. The increased rate of obesity in people with Down syndrome accounts for at least some of the increase in Type 2 diabetes. The symptoms include polydipsia (drinking increased fluids), polyuria (urinating more frequently), polyphagia (eating increased amounts of food), weight loss, and fatigue.

The onset of diabetes can be subtle, particularly in someone who has a reduced ability to perceive or to report the changes. Moreover, the sense of feeling poorly can contribute to behavioral changes or a depressed mood. In addition, urinary incontinence may occur because of the frequency of urination and this can be misinterpreted as a behavioral issue. This is also true for the need to drink increased fluids or to eat greater amounts of food in someone with untreated DM.

In addition, even after the diagnosis has been made, if the person's blood sugar goes too high or too low, behavioral changes may be seen. Particular attention must be given to prevent very low blood sugars. Very low blood sugars can result in significant behavioral changes, but, more importantly, can cause life-threatening problems.

At present, there is no recommendation to screen all people with Down syndrome periodically for diabetes mellitus. If, however, an adult with Down syndrome has a behavioral change or the new onset of psychological symptoms, a blood sugar test is usually indicated. Even if it is normal, some of the medications used for psychiatric problems can cause an increased blood sugar and, therefore, the blood sugar should be known before prescribing these medications (see Chapter 13 on medications).

DENTAL CONCERNS

Many adults with Down syndrome have significant tooth decay. Some of this is related to inadequate tooth brushing and flossing and some to misalignment of teeth (which is more common in people with DS). There may be genetic factors as well. In addition, gum disease is more common in people with Down syndrome. Pain, loose teeth, difficulty chewing, and other problems can occur because of the dental disease. Agitated behavior in response to dental pain is a common problem. Regular preventative dental care is very important. A good dental exam is imperative when there are concerning changes in behavior or emotional distress.

UNDER- OR OVERACTIVE THYROID

When the thyroid gland is not producing adequate thyroid hormone, the condition is called hypothyroidism (underactive thyroid). Nearly 40 percent of our patients at the ADSC have hypothyroidism. Some developed hypothyroidism when they were children but many didn't develop the condition until adolescence or adulthood. Hypothyroidism can cause numerous physical symptoms including constipation, dry skin, and weakness. When discussing mental health issues, it is important to note that hypothyroidism can also cause lethargy, depression, and even a decline in skills or dementia. The symptoms may be subtle. Therefore, because of the frequency of the problem and the subtlety of the symptoms, an annual blood test is recommended for people with Down syndrome (Cohen, 1999).

Often, treating the hypothyroidism is not the whole treatment for the problem, but is a necessary part of the treatment. Without treating the hypothyroidism, only limited improvement of the mental health problem is generally possible. Treating the psychological problem directly may also be necessary. For example, sometimes a depressed person who is found to have hypothyroidism will respond to treating the hypothyroidism and not require further medication. However, sometimes in addition to treating the hypothyroidism, the person will also need an antidepressant. Furthermore, even when someone responds to treatment with thyroid medication alone, if the dose needs adjusting, the symptoms may recur. It is important to do regular blood testing to confirm that the dose of thyroid medication is appropriate.

Hyperthyroidism (overactive thyroid) is also more common in people with Down syndrome, although nowhere near as common as hypothyroidism. Hyperthyroidism can cause weight loss, hyperactivity, anxiety, fatigue, and other personality changes. Blood tests for thyroid function are an important part of any assessment for emotional or behavioral changes.

GASTROINTESTINAL PROBLEMS

Gastrointestinal problems can be easily overlooked because most of the symptoms need to be reported by the person who is having them. These problems can cause significant distress without any external signs or findings. Peptic ulcer disease, gastro-esophageal reflux disease or GERD (heartburn), constipation, and other problems can cause discomfort that an adult with Down syndrome may express in a behavioral fashion if she cannot verbalize her discomfort.

During the physical, the practitioner should inquire about gastrointestinal symptoms such as diarrhea, constipation, and heartburn (making sure the adult with DS understands the terminology). If the patient can't clearly describe symptoms, it is sometimes necessary to treat her for a condition and see if it helps. One reason is that doing diagnostic testing to search for potential underlying gastrointestinal problems may be riskier than treating for the condition for a short time. For example, if there is a suggestion that some discomfort precedes a behavioral change and there is any history that suggests the possibility of GERD, treatment with medications to reduce acid in the stomach may be an appropriate adjunct therapy to treating the behavioral changes. This treatment might be tried initially instead of making a definite diagnosis by doing an upper endoscopy to look into the stomach. This test may be particularly difficult for some people with Down syndrome to comply with.

When assessing one young man with limited verbal skills for agitated behavior, one of the pieces of the history we obtained was that he was "fanning his chest" as if he were trying to cool off. Part of his successful treatment was using ranitidine, a medication to reduce the acid in his stomach to treat his apparent heartburn.

CELIAC DISEASE

Celiac disease is a gastrointestinal condition that is thought to be more common in people with Down syndrome. In this condition, there is sensitivity to gluten—a protein in wheat, barley, and rye. In people with celiac disease, an inflammation in the small intestine causes destruction of the villi, the small projections in the intestine that help us absorb food. This can cause a reduced ability to absorb food, vitamins, and minerals. It can be associated with diarrhea, poor weight gain, weight loss, over-eating, and fatigue. Some people may have constipation instead of diarrhea, probably because of large bowel movements secondary to undigested food. Many people with untreated celiac disease do not feel well. This can lead to irritability and contribute to a variety of behavioral, emotional, and psychological problems.

Celiac disease can begin at any age, so even if the person with Down syndrome has already been tested for celiac disease, it is worth repeating the test. Blood testing is used as the initial assessment for celiac disease. The blood tests include: anti-tissue trans-glutaminase antibody (or anti-endomysial antibody), anti-gliadin IgG, and anti-gliadin IgA. If the blood tests suggest celiac disease, the diagnosis is made by doing a small bowel biopsy that is collected by doing an endoscopy. Some families choose to eliminate gluten-containing foods from the diet based on the blood tests alone to avoid the endoscopy. However, the diagnosis cannot be definitively made without the biopsy.

Treatment of celiac disease requires elimination of gluten from the diet. In someone known to have CD, change in mood or increased irritation can be a sign that she has strayed from her diet.

Vitamin B12 Deficiency. Vitamin B12 deficiency appears to be more common in people with Down syndrome. At least some of this deficiency may be secondary to celiac disease. Vitamin B12 deficiency can cause a variety of psychological and neurological symptoms, including poor appetite, numbness, difficulty with balance, confusion, memory loss, and dementia. As has been described with several other physical health problems, correcting the vitamin B12 deficiency may not resolve the whole psychological problem. However, without optimizing physical health and treating the vitamin B12 deficiency, complete recovery is less likely. At present there is no recommendation to routinely screen all people with DS for vitamin B12 deficiency. However, we recommend testing each person who has neurological or psychological changes.

MENSTRUAL PROBLEMS

Menstrual difficulties can cause significant emotional changes as well. Most of our female patients manage their monthly cycle very appropriately. With the right training in hygiene, explanations that it is part of a normal bodily function, and support as needed, it becomes part of their routine. For some, however, menstruation continues to be a challenge and it can contribute to behavioral problems. When a woman with Down syndrome is experiencing menstrual problems, it is important to first consider whether there may be a significant problem such as premenstrual syndrome (PMS) or dysmenorrhea (painful periods).

Premenstrual syndrome or premenstrual dysphoric disorder (when the dominant symptoms are emotional) can be quite disturbing. Symptoms include depressed mood, mood swings, irritability, difficulty concentrating, fatigue, swelling, breast tenderness, headaches, and sleep disturbance. We recommend keeping a log of symptoms and the menstrual cycle to see if the symptoms are present in the premenstrual phase (approximately 7 to 10 days before the menses) and absent during the rest of the cycle. Treatment includes daily exercise, regular, balanced meals, avoiding smoking, regular sleep, stress reduction techniques, and counseling. A low salt, low caffeine, and low fat diet with frequent small meals of complex carbohydrates may also be beneficial. Vitamin B6, calcium, and vitamin E have also been used. Antidepressants and/or oral contraceptives can be helpful when the symptoms are more severe.

If the periods themselves cause discomfort (dysmenorrhea), anti-inflammatories can be of particular benefit. Ibuprofen (Advil, Nupren) and other anti-inflammatory medications block a chemical pathway that leads to increased discomfort. Acetaminophen (Tylenol) can help with discomfort but doesn't block the pathway and for many women does not work as well. Since painful periods may contribute to behavioral changes during that time of the month, treatment of dysmenorrhea may be a significant piece of the treatment for behavioral changes. Some women also get very significant improvement with the use of birth control pills.

MEDICATIONS

Medications can also be a source of health problems. Side effects from medications can contribute directly to psychological issues, create a sense of ill-health that leads to behavioral issues, or cause pain or other health problems that lead to psychological or behavioral problems. A thorough assessment of the medications includes reviewing when the symptoms began relative to starting on the medication, changing doses, or adding other medications or natural products. These are important aspects in determining whether medications are contributing to the problems.

SLEEP DISORDERS

Inadequate sleep, particularly if it is a chronic problem, has a huge effect on a person's ability to function in her daily activities. It can lead to irritation, problems controlling emotions, loss of concentration, attention problems, and apparent loss of cognitive skills. These difficulties are clearly apparent in our patients with sleep difficulties.

Sleep difficulties are very common in people with Down syndrome of all ages, and can include:

- ◆ Sleep apnea,
- ◆ Hypopnea,
- ◆ Restless, fragmented sleep, and
- ◆ Difficulties related to routines or sleep environment.

SLEEP APNEA

Sleep apnea is a serious health problem that is much more common in people with Down syndrome of all ages. If not treated, it can lead to heart and lung damage and can also contribute to behavioral or psychological problems.

In order to understand what sleep apnea is, it is important to know what normal sleep is. Normal, uninterrupted sleep consists of a cyclic pattern alternating between rapid eye movement (REM) sleep and non-rapid eye movement (non-REM) sleep. REM sleep is also called dream sleep. During REM sleep, many physiological changes are observed. For instance, there is a decline in chin muscle activity, generalized muscle relaxation except in the diaphragm, and irregular breathing. Consequently, with the onset of normal sleep, the pharynx (airway) narrows because of muscle relaxation, causing added resistance to air movement through the airway. During normal sleep, this causes reduced air movement and a slight increase in carbon dioxide in the body.

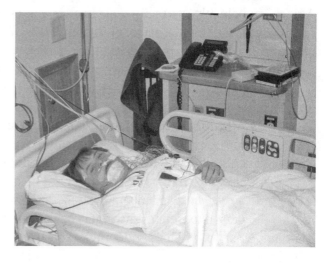

Sleep apnea is defined as a complete cessation of breathing from any cause during sleep, resulting in decreased oxygen in the blood or increased carbon dioxide (a greater increase than would be seen in normal sleep). The pauses in breathing usually last ten to twenty seconds, but can last as long as two minutes. In severe cases, more than 500 attacks of sleep apnea may occur during a night. In people with Down syndrome, apnea is most commonly caused by obstruction of the airway. Respiratory effort continues but the obstruction prevents movement of air into and out of the lungs. In children with Down syndrome, obstructed is frequently caused by large tonsils, adenoids, or tongue; small respiratory passages; or low muscle tone in the mouth and pharynx. In adults and adolescents, obesity is a more common cause, so if weight gain is a problem, this can be a clue that sleep apnea may be present.

Characteristically, a long history of loud snoring combined with restless sleep, excessive daytime drowsiness, and early morning headaches suggests the diagnosis of sleep apnea. There may also be difficulty concentrating, depression, irritability, and personality changes. We have even seen evidence of psychotic behavior that improved with treating sleep apnea. During obstruction, the person may aspirate secretions into the lungs, causing a cough or aggravating asthma symptoms. Shortness of breath and fatigue increase as the disease progresses. Sleep apnea also contributes to increased gastro-esophogeal reflux (heartburn).

Due to the high incidence of sleep apnea in people with Down syndrome, a history and physical exam should always include questions designed to determine whether apnea might be present. The doctor should inquire about how much the person with Down syndrome snores, restless sleep, daytime drowsiness, awakening during the night, whether the person's lips ever turn blue during sleep, and other symptoms of sleep apnea. Parents or other caregivers might want to videotape the person sleeping and bring it to the exam if they suspect apnea. If there is a possibility of apnea, the doctor should make a referral for a sleep study at a sleep disorders clinic or hospital. A sleep study involves attaching electrodes and other sensors to the body to measure breathing effort, the passage of air through the airways, brain waves, oxygen content of the blood, and the restfulness of sleep. The test generally requires staying overnight in a sleep lab but sometimes can be done in one's own home.

If sleep apnea is diagnosed, treatment depends on the severity of the disease, but may include:

- ◆ Attaching a sock with a tennis ball inside to the back of the pajama top, to prevent the person from sleeping on her back (if apnea only occurs when the person sleeps on her back);
- ◆ Use of CPAP or BIPAP, which are means of delivering pressure to the airway to keep it open throughout the breathing cycle (and requires the person to wear a mask over the mouth and/or nose when sleeping);
- ◆ Surgery such as widening of the airway or a tracheotomy.

Jim, 34, was experiencing increasing self-talk, paranoia, agitation, aggressive behavior, and a decline in skills. During an evaluation at the Center we also found that he was falling asleep at work, snored loudly, and made loud snorting noises when sleeping that seemed to occur when he started breathing again after a pause in his breathing. A sleep study was recommended and the diagnosis of sleep apnea was confirmed. With treatment of the sleep apnea, his behavioral and psychological issues improved. With supportive counseling, he returned to his typical level of functioning.

HYPOPNEA

Hypopnea is similar to sleep apnea. Instead of cessation of the air flow during sleep, however, there is reduced air flow, due to narrowing or obstruction of the airway. In people with Down syndrome, sources of this obstruction are similar to those in sleep apnea. If the airflow is reduced enough, oxygen levels drop and carbon dioxide levels rise, resulting in many of the same symptoms that sleep apnea causes. Signs of hypopnea can include snoring, labored breathing, odd sleeping positions such as sitting up during sleep, etc. Again, diagnosis is made with a sleep study.

ROUTINES AND ENVIRONMENT

Abnormal sleep can be a problem even if there isn't apnea. If a person does not get into a good sleep routine, poor sleep may result. As discussed in the section on "The Groove" (Chapter 9), routine is important to many people with Down syndrome. For sleep, the downside to the groove is that without a set pattern of getting ready for bed, a person with Down syndrome may have a difficult time settling down and falling asleep. The upside is that once a bedtime routine is established, it can generally be successfully followed night after night.

Sometimes sleep disturbance is more of a social problem. Noise from roommates or other activity in the house may keep a person awake. This is generally more of a problem in group residential facilities where staff may have other duties at night that can make noise and be disturbing. However, we have seen this in a number of our patients who live in their family home as well. Many people with Down syndrome seem to be "light sleepers," and when other members of the family have different schedules, their activity may wake the person with Down syndrome. In addition, inadequate supervision and too much independence at night may contribute to inadequate sleep. The women who lived in a group home and developed impaired skills after too many late nights are a fine example of this (see Chapter 7). However, too much independence can be a challenge for our patients who live at home as well. Some of our patients need assistance making a scheduled routine for sleep and may need "refresher" courses periodically to stay on the schedule.

RESTLESS, FRAGMENTED SLEEP

Even when all the above causes of sleep difficulties are eliminated, many people with Down syndrome have restless, fragmented sleep. Studies have shown that for unknown reasons, they may move all around the bed, fall out, sit up, lean their heads against the wall, or wake up frequently during the course of the night. These types of chronic sleep difficulties can lead to problems with irritation, attention, and emotional control. Parents and caregivers should be aware of these sleep difficulties as a possible source of behavioral problems, although there is no specific treatment for them. Sometimes a trial of medication that produces sedation might be beneficial.

ALLERGIES

Allergies can be a significant contributor to behavioral challenges or psychological changes. While further research is needed to determine whether there is a direct link between allergies and behavior, it is very clear that there is an indirect link between allergies and behavioral changes. The sense of poor health or feeling poorly can lead to irritability and mood changes. We have seen adults with Down syndrome who have more behavioral challenges during the time that their allergies are symptomatic. An assessment for allergy symptoms and a possible link to behavioral changes is therefore an important part of the history and physical exam.

SENSORY ISSUES

Some people with Down syndrome seem to be more sensitive to stimuli around them. They may be sensitive to noise, touch, temperature changes, and other sensory input. As indicated above, most seem to be less sensitive to pain.

With hearing loss, some people experience a phenomenon called recruitment. They generally hear poorly at lower levels of sound. As the sound gets louder, at some point enough hearing cells have been "recruited" and suddenly the person can hear at that loud level. This can be very startling and frightening.

Many of our patients also tend to have an increased sensitivity to touch. This is common in people with autism, and in our patients who have both autism and Down syndrome, this is a particular problem. However, it is an issue for many people with Down syndrome without autism as well. In particular we have noticed that many of our patients are reluctant to use moisturizing cream for their dry skin. They don't like the sensation of the cream.

For some people with DS, it seems that the issue may not be so much a heightened sensitivity as an inability to filter out sensory input. Some of our patients seem to be sensitive to activity going on around them that others might just "tune out." This can lead to sensory overload. As noted in Chapter 4, many of our patients are very sensitive to activities that are going on a distance from them that do not involve them.

This awareness of activity is present even when the person doesn't appear to be paying attention. For example, in the exam room when the conversation moves away temporarily from the person with Down syndrome and we are speaking with the family, the person with Down syndrome will often appear not to be even paying attention, perhaps reading a magazine or playing a video game, when suddenly she makes a comment that clearly indicates she is hearing and understanding the conversation very well.

Loud noises, overly stimulating environments, and other "sensory overload" can cause the person to become upset, agitated, anxious, or depressed. In addition, she may be aware of events that others may not realizes she is aware of. We often hear, "She doesn't even seem to be paying attention to the noise around her" or "She was not aware of the event because we never told her." However, the stimulation or awareness is usually occurring even if the person makes no sign of being aware.

These sensory inputs can be a source of behavioral and emotional problems and should be considered in the evaluation.

ALZHEIMER DISEASE

Alzheimer disease is a progressively degenerative neurological condition that affects the brain. Alzheimer disease is a form of dementia (a persistent impairment of a prior level of intellectual functioning). There is progressive destruction of brain cells, especially in certain parts of the brain. People with Alzheimer disease experience progressive impairment of memory, cognitive skills, and skills of daily living, as well as psychological changes. There is presently no cure for Alzheimer disease, but there are some treatments that can, at least temporarily, reduce its effect.

Research is inconclusive as to whether Alzheimer disease is more common in adults with Down syndrome. However, we do know that the disease can occur earlier in people with Down syndrome than in other people—often beginning in the 50s (and sometimes in the 40s) instead of the 60s or 70s. As we mentioned before, many cases of suspected Alzheimer disease turn out to be something else; still, doctors should assess for it in adults with Down syndrome. It is a diagnosis we particularly consider if the person is over the age of 35. The youngest person we diagnosed with Alzheimer disease was in his late 30s. Alzheimer disease is addressed in detail in Chapter 23.

ATTITUDE TOWARD HEALTH PROBLEMS

If an adolescent or adult with Down syndrome is aware that she has a significant health problem, it is important to assess her attitude toward her condition. This is because one of the possible secondary psychological impacts of illness relates to how we explain what is happening to us and what will potentially happen to us. If we understand the implications of the illness and the treatment, we can be empowered to be a participant in the treatment process. For a person with limited intellectual skills, the inability to understand the process can limit her opportunity to participate in it. For example, we often encounter this problem when people need physical therapy but cannot comprehend that the mental and physical challenges of therapy are needed to achieve improved health (e.g., regaining mobility in an arm or leg after a fracture and casting). These individuals are often less able to participate adequately in the therapy.

We have often seen people with Down syndrome who understand that something is happening to them but either cannot understand what it is or are not able to discuss it. Fears about the possible implication of the illness can be an issue for people with Down syndrome, even if they do not express this fear verbally. For example, if a person with Down syndrome saw someone in the hospital who required oxygen and subsequently died, this could lead to a markedly exaggerated fear of the need for oxygen in the event of her own illness. Her inability to verbalize this fear or to understand how her own illness differs from the deceased person's can have a negative impact on the treatment and lead to problems such as anxiety or depression.

Some of our patients are very capable of expressing their feelings about their condition. They may share these feelings in the practitioner's office or they may give a clue about their feelings to someone else through the course of their day. This is important information for the practitioner to have, whether he obtains it directly from the patient or the family. Sometimes, however, it is necessary to try to put yourself in the person's shoes and ask, "Would I be frightened or anxious in this situation?" If so, then it is usually safe to assume that the person with Down syndrome may also have those feelings. Avoidance and denial are mechanisms that most people seem to use on some level in dealing with health problems. These should be considered when deciding on the treatment approach for people with Down syndrome as well.

CONCLUSION

Medical or physical conditions are often a part of a psychological or behavioral problem. To treat the psychological or behavioral issue without addressing the medical problem will generally result in a less than satisfactory outcome. We have seen many people with Down syndrome who had psychological symptoms that were at least partly due to a physical problem. A high school student who was crying and laying his head on the table, especially at school, was found to have atlanto-axial instability. A thorough medical evaluation of an agitated adult led to the diagnosis of an atonic (poorly contracting) urinary bladder. He was experiencing pain from an over-filled bladder that he couldn't empty. Another adult with Down syndrome who was having difficulty maintaining his weight and had a lack of interest in activities was found to have celiac disease. These, and many other people, have had significant psychological issues for which at least part of the treatment was caring for an underlying physical problem.

Careful attention to potential physical or medical conditions is essential for diagnosing and treating behavioral and psychological conditions. Addressing the physical and medical conditions can reduce discomfort and improve diagnosis and treatment of behavioral and psychological conditions.

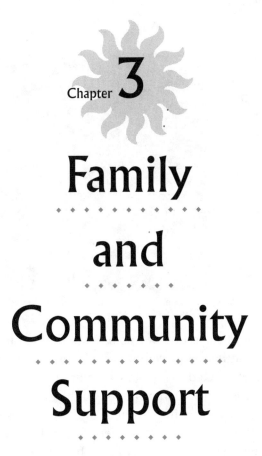

Chapter **3**

Family
and
Community
Support

In the Introduction, we introduced you to Joe. Joe is healthy, physically and mentally. This did not occur in a vacuum. Joe has a supportive family and a community that cares about him. In turn, Joe supports his family and gives back to his community. These are critical aspects of Joe's success.

FAMILY

Family is generally very important to people with Down syndrome. Just as for other people, it is a place of grounding, a group that loves and is loved, that supports and is supported. There is a commonality. There is a bond. Without this bond, people generally have a sense of something missing. As one mother said to me, "When I die, the best thing I can do for my son is arrange for someone who will advocate for him without being paid to do it." This was not a slight to the staff who cared for her son, but recognition of the importance of family. That certain bond of love that comes from family is still important, no matter how many other people are there for the person.

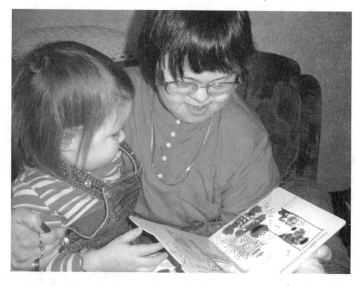

The definition of family has changed a great deal over time. It is not in the scope of this book to define family or to comment on the different types of families. However, it is critically important for the person with Down syndrome to be connected to people who mutually view one another as family. Maintaining a constant presence of some people in the life of a person with Down syndrome is the key. It is particularly important to anticipate these needs as parents age and die or staff at a group facility turn over. Identifying others who have a committed, ongoing relationship with the adult with DS help broaden the sense of connection as well as to soften the impact of possible future loss.

The importance of family is magnified for our patients who live in a residential facility and have no contact with their families. This can become particularly evident at holiday time. As the other residents go home to their families, they feel a sense of absence in their life. Family is important whether the person lives at home or in a group home.

Family is not just a group that supports the person with Down syndrome. It is also the main group that the person with Down syndrome can support. We repeatedly see dramatic mental health benefits for people with Down syndrome who have opportunities to help others. The family home is the first place a person with Down syndrome can learn this behavior as a young person (and be encouraged to do it). It is also where he can continue to use and improve these skills. To care for others is a tremendous motivator and contributes to the development of a sense of self-esteem. Unfortunately, many people with Down syndrome spend their entire life "being done for" and don't get an opportunity "to do for."

To Live at Home or Not?

Many adults with Down syndrome continue to live at home throughout their lives. We are often asked, "Is this the best choice?" There is not a single answer to that question.

For some of our patients, living at home with their parents and/or siblings is the best choice. For others, living in a residential setting or in their own home or apartment is best. Some who live at home would be better off living in a residential setting or their own place and vice versa. It depends on the person, the setting, the needs of the family, and many other factors. Sometimes families can only determine the best choice by trying something else and deciding that the original choice was the best fit.

ADVANTAGES OF LIVING AT HOME

Elizabeth, 31, was evaluated at the Center for a depressed mood and a desire to move back home. She had moved to a residential facility four years prior. Although it was a wonderful place where a number of our patients live, Elizabeth expressed concern that she was missing out on family activities. Elizabeth comes from a large ethnic family whose members live close to each other, see each other frequently, and are very involved in each other's lives. She was less able to participate in these activities and it made her unhappy.

Due to a shortage of residential placement openings, Elizabeth and her family had waited a long time for her to be able to move to her residential facility. They were reluctant to "give up her spot" unless it was the right thing to do. We discussed the issues and the options with Elizabeth and her family. We evaluated her to see whether she was depressed and whether that was causing the problem. She wasn't. She was just unhappy about the situation. In the end, Elizabeth and her family decided that she would return to live with her family, and that was the best decision for them.

Living at home has many advantages. There is a familiarity to the routine, the expectations, and the opportunities. At the same time, increased or different expectations and opportunities can be developed as the person ages and his skills and interests change. He can participate in housekeeping chores, have an outside job, and have his own friends just as other family members would.

There is a sense of safety and support at home as well. Safety can be a concern for people with Down syndrome. Families have realistic concerns about how others may treat their family member with DS. As addressed later in this chapter, a balance has to be found between safety and helping the person with DS to optimally develop his skills. With attention to these two needs, we have seen many families and ensure that their home situation is one that offers safety, support, and opportunity for the adult with Down syndrome.

Living at home will also likely give the person with Down syndrome more opportunities to support his family. As indicated above, this can be very beneficial for him and the other family members. In fact, we have seen a role reversal in many families. As the parents age, their son or daughter with Down syndrome takes on greater caregiver functions. This can be of tremendous value to the parents and the person with

Visual Supports

One of the advantages of living at home is that the same people support the adult with Down syndrome on an ongoing basis. With this constancy, family can learn about the person's needs, means of communication, desires, schedules, etc. With an active effort to use previous knowledge of the adult and build on it, this can be a dynamic learning process for both the person with DS and his family.

One way for families to build on this information is to use visual supports. For example, as discussed later in this chapter, picture schedules can be a very effective way to help the person with DS develop a sense of order to his schedule. They also communicate to others what his expectations are for his schedule. If a change is anticipated, discussing and negotiating this with the person with DS prior to the time of the change can reduce the stress of the change.

Another very helpful tool is a book about the person with DS. The book can include a variety of sections, including "Who I am," health history, likes and dislikes, schedules, means of communication, etc. This can be a very helpful way for each family member to recognize the needs and wants of the person with DS and to support him. These books are even more helpful in communicating this information with non-family members such as employers, recreation directors, etc. who come in contact with the person with DS. These books can also be invaluable if the person moves to a different setting.

If the adult moves to a group home, we encourage continued use of these books or the development of some other tool to communicate this information to staff. We also encourage the person with DS to participate in the process of deciding what is included. The information can then be used to optimize communication by those who support or come into contact with him.

Down syndrome. On the other side of the coin, we have seen many families who feel a sense of purpose because of their adult son or daughter with Down syndrome. As described by many parents, their continued caregiver role for the person with Down syndrome keeps them "young and active."

One practical concern families have is what happens if/when the parents of the person with DS die or become unable to care for him. Clearly, families need to make a contingency plan ahead of time. These plans might include: the person with Down syndrome moving in with siblings; siblings moving into the family home; the adult moving to a residential facility; donating/selling the family home to a residential facility with the contingency that their son or daughter will continue to live in the home supported by the residential staff; and others. The option of being able to continue to live in the family home has been a very good choice for a number of our patients. The continued familiarity and the sense of continuity and constancy can be very steadying in the face of the other changes.

ADVANTAGES OF LIVING AWAY FROM HOME

For an adult with Down syndrome, there can also be some disadvantages to living at home and some advantages to living in a residential facility or his own apartment or home. Chief among the disadvantages to living at home are the risks of isolation and overdependence on the family.

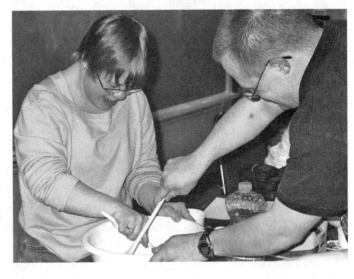

In some cases, an adult with Down syndrome who lives at home may become more isolated. Perhaps the only non-family members he comes in contact with are his parents' friends. As his parents age, they may leave the home less or have fewer people to the house, and this may also create isolation.

A continued dependence on family may also occur. The familiarity with routine discussed as a positive above may also be a negative if family members continue to do tasks for the person with DS that he could do or learn to do for himself. He may not develop skills or may lose skills if family members do too much for him. Families often have to make a concerted, conscious effort to help the adult with Down syndrome continue to develop his skills. If they don't, the person with DS may not get enough mental stimulation. This can be particularly significant if his home life is isolating as well.

Roger, 43, lived with his mother, who was in her late 80s. She had a number of health problems that limited her ability to leave the house or to participate in activities. Roger was helpful to his mother and felt good about the care he was able to provide. However, he did not have opportunities to work, socialize with others, or participate in community or recreational activities. When his mother died, Roger went to live with his sister, who lived close to the Center (1500 miles from Roger's former home).

Roger's mother and his family had not made any real plans for him in anticipation of her death, and unfortunately, his sister could not really care for him. One particular struggle was that Roger had developed a very set routine with his mother and he was resistant to change. For example, he had an extremely rigid and limited diet that was not healthy. Eventually, Roger moved to a residential facility. He gradually adjusted over several months, but developed depression in the interim and required antidepressant medications.

Roger's situation illustrates a number of potential problems that deserve consideration. Roger and his mother had developed a very set routine that was functional in their home. However, nobody considered the possibility that Roger would move out in the future, and, therefore, no efforts were made to help Roger build in some flexibility. When his mother died, Roger had to deal with her death, a long-distance move, and living with his sister who could not care for him. All these changes occurred simultaneously. Shortly thereafter, he also had to deal with moving to the residential home. It was a nice home with a few other residents and a very supportive staff, but it was another change.

We have often found that it is advantageous for the person with DS (as one mom put it) "To make the move before he has to." If the ultimate plan is for the person with DS to move to a residential facility if his parents are unable to care for him or when they die, there are advantages to making this move prior to the time it becomes necessary. One advantage is that he will not have to deal with the stress of the move at the same time he is dealing with the stress of his parents' incapacity or death. Another advantage might be that an urgent situation could be avoided. At the time when the parents die or become unable to care for him, the choice of living arrangement (residential facility, apartment, home, etc.) may be unavailable. This can lead to rushed, anxiety-provoking efforts to find a place and may necessitate multiple moves that can add to the stress.

Staff Turnover

The issue of staff turnover requires further comment. For people living in a group home, the staff often becomes like family. This is especially true if the person does not have other family involved in his life, but is also true even when the person's family is still very involved. When a staff person leaves employment at the facility, it can be very much like a member of the family leaving. It can be quite traumatic. We have often wondered what it would be like to have our families turn over every six months. It is clear to us that we ask the people with the least intellectual ability to deal with greater change than most of the rest of us could cope with. The challenge is to create as much constancy in the "family" as possible, to appreciate the stress that occurs because of these changes, and to be supportive.

It might be easier and more reassuring if we could give a quick, one-word answer to the question, "Is this the best place for him to live?" However, to no one's surprise, this is not the case. There are many issues to address that are unique to each person with Down syndrome and to each family. Perhaps even more troubling for families and people with DS is the situation in which they have concluded that a setting other than the family home is best but the setting or the appropriate support system is not available. That issue obviously is one of the factors in the decision.

Each person with Down syndrome and his family assesses the issues they value and their goals along with the available resources. Safety, independence, continued learning and growth, accessibility to family, available residential settings, ability to live independently in an apartment, available support systems, and many other factors are all weighed. The setting that is chosen is then optimized to support the values and achieve the goals. For many reasons, there are different right answers for different people with DS and their families.

PEERS

In addition to family, people with Down syndrome need friends and peers. Having a variety of friends with varying interests is a reasonable goal. However, it is important to remember that most of us have friends who have similar interests and are usually of

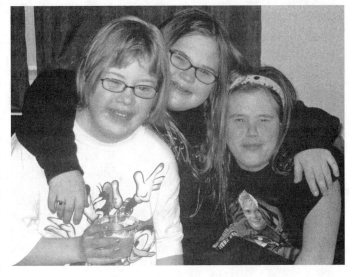

similar intellect. A member of the audience at one of our conferences stood up and suggested that people with Down syndrome have "the right to congregation as well as the right to integration."

Particularly with the improved opportunities for people with Down syndrome to be more fully integrated into society (especially in school), it is important not to discount the value of having peers with a similar level of intellect. Often as children with Down syndrome get older, both they and their classmates become more aware of the differences between them. While we are not advocating limiting these friendships, we *are* advocating not fostering them exclusively at the expense of friendships with other people with intellectual disabilities. Without these friendships, we have seen a number of people with Down syndrome find themselves "between two worlds" and feeling as if they do not fit in either one.

In addition, steering an adult with Down syndrome away from others with disabilities or only toward people without disabilities has posed challenges for some of our patients that weren't anticipated. The message that may be heard is that a person with Down syndrome shouldn't associate with people with intellectual disabilities. Since he has an intellectual disability, he struggles with his own identity. If he shouldn't "like" others with disabilities, he cannot like himself, since he has a disability. For some of our patients, this has become a true existential crisis. This is further discussed in Chapter 7.

Having friends with and without disabilities adds richness to life. We were so impressed by a young woman with Down syndrome who presented at a conference where we were also presenting. She told us of her "Rolodex." She had a card for each friend and acquaintance. When she wanted to plan an upcoming activity, she went through the Rolodex one by one until she found the person or people that she wanted for the activity. Her family promoted wonderful social interaction skills from an early age.

RECREATION

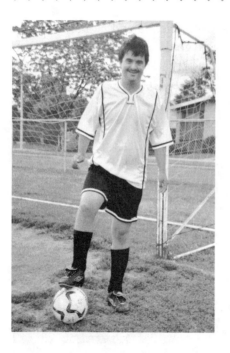

Recreational activities are an important part of the lives of people with Down syndrome. In addition to being part of the enjoyment of life, they are important for the promotion of both physical and mental health. They not only promote health but also play an important role in restoring health when there is an illness.

Participation in activities, hobbies, travel, and community events promotes a sense of well-being, helps develop self-esteem, and helps a person develop and improve social skills. We often recommend interesting events that promote both physical and mental stimulation such as walking around a museum. People with Down syndrome often learn by the example set by others, and some are great "imitators." Therefore, participation of family, friends, and care-providers in these events is a wonderful motivator. For example, we have run a group at our Center in which one of our staff members was "part of the group." She did the exercises, she learned about and practiced good nutritional habits, and she participated in the discussion right along with our patients. Rather than just being a leader, she was a participant and an example and the group flourished.

The "imitation" behavior of some people with Down syndrome can also, unfortunately, contribute to a reduction in activity level. For example:

> Luke was a 47-year-old man with Down syndrome whose father
> developed severe lung disease and required oxygen therapy all the time.
> The father stopped going out of the house except on rare occasions and
> he sat in the living room most of the day in his pajamas. Luke's activities

decreased as his father's activities decreased. Luke's father had been a major source of activities outside the home for Luke. Luke reached a point where he refused to leave the house. He began sitting in the living room most of the day in his pajamas. He even went a step further than his father did because he would only wear blue pajamas.

The reduction of activities is not always related to an illness in the family. As parents naturally slow down with age, they may become less active outside the home, and the person with Down syndrome often becomes less active as well. This can lead to less involvement in enjoyable activities, as well as isolation from friends and peers. We have seen this contribute to the onset of depression in a number of our patients. The problem can be compounded if the parent develops dementia. When a parent develops dementia, it is not just physical activity that decreases, but also mental stimulation.

Wes was a 45-year-old man whose mother developed Alzheimer disease. Although her mental capabilities were declining, she and Wes still lived by themselves. Wes stopped going to work as well as to many activities outside the home. Initially, Wes took on the caregiver role. However, as the situation became overwhelming for him, he too began to decline. He initially appeared to have Alzheimer disease himself, but it later became clear that he was depressed. Wes responded to counseling, assistance in the home for both him and his mother, and antidepressant medication. As his mother further declined, Wes moved into a group residential facility.

At a younger age, the possible impediments to recreational activities may appear to be much less dramatic, but the consequences may be just as damaging. As the person with Down syndrome ages out of the school system, often fewer activities are available. Therefore, it is critical to help the person develop skills that will serve him well in adulthood when he is still a child. A planned transition from school to adult life is important. It is imperative that social opportunities be included in the planning. Each person's needs are unique, and a careful assessment of skills and personal preferences is important to determine what activities will best suit the person.

It is beyond the scope of this book to go into great detail about locating and taking advantage of recreational opportunities for adults with Down syndrome. However, if you are concerned that your adult child is getting too little mental and physical stimulation, here are some places to begin gathering information about opportunities in your community:

- ◆ The local ARC or Down syndrome support group;
- ◆ A local chapter of Easter Seals;
- ◆ Special Olympics;
- ◆ Your local community college (many have programs or courses aimed at students with developmental disabilities);
- ◆ Community recreation center;
- ◆ Special recreation programs.

EMPLOYMENT

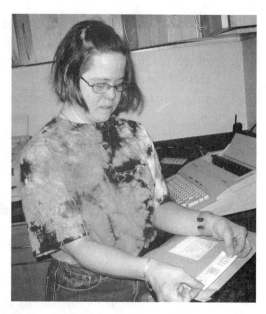

Employment is an important part of daily life for many people. In addition to providing one's livelihood, it can be important for self-esteem and help provide a sense of purpose and direction.

Just as it is important to help adults with Down syndrome to select recreational activities, it is also important to consider personal preferences when looking for employment. The ability to choose and the ability to have an impact on choices being made are significant.

> *Cyrus, 24, had graduated from high school and was working in a workshop. He seemed to be doing well. However, he began to have significant behavioral challenges at the workshop. These challenges had never been a problem before. Cyrus became depressed. Although he had pretty good language skills, he had difficulty verbally expressing his emotions.*
>
> *Through counseling and talking with his family, Cyrus was eventually able to verbalize that he was unhappy with the workshop. He seemed to be asking himself, "Is that all there is?" He felt limited by the workshop. His mother had spent a great deal of effort helping get the program up and running, which contributed to even more communication problems with regards to Cyrus's unhappiness. He seemed to have a sense that he had not had an impact on the decision to work there. As the problem became clear, he transferred to a different workshop. It really was not significantly different from the one he left. The difference was that he had had an impact on the decision. Cyrus was much happier in his new setting.*

Like other people, adults with Down syndrome have a varied range of interests. Some people with Down syndrome enjoy a repetitive job that fulfills their need for order and regimen. Some want to feel needed and achieve this by doing things for others. Still other people with Down syndrome have the desire and skills to handle a job in the community. There are often fewer other people with intellectual disabilities working at these jobs. However, they find the job more attractive and rewarding than the opportunity to socialize with peers at work. For others, a setting where there are more people with intellectual disabilities is a better fit. Sometimes these jobs might appear to be less interesting. However, to the person with Down syndrome, the job may be more interesting than a job in the community. Also, the opportunity to be with peers might be the most attractive aspect of the job. The key is personal preference.

Employment, like activities, is ideally more than simply just "something to do." It is an opportunity for learning and developing a sense of accomplishment and worth. An assessment of skills and capabilities must be part of the job selection process to ensure that the person ends up in a job where he can learn and become more accomplished. The job then has to be taught and organized in such a way that the adult with Down syndrome can be successful.

> *A young woman with Down syndrome, Barb, was a fantastic bagger at a grocery store. She learned the rules ("bread on the top," "be careful with the eggs," etc.) and was able to do the job very well. However, another part of her job was "facing the shelves." This task involves pulling the items on the shelves forward to make them more accessible and visible. In a store that covers thousands of square feet, this can be an overwhelming task. The manager was aware of this and helped Barb break the task down into pieces. Barb did a magnificent job. While many of the other people in the store found the task repetitive and boring, Barb relished the order and preciseness.*
>
> *Unfortunately, when a new store manager started, he did not appreciate Barb's need to have the task broken down into pieces. When he only directed her with, "Face the shelves," Barb became overwhelmed by the enormity of her responsibilities. She became immobilized and could not even perform the tasks she previously did well. This led the manager to believe she was being insubordinate and caused her to lose the job.*

A rewarding job that pays well is a wonderful, achievable goal for many people with Down syndrome. Depending on an adult's skills and the availability of jobs, however, this goal might not be achievable. If the right job is not possible, we recommend reassessing priorities. This might include a decision to eliminate the moneymaking aspect of the goal or at least reduce it on the priority list. One of the ways that some of our patients and their families have put this reassessment into action is to do volunteer work instead of, or in addition to, a paying job. Many people have developed an improved sense of accomplishment and self-esteem through volunteer work. In addition, often the person can learn new skills that can later be used in a paying job. Also, volunteer opportunities often bring the person out into the community and may lead to other opportunities for employment. Further information on employment can be found in the chapter on self-esteem, Chapter 7.

SELECTING APPROPRIATE ACTIVITIES

The choices made regarding jobs, recreational activities, and residence can be difficult to make. Is the choice appropriate? Will it help foster independence and personal growth? Is it safe? Does the adult with Down syndrome have the skills to be successful? These are all challenging questions to be considered.

Helping a child develop independence is an important part of parenthood. While it can be argued that most of us are not truly completely independent, people with Down syndrome will generally have a greater degree of dependence throughout life. The ongoing challenge for families and care providers is to help the person with Down syndrome achieve maximal independence. On a day-by-day basis, providing opportunities to develop skills and having appropriate and realistic expectations are key aspects to assisting a person with Down syndrome increase independence.

It is truly a challenge to help someone develop increased independence. Skills need to be learned and practiced; regular, ongoing assessment of skills must be done so that reasonable expectations can be made and an appropriate level of independence can be provided; safety issues must be addressed and monitored.

Teaching and practicing skills or activities of daily living usually is, and should be, part of training, both at home and at school, during childhood. This training should continue into adulthood. Generally, adults with Down syndrome can continue to learn

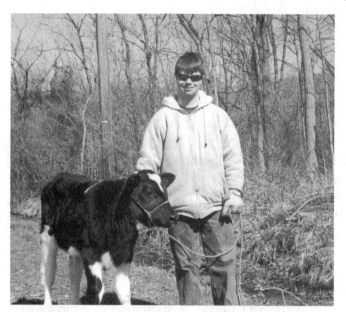

throughout life. The training should not only include how-to-do skills (e.g., brushing teeth, washing dishes, traveling on public transportation). To be truly independent, a person needs to learn how to schedule and organize his time and activities. This is often a bigger challenge for people with Down syndrome. For many of our patients, schedules and calendars are helpful. Many do well when pictures of the activities are used rather than written words. Even some of our patients who read find schedules or calendars with pictures easier to use. Actual photographs often are better than schematic drawings. Calendars and schedules can usually be pretty easily made at home. In addition, there are some commercially available products. (We use the Boardmaker™ software program from the Mayer-Johnson Company; www.mayer-johnson.com.)

At school and work, there is generally some sort of ongoing evaluation of skills. Families usually evaluate skills on a less formal basis. Evaluation is key to the process. Regular assessment helps determine when the person is ready for greater independence.

Safety concerns are clearly a major hurdle for a person with Down syndrome who is developing independence. Safety issues not only make it logistically more difficult to help a person develop greater independence, they also make it difficult for families and care providers to be willing and ready to allow it to happen. Clearly, safety concerns prevent some families and care providers from allowing adults with Down syndrome to gain more independence. This problem should be openly discussed so that family, teachers, care providers, and other professionals can develop strategies to address the concerns. Occupational therapists can be a good resource to help evaluate skills and develop ways to increase independence.

Too little independence is clearly a problem. It stifles growth and development of skills and can lead to a sense of frustration. Too much independence is also problematic. The individual can become overwhelmed and actually perform at a level lower than his skills. This is further discussed below in the section on the "The Dennis Principle."

Expectations can have a major effect on an individual's ability to become as independent as possible. When expectations are too low, they can limit growth; when they are too high, they can be confusing and cause the person to "shut down" or give up trying. This can lead to depression (discussed in Chapter 14), obsessional slowness (discussed in Chapter 16), or other mental illness.

Once again, regular evaluation is needed to determine appropriate expectations. Adjustment of the expectations is the natural next step as the person's skill level changes. The key is to find the appropriate level of expectation and adjust it upward as the person develops. Again, the hurdle to overcome is finding the balance between appropriate expectations and safety. Some "falling down and skinning one's knees" is necessary for achieving the desired growth and optimal skill level.

THE DENNIS PRINCIPLE
◆ ◆ ◆ ◆ ◆ ◆ ◆ ◆ ◆ ◆ ◆ ◆ ◆ ◆ ◆ ◆ ◆

In business, the Peter Principle describes the phenomenon in which a person is recurrently promoted until he reaches a position for which he is not qualified. We have seen a similar phenomenon for a number of our patients. We have named it the Dennis Principle (not because Dr. Dennis McGuire has reached a position for which he is not qualified, but rather because he was the first to describe it).

A number of our patients with Down syndrome have been recurrently "promoted" to less restrictive residential or work environments until they have reached a level that they cannot manage. Often we find that they can manage the actual tasks. For example, they can cook for themselves at home or can do the actual job at work. However, they may not be able to develop a plan to use these skills without assistance or direction. In addition, when they reach the level they cannot manage, the emotional challenge can overwhelm their coping skills.

Sometimes the issue is that the adult lacks the self-initiation skills to use the appropriate behavior. Other times, difficulties revolve around dealing with roommate issues or interpersonal problems. Often the issue is not knowing how to use "downtime" or relaxation time. The person may be unable to decide on and initiate a recreational activity when there isn't a structured event. This can lead to isolation, frustration, or unhappiness if he spends too much time without anything to do. He may not have the skills to use his time in a fashion that allows for healthy relaxation.

If these issues are not addressed, the situation can become progressively stressful and the adult may become depressed. Some people have become overwhelmed and have experienced a decline in skills in several areas, even to the point of not being able to do the tasks they could previously do.

In Chapter 7 we describe three women who were staying up late to watch movies and eat large amounts of food. They were depressed, fatigued, and experiencing a decline in their job performance. One woman had declined so greatly that the staff of her group home thought she was developing Alzheimer disease. The women were making poor choices with their high level of freedom. This was addressed with the women, their families, and the staff of the group home. The resultant changes in assistance for the women succeeded in getting them back on track.

Sometimes it is a matter of helping the person write down a schedule. For example:

> Brad, 25, had previously been very active in sports and was quite skillful in several. However, when he was brought to the Center, he was no longer involved in sports, was gaining weight, and was falling asleep at work. He was also having some interpersonal issues with his roommate.
>
> Brad had recently moved from his family home to an apartment with a roommate. He had previously cooked, cleaned, and attended several activities after work and in the evening. He was doing very few of these activities in his apartment, and his new sloppiness was causing conflicts with his roommate. The problem resolved over several weeks after the development of a written schedule. He was capable of all the tasks on the schedule and enjoyed doing them. However, he was not able to initiate the schedule without some assistance and needed a written plan to follow. (When he had lived with his family, the structure of the family schedule and subtle cues from his family had enabled him to do what he needed and wanted to do). Brad, like many people with Down syndrome, needed consistency and repetition (see Chapter 9, The Groove). He felt supported and much more at ease with the new schedule that he helped devise with the help of the staff.

The Dennis Principle points out the need to try to assess not only "task abilities" but also the ability to self-initiate activity (including recreational or relaxation activities) and the need for some reminders. The reminders do not necessarily have to come from another person. In fact, a system that does not rely on another person for reminders promotes greater independence. Printed or picture schedules or calendars are quite helpful for many people with Down syndrome. The person with Down syndrome becomes more personally responsible for emotional and interpersonal issues when he moves into a more independent setting. The Dennis principle stresses the importance of assessing, and, if necessary, assisting the person with Down syndrome with these responsibilities. Assessing the needs before the change and reassessing the situation after the move can help reduce the stress and improve the likelihood of a successful adjustment to the new situation.

CONCLUSION

Family and friends are commonly recognized as essential people in our lives. Interactions with family and friends are just as important for people with Down syndrome. The key is to encourage and assist in the development of these relationships from a young age. Similarly, decisions about where the person with Down syndrome will live, recreational activities, and employment must all be made carefully, with an eye toward mental health promotion.

Chapter **4**

What

Is

Normal?

Understanding "Normal," "Usual," and "Common" Behavior in People with Down Sndrome

"Is this behavior 'normal'?" "Why does my son do that?" "Do other people with Down syndrome also do that?" These are questions families and caregivers of people with Down syndrome often ask us.

Although the assessment process described in Chapter 1 can ideally provide answers to questions like these, we realize that: 1) getting a thorough mental health assessment might not always be feasible; 2) you may not have access to healthcare professionals who know the answers to these questions; and 3) you just may want to be reassured that your son or daughter is fine without getting an assessment.

This chapter will help you understand the continuum of behavior that ranges from normal to abnormal, the strengths and weaknesses frequently seen, and the common characteristics of people with Down syndrome. These factors all need to be considered when deciding whether behavior is "normal" for someone with Down syndrome.

Normal vs. Abnormal Behavior

There are clear definitions for abnormal behavior and psychological problems. *The Diagnostic and Statistical Manual of Mental Disorders,* 4th edition (DSM-IV), published by the American Psychiatric Association, clearly describes the diagnostic criteria used in the United States. (Other countries use a similar manual called the *International Classification of Diseases.*) To be diagnosed with a particular mental disorder, someone must have a certain number of the symptoms listed for that disorder and for the specified amount of time. However, even in the general population, there is room for interpretation. Clinical assessment is important and the clinician uses his judgment to determine how behavior meets (or doesn't meet) the criteria.

The DSM-IV criteria are less clear when describing a person with an intellectual disability, since these guidelines were written for people without intellectual disabilities. The typical (or normal) behavior, the developmental stage, communication skills, and other aspects of a person with Down syndrome are different from those of a person without an intellectual disability. Therefore, there is more room and need for interpretation of the criteria when applying them to a person with Down syndrome.

Particularly in light of the need for interpretation of behavior when it comes to applying the criteria for abnormal, behavior should be looked at as occurring on a continuum from normal to abnormal. At one end of the spectrum is behavior that is clearly abnormal and at the other end is the behavior that is clearly normal, but there is a vast middle ground in between. The same behavior may in one context be normal while in another be abnormal. For example, it is normal for an adult to cry and feel very sad after a loved one dies, but it is not normal for an adult to cry throughout the day merely because little things are going wrong.

Developmental Age

When trying to interpret behavior on this continuum, the first task is to define normal (or typical). When defining normal, a number of issues must be considered. It is particularly important to look at the developmental level of the person.

Psychological testing (including IQ testing) is often done as part of an assessment of a person with Down syndrome. Often at the end of the written report, a developmental age is written (for example, 6 years 7 months). This developmental age means that the person's skills, taken as a whole, are about what you would expect for a typically developing person of that chronological age. This is a reasonable place to start when assessing what might be normal for the person. As will be outlined in more detail in other chapters, there are behaviors that are normal for a person at each developmental stage. These characteristics would not be normal for a person without an intellectual disability at the same chronological age (who is at a developmental age that is the same or closer to his chronological age). For example, it is very normal for a 4-year-old to have imaginary friends. When one of our daughters was 4, she regularly invited Barney the Dinosaur to our dinner table and insisted we set out a plate for him. A 4-year-old would not be treated for a psychotic disorder for this behavior. On the other hand, if her father had insisted on inviting Barney to dinner, one would assess his behavior differently.

The importance of understanding who the person is and where she is developmentally is of critical importance. If the person with an intellectual development similar to that of a 7-year-old, for example, displays behavior that is normal for a 7-year-old, the behavior may be normal, developmental stage-appropriate behavior. For example, it is normal for young children to talk to themselves and to have imaginary friends. It is also normal for a 23-year-old with Down syndrome to talk to herself if she is at the developmental age of a young child.

In our experience, many adults with Down syndrome have developmental ages ranging from about 4 to 11 or 12. You must always have an idea of an adult's developmental level and behaviors that are appropriate for that developmental age before determining whether her behavior is normal or not.

An important caveat when looking at developmental ages for people with Down syndrome: You must not forget that this score is, in a sense, an average of the different aspects of the person's personality.

If you put your head in the freezer and your feet in the oven, on average your body temperature may well be normal. However, you aren't very comfortable. An average score can be misleading. While the person may have a developmental age of 5 years 6 months, some aspects of her personality may be closer to someone 4 years old and others may be on a much older level, even consistent with her chronological age. The key is to not put all the focus on the developmental age without considering the whole person. While her social skills may be closer to age 4, her social aspirations may be similar to those of a person who is 22 years old. While she has many skills at a level comparable to a 13-year-old's, her judgment may be closer to a 7-year-old's. Without acknowledging these possibilities, expectations can be too high or too low. It is challenging to develop an understanding of the multiple aspects of her personality and to assist a person with Down syndrome in optimally developing in each of them. However, you are much less likely to succeed if you only look at the person as having skills and abilities at the level of the "average" developmental age.

Understanding developmental age is an important part of helping a person with Down syndrome optimally develop her skills. Psychological testing provides insight into developmental age. However, care must be taken to appreciate the whole person as well as to understand the behaviors and characteristics that are commonly seen at each developmental age.

COMMON CHARACTERISTICS

◆ ◆

Robert, a 36-year-old man with Down syndrome, came into the office for the first time. When discussing his family history, he suddenly started crying that his father had died. After further discussion, we learned that his father had died 15 years prior. Robert has an excellent memory and to him, there is little if any difference between several weeks ago and several years ago. In addition, as for many people with Down syndrome, the concept of time is difficult for him. With an understanding of these concepts, Robert was comforted and reassured and the interview continued. There was no need to consider the diagnosis of prolonged grieving or even depression.

In addition to considering developmental age when determining whether behavior is normal for a person with Down syndrome, many aspects of the person's personality must be taken into consideration. The first consideration is that the person has Down syndrome. (What are common or typical behaviors for a person with Down syndrome?) However, care must be taken not to make this consideration the only one taken into account. Many families have shared with us that this was the only consideration when their family member had a change in behavior. After presenting their concerns to a healthcare professional, they were told, "It's just the Down syndrome," as they were politely dismissed from the office. This approach is neither correct nor helpful; neither is the other extreme of not considering that the person has Down syndrome and an intellectual disability.

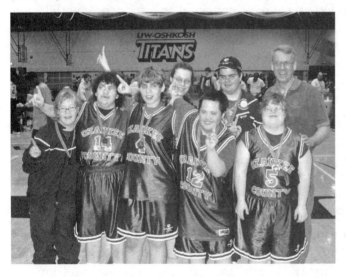

Many behaviors are commonly seen in people with Down syndrome. They are considered normal within the context of the person. In this section we will discuss a number of characteristics that are common in Down syndrome that should *not* be taken as evidence of mental health problems. These characteristics include:

- ◆ Differences in emotional response and development
- ◆ Language delays
- ◆ Self-talk (talking to oneself, also called private speech by some researchers)

◆ Tendency toward sameness or repetition
◆ Lack of flexibility
◆ Concrete thinking
◆ Difficulties understanding time concepts
◆ Slower processing speed
◆ Memory strengths and weaknesses

DIFFERENCES IN EMOTIONAL RESPONSE AND DEVELOPMENT

THE MYTH OF PERPETUAL HAPPINESS

"Individuals with Down syndrome are always happy." Although this is a commonly believed stereotype, it is a myth. The corollary to that myth, which is equally incorrect, is that people with Down syndrome have no stress in their lives (thus, the reason they can be happy all the time). In reality, people with Down syndrome have a wide range of emotions. Their emotions can reflect their inner feelings, as well as the mood of the surrounding environment. Sometimes the emotion is a result of the stress the person is feeling.

The notion that all people with Down syndrome are happy all the time evokes a positive image of people with Down syndrome. While it may be beneficial in light of all the negative stereotypes, it sets up unrealistic expectations for behavior. This can lead to misinterpretation of behavior, since, as Chapter 6 discusses, people with Down syndrome often have difficulty verbally expressing their feelings. We have heard many people express concern when a person with Down syndrome is not happy. In the backdrop that all people with Down syndrome are happy all the time, it is assumed that something is "wrong" with the person with Down syndrome when she is not happy.

The range of emotions for people with Down syndrome is typically wide. Rather than being narrower, the range may be even wider in some individuals. People with Down syndrome certainly express sadness, happiness, anger, indifference, and other normal emotions. Generally, we have found that our patients have a high degree of honesty when it comes to their emotions. They tend to show or even exaggerate the emotion they are feeling. This can be a very positive trait when it comes to optimizing communication. Unfortunately, it can also lead to tactless remarks or socially inappropriate or unacceptable behavior:

> Joe, a 27-year-old man with Down syndrome, had a job bagging groceries at a local grocery store. When customers would rush him or upset him, he would voice the anxiety and agitation he was feeling. This behavior offended some customers, who complained to the manager. Joe was fired.

The problem was not that Joe was unhappy, but that he inappropriately expressed his unhappiness. Negative emotions are just as "normal" in people with Down syndrome as they are in other people.

SENSITIVITY AND EMPATHY

Mark, 15, was with his parents at a school conference. The focus of the conference was expectedly on Mark. Suddenly, he changed the flow of the meeting by asking his teacher, "How are you doing? You seem upset." His parents, who had not noticed a problem, were somewhat startled by his interruption and confused by his apparent lack of understanding of the purpose of the conference. The teacher paused, became teary-eyed, and then told Mark and his parents that a close relative had recently died. She thanked Mark and spent much of the rest of the conference discussing Mark's empathy and compassion for others.

There can be some positive aspects to the honesty of expression of emotions. This is particularly true when accompanied by the real sense of empathy many adults with Down syndrome possess. Often adults with Down syndrome excel at sensing the emotions of other people.

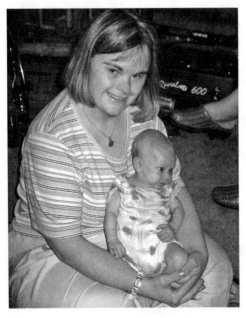

At times the strong sense of empathy and the honest expression of emotions is like a mirror. The emotions of a person with Down syndrome can be a reflection of what is going on around her. In particular, the emotion expressed can reflect the emotion of the person she is with. In a setting with people who are treating her kindly, this characteristic can be very positive. However, when those around her are expressing negative emotions, she may express similar negative emotions.

This is important for family and caregivers to be aware of and to accept. The question, "Why has Mary become so angry?" cannot be answered in a vacuum. In other words, an assessment of changes in the environment is essential. A child counselor and colleague used to describe it like this: "When families bring a child to the office and drop him at the curb and say, 'fix him,' you know you are going to have a real challenge." If families and care providers are unwilling to evaluate (and, if appropriate, acknowledge) the role the environment may play in the behavior change, the treatment will be more challenging and less likely to succeed.

The person with Down syndrome may reflect the emotions of a variety of settings. The emotions she expresses in one setting may actually be in response to something that occurred elsewhere. For instance, anger you see at home may actually be in response to something that occurred at school or work. In addition, physical health or biological issues may be contributing to her behavior or emotions. Therefore, any given environment may contribute little or nothing to a behavioral or emotional change. On the other hand, the environment may play a large role. Therefore, assessing each environment and reviewing the importance of this issue with people in each environment is an important part of the healing process. For example:

Jeff came home from work very upset and agitated. When this continued for over a week, his family contacted the ADSC. We called his worksite, but his supervisor could not explain the change in Jeff's behavior. There were no problems among the individuals in Jeff's work group and the staff had not observed anything unusual or problematic for Jeff. After some investigation, we found out that Jeff was upset about a coworker who was having frequent outbursts and crying spells. Interestingly, this man was in a separate room some distance from Jeff (over 200 feet). Jeff actually had no contact with him during the course of his day. Still, he seems to have picked up or absorbed the other man's tension and was greatly affected by it.

We have found that many people, like Jeff, may not always be able to filter out the emotions, stressors, tensions, and conflicts of others. In short, if someone with Down syndrome is showing emotions that do not seem to fit the situation, do not jump to the conclusion that she has psychological problems. Consider first: is she mirroring the emotions of those around her? Is she displaying extreme sensitivity to the events around her? Do her emotional reactions seem exaggerated? All of these are "normal" for people with Down syndrome. That is not to say that she may not need some help handling her emotions. For instance, people around her may need to work harder to display positive emotions around her or she may need to learn when it is tactful to be honest about negative emotions.

SENSITIVITY TO CONFLICTS BETWEEN OTHERS

We have found that people with DS may be very sensitive to conflicts or tensions between significant others in their lives. Depending on the type and degree of conflicts, they may be severely affected by these types of conflicts. For example:

Mary, a resident of a small group home, was brought to the Center when a mild habit of scratching her skin became a more serious problem of digging deep cuts in her neck and arms. Even though she had been very social and capable, she developed symptoms of a major depression, including a loss of appetite, restless sleep, sad mood, loss of energy, fatigue, and a loss of interest and participation in activities that she had formerly enjoyed. In her own words, she was "really down." When we questioned her group home manager, who brought her to the appointment, she complained that Mary's mother was the cause of her problems because she was overly protective. An example she gave was that Mary's mother would not allow her to go on outings that staff felt were beneficial for her. When we called her mother, she in turn complained that the house manager was trying to turn Mary against her and this was the reason that Mary was under so much stress.

After further exploring the situation, we found that the conflict between Mary's mother and staff had existed for some time. It turns out that neither the mother nor the house manager was necessarily wrong in what they wanted for Mary—they just held contrary opinions about what was best for her. For her part, Mary was extremely torn and stressed by this conflict because she loved her mother but also felt very close to her house manager. As the situation escalated and became increasingly intolerable for Mary, her agitation and depression increased.

We have seen similar problems with people caught between two parents in conflict, such as when parents were having serious marital problems or having a contentious divorce. In fact, asking the person with DS, or anyone, to take sides against people they love or who are important to their well-being is extremely dangerous. The stress that this creates invariably causes changes in mood and behavior in the person.

In theory, the solution to these problems is fairly simple. The person with Down syndrome must be removed from her position in the middle. This is possible if she is not asked to side with one parent or caregiver over the other. For example, in Mary's case, the ADSC staff relieved Mary of her position by becoming the intermediary in the conflict and working out a solution that was agreeable to both parties. For example, her mother and house manager agreed to a compromise which allowed Mary to go out in the community, which is what her house manager wanted, but with a staff person accompanying her, in deference to the mother's safety concerns. In time, many other issues were also resolved in this way with the help of mediation from the ADSC staff.

Although Mary's problem was solved fairly readily, resolving conflicts may not always be simple, such as when people are in the middle of a contested divorce. In these instances, it is still critical to get the person with DS out of the middle. What is most successful is to set up firm ground rules to free the person with DS from taking sides. One absolutely essential rule is for each parent to refrain from commenting about the other parent in front of the person with DS. Rules about how and when the person with DS makes transitions between his mother's and father's households are also of critical importance. Even when there are court-ordered visitation schedules, the rules surrounding this process must be carefully and meticulously reviewed with both parents. The reason is that whatever anger remains between parents will often be expressed in this process. Examples include late pick-ups or drop-offs, subsequent phone calls, and, of course, angry comments about the other parent directly to or within earshot of the son or daughter with DS. Moreover, the reason for these rules must be stated very clearly to each parent: Either you do this or you are responsible for the extreme stress and mental or behavioral changes that will be expressed by your son or daughter.

In some cases, the anger between parents is too strong and the only solution is for the person with DS to move to a neutral environment, such as a group home. This does not solve the problems completely but it does limit exposure of the person with

DS to the tension. Once the pattern of transitions is established, the person with DS is free to respond to each parent without fear or concern of hurting the other. In time, people are able to go back to their normal lives unencumbered by the intense burden one often feels when experiencing this process.

DELAYED MATURATION

Throughout the lifespan, there are periods when certain emotions tend to be more prominent. This is as true for people with Down syndrome as it is for others. One aspect that is different for people with Down syndrome is the timing. For example, many families report that their son or daughter in his or her early 20s wants to be left alone and is asserting him- or herself more. This can be seen negatively as depressed or agitated behavior. However, frequently it is all put in perspective when one question is asked: "Do you recall what your other children were like when they went through their teenage years?" This is typical adolescent or teenage behavior that is often, but not always, seen at a later age in people with Down syndrome. See Chapter 10 for more information about this delay in maturation.

DELAYED GRIEF RESPONSE

People with Down syndrome often have a delayed grief response. For example, when a family member dies, the person with Down syndrome may initially seem to be unaffected. Typically, she will begin to grieve approximately six months later. It is not completely clear why this delay occurs. However, it most likely has to do with slower cognitive processing (see below). It may simply take people with DS longer to recognize and understand that a loss has occurred (that the loved one is truly gone, etc.). Understanding and anticipating this response can help prevent problems and prepare family and care providers to help with the grieving process when the time comes.

LANGUAGE DELAYS

Language limitations in adults with Down syndrome can also lead to misinterpretation of their behavior. Many people with Down syndrome have language deficits. Often their expressive language skills are lower than their receptive language skills. That is, many people with Down syndrome understand what is going on around them, but are unable to express their concerns. This can be a real emotional challenge. It can lead to frustration, irritation, anger, and other emotional changes. Interpreting behavior change in light of this challenge can greatly improve the understanding of the behavior. Because language skills are often a major challenge for people with Down syndrome, we devote Chapter 6 to exploring them in depth.

PROCESSING SPEED

The ability to process data rapidly is an increasing demand of a world whose pace of activity is accelerating. Many people with Down syndrome have a limited ability to rapidly process data. In addition, they have a limited ability to shift processing speed in different situations, which can be even more problematic. Many people with DS find it a struggle when a situation demands a sudden acceleration in the pace of activity. Responding to an urgent situation can be very distressing. This limits adaptation to different settings. For example:

> *Neal, 17, was having difficulty in school due to his problem switching classes. When the bell rang and the other students moved to their next class, Neal would not move. After discussing the situation with Neal and his family, it became clear to us that Neal required a short period of time to process the need to adjust from the quiet classroom where he was seated to the active, noisy hallway. A verbal warning about five minutes before the bell gave Neal time to prepare for change in activity.*

The fact that people with Down syndrome have a limited cognitive processing speed may seem evident based on their intellectual disability. However, in practice, others who are interacting with people with Down syndrome often don't appreciate this. This is a particular problem in fast-paced places of business and with employers and can lead to difficulties in the work place or in the classroom, particularly an inclusive classroom.

In the Center, we see this manifested when we ask questions about a person's health. Over the course of the interview, we ask multiple questions. Not only may it take a moment or two for the person with DS to answer, but some of our patients are also quite fatigued by the end of the appointment. They have spent a great deal of mental energy thinking about and answering the questions.

When asked a question, people with Down syndrome often pause before answering. This can lead to misinterpretation of their behavior and problems in interacting with others. Often others interpret the pause as meaning that the person with Down syndrome is ignoring what they said, is insolent, or has an attention problem. This has led to problems for many of our patients, especially at work or school. It can be a source of friction between the person with Down syndrome and her boss, teacher, or fellow employees.

In addition, if multiple directions are given before the person is able to process them, then she can become frustrated. We have seen or heard about many people with Down syndrome who stop attempting to process in that situation because they have become overwhelmed. The employer may also become frustrated and lose patience. This can lead to agitation and strained interaction between the two people.

These types of misunderstandings are a common source of conflicts at work or school and can lead to loss of employment or disciplinary issues. Interestingly, this type of issue is a more common cause of job loss than lack of skills to do the job (Greenspan and Shoultz, 1981). Understanding and appreciating the challenge of slower processing and providing information at a rate that the person with Down syndrome can process will lead to a much healthier situation and less frustration and conflict.

MAKING ACCOMMODATIONS FOR PROCESSING SPEED

In light of these issues with slower processing speed, how can others optimize interaction with a person with Down syndrome?

- ◆ Understand that this is a potential issue. Being prepared to adjust one's approach is the first step.
- ◆ Be careful not to view this as a "behavioral" issue. It may be that the person is slower at processing the information rather than insolent.
- ◆ Anticipate that she may need a period of time to process the information. Start the request soon enough so that she will have that time.
- ◆ Get her attention. Wait for a response from her such as "What?" or "Yes" to indicate she is acknowledging you have her attention.
- ◆ Make the request or give the directive in an understandable fashion and confirm that she understood.
- ◆ Give her the time she needs to process the request.
- ◆ After an appropriate period of time (this varies from person to person but it may be several minutes, depending on the request), check with her to make sure she understood or that there is no impediment to her proceeding (rather than making the request repeatedly or louder).
- ◆ Bear in mind that many people with Down syndrome will just stop their effort to comply if there is an impediment rather than try an alternative approach or ask for assistance.
- ◆ Try to find alternative ways of communicating (to speak to the person's strengths). For example, many people with DS benefit greatly from visual images that may augment or accompany a verbal communication or instruction. After all, visual images are useful in any teaching situation. This is why presenters or teachers use blackboards, slides, or other visual aids when teaching. For people with DS, this may be especially useful because so many are visual learners (see Chapter 5). For example, we consistently hear from job supervisors that even complex, multi-step tasks may be learned and repeated reliably if the task is broken down into smaller steps that are shown to the person with DS.

TIME REFERENCE

Understanding the concepts of past, present, and future is something most people take for granted. Since these concepts are abstract, however, they are difficult for many people with Down syndrome to understand. This can lead to confusion for both the person who doesn't understand and for the people around her. When taken in context of the very strong memory (see Chapter 5) that many people with Down syndrome have, this can lead to even further confusion. Recall the example of Robert at the beginning of the chapter, who reacted as if his father had just died when questioned about him, when, in reality, he had died 15 years ago. The understanding of past and present seemed to be different for Robert than for people without Down syndrome. For him, a very strong memory made past events seem as real as present events.

Often we find a less clear line of distinction between past and present than we would expect in someone who doesn't have Down syndrome. For the person with Down syndrome, the understanding of many concepts is much more concrete and the concept of time is too abstract.

This decreased sense of the difference between past and present can lead to much confusion in conversation with other people. Some of our patients have even been diagnosed as psychotic by other practitioners because the person with Down syndrome appeared to be disconnected to the reality of the present. Most often we have found this type of misdiagnosis to be due to miscommunication and to the practitioner's unfamiliarity with the way people with Down syndrome sense time. As noted before, when this characteristic is taken in the context of a very strong memory, the person with Down syndrome can recall far-off events and may seem to have a disconnection with the present.

If an adult has limited communication skills, this problem is exacerbated. It can be very difficult to ascertain if she is talking about an event that occurred recently or in the distant past. This can, for example, make it very difficult to get an accurate history regarding symptoms:

> Carol, 25, has very limited verbal skills and usually speaks in one- or two-word phrases. She was complaining of ear pain. A thorough evaluation revealed no underlying problem. After further discussion, it seemed that this was more of a complaint of her past medical history of frequent ear infections.

Sometimes the misunderstanding may be due more to language usage of past and present tenses than to a true lack of understanding of time. Dr. Libby Kumin, a speech-language pathologist with a special interest in Down syndrome, theorizes that some people with Down syndrome never learn to use verb endings correctly because hearing problems in their formative years prevent them from hearing the final –s or –ed on verbs. Others do not master irregular verbs due to language learning difficulties and may answer questions such as "What did you do this weekend?" along the lines of "Saturday I eat dinner with my Mom." In context, the listener can figure out that the person is speaking of a past event, but a less careful listener could be confused (Kumin, 2003). As indicated, this different time reference can affect interactions with other people. The biggest problem for people with Down syndrome occurs when someone assumes they understand time and time references in a "typical" or "usual" fashion. This leads to misinterpretation of what they say and sometimes to disagreements or misunderstandings, and can lead practitioners to make an inaccurate diagnosis on the basis of an apparently altered thought process.

Based on these findings, we have some recommendations for optimizing communication:

◆ Appreciate that someone with Down syndrome may have a different understanding of time. Knowing that she may be speaking in the present tense about a past event can lead to further questions to prevent confusion.

◆ What are the person's overall language skills? Have you previously heard her use past tense or words like "yesterday"? If not, when she is speaking in present tense, she may actually be speaking about the past.

◆ If possible, help the person put the event in the time context of another event. For example, ask, "Did it happen when you were in school? When you were working at the grocery store?" Particularly if the person says she doesn't know, look for other clues about when the event occurred. Parents are often very helpful in helping answer this question. For example, "I know that is a past event because she referred to Sally, who was a high school classmate."

Awareness of "Clock Time"

An interesting paradox is the incredible ability of many adults with Down syndrome to "know the time." This is often demonstrated in grooves (see Chapter 9). Sometimes people with Down syndrome are very inflexible about times in their routines, insisting that meals, breaks at work, televisions shows, etc. occur at set times. Many people who follow set time schedules cannot "tell time," yet have an internal clock that is often extremely accurate. We have learned to pay close attention to time at the Adult Down Syndrome Center because people can be less tolerant of our questions and procedures when we intrude on their lunch time.

Inflexibility about time can also cause problems in employment settings. For example, in the early days of the clinic, we employed a young woman with Down syndrome, Jean, who did an excellent job of data entry. At the time, we had limited space and Jean had to share a small office with two other employees. One afternoon, Jean suddenly got up and literally climbed over both staff members to leave the room. She then left the building and caught her bus home. The staff members were surprised to find that she had not saved her work or turned off her computer before leaving. When questioned about this later, Jean could not understand their surprise. She explained that it was 2:30, which was "time to go home." Fortunately, Jean was able to learn a different routine, which included finishing her work activities appropriately in anticipation of quitting time.

CONCRETE THINKING

Most of us who are past the age of 12 or so can think both concretely and abstractly. Using our five senses gives us a concrete understanding of the world. However, it can be more challenging to think beyond what we can perceive with our five senses to think abstractly or theoretically. People with Down syndrome often think in a very concrete manner and frequently cannot think well abstractly.

> *Eugene was in the office for a complete evaluation, which lasts approximately three hours. After seeing the social worker, the audiologist, and the nutritionist, he was now seeing the physician. One of the standard questions asked is about appetite. As the time was approaching noon, Eugene's response was, "I am hungry." The question was rephrased in several different ways in an effort to understand Eugene's appetite in a general sense, but the answers only became more emphatic as to his present state of hunger. His mother explained his eating habits and we moved on to the next question (and as quickly as possible, to lunch).*

The concrete nature of the thought processes of most people with Down syndrome is very functional and can be very precise if allowed to flourish in an appropriate setting. Often people with Down syndrome do wonderfully in jobs that have concrete tasks. In fact, we find that most often when a person with Down syndrome has problems at work, it is not because she can't do the tasks. Often, she does the task extremely well and is a model employee because her concrete nature helps her to do it well repeatedly. While the physician struggled with Eugene to get the answer to his question, the inability to answer the question as asked had no real impact on Eugene (other than to slightly delay his lunch). On the other hand, Eugene is the best employee in his mail service job. He is responsible for delivering mail in a six-story office building. He goes from the mailing center in the basement to the sixth floor and precisely moves from floor to floor delivering the mail. In a concrete world, he flourishes.

The challenge for many people with Down syndrome comes when a task changes and they must take what they have learned and apply it to a new situation. For example:

> *Luis works at a job about ten miles from his house. He takes a bus about four miles, transfers to another bus and rides it about six miles, and then walks the last three blocks. He does very well in getting back and forth to work on time. One day, however, there was construction on one of the streets that his bus usually traveled on. The bus had to take a detour a block east, go north two blocks, and then return west to the street the bus usually travels. Luis recognized as he traveled north on the new street that he was not on the usual route. He got off the bus and became lost. While his concrete thinking required for the daily trip was excellent and he was able to manage public transportation very well, the abstract thinking required by the change in route was difficult for Luis.*

ABSTRACT VS. CONCRETE LANGUAGE

Communication is often spoken in a concrete way, when, in fact, it is meant to be interpreted using abstract reasoning skills. For instance, a young woman with Down syndrome was working in an office and was encouraged to "call any time" if she had questions. After she made a few 3 a.m. phone calls to the home of a coworker, the true meaning of "call any time" had to be clarified. Another office worker has trouble with tasks like these, which require abstract language skills:

◆ Answering the phone and differentiating telemarketing calls—which should be screened out—from legitimate calls—which should be transferred to the appropriate coworker;

◆ Understanding that when colleagues ask her what she did on the weekend, they do not want to hear a lengthy hour-by-hour report, but a quick summary;

◆ Recognizing and weeding out duplicate names when entering customer names into a computer program that is used for generating mailing lists (e.g., not realizing that Thomas Dooley, T. Dooley, and Tom Dooley are probably one and the same person, especially if they live at the same address).

These kinds of misunderstandings are often the source of significant problems in the work place.

GENERALIZATION SKILLS

The tendency towards strength in concrete thinking and weakness in abstract thinking also makes it difficult to take what is learned in one setting and apply it to another—that is, to *generalize* skills. This is frequently a problem where money or other math skills are involved. For instance:

> *Rosa was learning money skills at school. The teacher worked with her on several occasions, sitting at a table in a room. She could identify each coin and its value and add coins up to get a total value. However, after walking down the hall 30 steps to the soda machine, Rosa was unable to add up coins to reach the 60 cents that were needed to make a purchase. After additional training, she was finally able to purchase her own drink.*

Similarly:

> *Valerie, who is employed as an office assistant, is able to count quite competently. However, if she is photocopying a long document for a coworker and the pages get out of order, she is unable to correct the pagination herself. She usually ends up in tears if she struggles with the jumbled-up pages too long.*
>
> *Valerie also has trouble generalizing her excellent reading and writing skills to help her perform her job. Often when she is having problems*

remembering how to do something, a coworker will prompt her to write down the steps involved. Afterwards, Valerie can usually follow the written instructions and complete the task independently. However, it never occurs to her to write needed information down for herself, even when it is something (such as state abbreviations) that she repeatedly asks her coworkers for.

Problems with generalization can lead to problems at work and school. Others may assume the person with Down syndrome is deliberately pretending she doesn't remember how to do something in one setting that she could do in another.

WHAT HELPS

What may seem to be an obvious logical next step may not be obvious to someone with Down syndrome. This can lead to misunderstandings, communication difficulties, and even "behavioral issues." (Either the inappropriate response is interpreted as a "behavior problem" or the person with Down syndrome may become frustrated and her behavior may change.) If the task is broken down into concrete pieces, however, the person is often quite capable of managing the tasks with little, if any, confusion and "behavioral issues."

We have found that one particularly beneficial way to assist many people with Down syndrome make sense of abstractions is to help them visualize the tasks by providing pictures. We also find that schedules (often with pictures) are quite helpful. For example, breaking the bedtime routine into a schedule of concrete tasks is beneficial. We encourage the person with Down syndrome (with the help of her family or care provider) to select approximately five or six tasks that need to be done before bedtime. These tasks are selected out of a series of pictures. The picture corresponding to each task is then pasted on a small piece of cardboard in sequential order. This serves as a reminder. For other people, a system that allows them to check off boxes as tasks are completed is a better way to manage the bedtime routine. Interestingly, even some of our patients who generally function independently and would seem not to need this assistance may benefit from this type of system.

We have found that providing pictures can be helpful in other areas as well. Coming to the doctor's office frightens some of our patients. We have made a book with pictures of a visit to the office. As the person looks through the book, it makes it less abstract and more concrete, and generally, less frightening. Likewise, to assist patients in taking more responsibility for their own care, we have found it helpful to develop patient education materials that have pictures that guide the person through self-care. While it may be initially more time consuming to make schedules and directions with pictures, it does give the person with Down syndrome more opportunity to direct her own care. It also reduces the confusion that can occur when the directions are only provided verbally. In the long run, it will probably also save time in completing daily tasks.

Including information in this book to help the person with Down syndrome work through issues related to concrete and abstract thinking (and, thus, help her be more independent) is extremely important. Being successful in self-care can lead to a great sense of accomplishment, improved self-esteem, and increased interest in caring for oneself (see Chapter 7). A personal sense of good health is an important part of mental health. In contrast, confusion about what is being asked or is expected can lead to an escalating set of problems. The loss of a job, the loss of self-esteem, and other negative effects can lead to more severe mental health issues.

Problematic issues related to concrete thinking are very important to recognize, particularly when it comes to promoting mental health and preventing mental illness. In a world that demands both concrete and abstract thinking, it is very important for those assisting a person with Down syndrome to consider these issues. The goal is to present the tasks of daily life in a way that capitalizes on strengths in concrete thinking but does not penalize for the limited abstract nature of the thought process.

Self-Talk

Another behavior that we frequently encounter is self-talk. As described in detail in Chapter 8, self-talk is very common in people with Down syndrome. We became particularly interested in this topic when we found a great number of our patients being treated by other practitioners for psychoses. Talking to themselves seemed to be the major reason these misdiagnoses were made. While self-talk can be part of the diagnostic criteria for psychoses, these major psychiatric disorders are characterized by delusions, hallucinations, withdrawal from reality, paranoia, unusual affect, and an altered thought process. Self-talk without these other symptoms is not a psychotic disorder. When we assessed all of our patients for self-talk, we found that approximately 83 percent of them talked to themselves and that many of the other 17 percent did not speak at all. Without understanding or appreciating this finding, it can lead to over-diagnosis of "abnormal."

As mentioned above, self-talk is developmentally appropriate for many adults with Down syndrome, since many typically developing children under the age of 6 or so talk to themselves.

A similar behavior that is often appropriate for an adult's developmental stage is the use of imaginary friends. This too can lead to inaccurate diagnoses if the developmental stage of the individual is not considered. Self-talk, imaginary friends, and fantasy lives are addressed further in Chapter 8.

Tendency Toward Sameness and Repetition

Another truly fascinating aspect of the personality of many people with Down syndrome is the tendency to prefer sameness or repetition. We call this "the groove." The groove has many advantages, such as helping a person maintain order in her life and optimizing use of her skills. However, the lack of flexibility can make it difficult to deal with the realities of the changes and inconsistencies of life. In addition, if others do not understand this tendency, it is easy for conflicts to develop, because dealing with apparent inflexibility can be disruptive for people who have less "groove."

Because so many adolescents and adults with Down syndrome have "grooves" that can be misinterpreted as behavior problems, we discuss the issue in detail in Chapter 9.

KEEPING SIGHT OF THE CONTINUUM

Understanding what is normal or typical for people with Down syndrome helps define the continuum of normal to abnormal. This understanding gives a reference point for comprehending behavior in adolescents and adults with Down syndrome. Looking again at some of the issues discussed above will illustrate this principle.

Looking at the tendency toward sameness or repetition, the normal (or typical) behavior for a person with Down syndrome is "the groove." Abnormal is taking the groove to such an extreme that it interferes with the ability to function efficiently in daily life. Grooves can be quite useful if others in the environment recognize this ten-

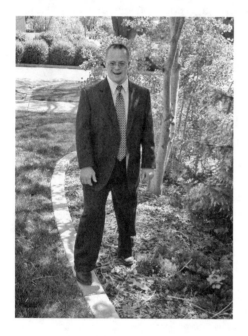

dency and are willing to work with the behavior. However, if the tendency prevents functioning in daily life—either because of the degree of compulsion or the inability of others to work with the tendency—obsessive- compulsive disorder may be diagnosed (see Chapter 16).

Similarly, with grief, depending on the degree of the problem and the environment in which the person is grieving, the reaction may fit somewhere on the continuum from normal grieving to depression.

Self-talk is another behavioral aspect that can fit on a continuum. As indicated, self-talk is a common behavior in adults with Down syndrome, but self-talk can also be a feature of psychoses. A careful assessment of the nature of the self-talk, associated symptoms, environmental circumstances, and the person's functioning, as well as the presence or absence of self-talk prior to the present concern, is necessary to understand where the self-talk fits on the continuum.

Another aspect of the continuum that is important to understand is that complete absence of the particular behavior is not necessarily healthier than the presence of the behavior. In other words, because "too much" of a particular behavior meets the criteria for a particular psychological problem (e.g., psychotic disorder), the complete absence of the behavior is not necessarily the goal. For example, families and caregivers often ask whether self-talk should be suppressed. As is discussed in more detail in Chapter 8, people with Down syndrome often use self-talk as a means of talking through problems.

Therefore, to suppress the self-talk may actually hamper the healing process. In this situation, eliminating self-talk is neither healthy nor the goal of therapy.

While it is important to consider these "typical" behaviors in light of the continuum, it is equally important to avoid the trap of "blaming everything on the Down syndrome." A typical behavior that has become problematic may no longer just be "typical behavior of Down syndrome." It is necessary to assess whether it has become a psychological problem. This is optimally achieved by understanding the individual's behavior throughout her life, particularly if she has undergone a change in behavior. Developing an understanding of the person before the change, assessing the period of her life, evaluating the environment, and other assessments as outlined in Chapter 1, will help delineate the causes of a change in behavior. This evaluation will help clarify whether this is common or typical behavior for a person with Down syndrome, where it fits on the continuum, and whether further assessment and treatment is indicated.

Evaluating behavior with an understanding of the continuum has a number of advantages. It provides a framework for appreciating and acknowledging the unique qualities and common behavioral characteristics of people with Down syndrome. It stresses the importance of the role the environment plays in supporting the person with Down syndrome in developing mental health. It also provides a structure to assess when behavior is abnormal and further intervention and treatment is necessary.

Chapter 5

Memory

* * * * * * * * * *

While at the Adult Center, the mother of a 32-year-old woman with Down syndrome commented that she and her daughter, Kristin, had recently visited their native country of Romania. This was their first opportunity to visit family and friends since they immigrated to the U.S. 16 years ago. What surprised the mother was that her daughter remembered their native country far better than she did. For example, even after 16 years, Kristin recognized scores of relatives (even those they had seen only occasionally). She also recognized the neighborhoods these relatives lived in, and even the location of their houses. Perhaps most surprising to the mother was Kristin's ability to remember the details of family events that occurred 16 to 25 years in the past, while they still lived in Romania. This was particularly the case when she was shown photographs of these events by her relatives.

We frequently hear from other families that their family member with Down syndrome has similar memory skills. We have found that, like Kristin, people with DS often have exceptional memory for things they have seen or experienced visually. We will discuss this skill and related issues in this chapter.

As Chapter 3 discussed, there are many cognitive and behavioral characteristics that are normal for someone with Down syndrome but not necessarily normal for someone without. Many of these involve abilities that might be considered "deficient" or a bit odd. But many people with Down syndrome actually have some abilities that might be considered relatively advanced. One of these abilities is in the area of memory. In some respects, many people with Down syndrome actually have better memories than other people do. In other respects, they don't. Since a great deal of research has been done into the ways in which memory is poorer in Down syndrome, we will only touch on those areas here and focus primarily on the areas of memory in which people with Down syndrome excel.

OVERVIEW OF MEMORY ISSUES

Given that almost everyone with Down syndrome has some degree of mental retardation, it is not surprising that Down syndrome is usually associated with some difficulties with memory. Areas that are usually impaired by Down syndrome include:

Working Memory: Working memory is a critically important form of short-term memory that allows people to do immediate tasks in their day-to-day lives. Our working memory enables us to hold information in our mind long enough to complete a task. There are two types—verbal and visual-spatial working memory, which are governed by different parts of the brain. This type of memory does not necessarily have to be stored for future use. However, whatever is learned in this process may be stored in long term memory (similar to storing data on a diskette or the hard drive of a computer). People with Down syndrome have definite deficits of verbal working memory and some related problems with visual working memory.

Verbal Working Memory: This is the ability to remember words and numbers that are spoken aloud. An example of a deficit in this area is having difficulty remembering a phone number long enough to dial it. A second example is having difficulty remembering the sounds associated with letters and words (phonetics), which may then impede language usage. This memory deficit does not appear to be related to either hearing or speech problems (Jarrold, C., Baddeley, A.D., 2001). Because so much of our daily experience is mediated by verbal language, the inability to remember verbal messages may cause problems functioning in the world. This may delay expressive or receptive language development and use (Buckley, S., Le Prevost, P., 2002). This kind of deficit can also affect how a person's behavior is viewed. For example, if someone cannot remember a series of instructions given to him verbally, he may be considered oppositional or less competent than he is.

Dependence on Concrete Thought: As discussed below, many people with Down syndrome have above average visual-spatial memory. However, the benefits of visual memory may still be relatively limited. This is because people with DS depend on concrete rather than abstract forms of thought. This may prevent them from learning from past experiences stored in long-term memory. The reason for this is that abstract thought allows one to see the relationship between things and not just the individual (concrete) case. In the absence of this, the person is often not able to use a past visual memory to help deal with his current situation.

For example, people with DS can learn how to ride a bus on a specific route by initially watching and copying a family member or mobility trainer (a staff person who teaches people how to use public transportation). However, if the route changes due to road construction or the like, the person may not be able to cope. We have heard about several people in this situation who have simply gotten off the bus. Although they could "see" the original route in their memories, they could not "envision" that another way was possible. They also could not use their experience with learning the route the first time to help them adapt (even temporarily) to a new way. These individuals had to be retrained to use the temporary route. They did not have to be retrained to use the old route, however, once the construction was finished. Their ability to recall and use a visual memory of the old route was still strong. It seems then that past events may still be used effectively, if there is no change to the original event.

Now, we can still use the person's visual skills to teach a host of adaptive skills (see below) and enhance learning by pairing visual skills with verbal stimuli. At the Adult Center, we also frequently succeeded in using visual images to teach more adaptive behavior (see Chapter 13 on modeling). But we still need to manipulate the images for people with DS and not depend on them to do so on their own.

This is not to say that people may not be able to find different ways and means of learning and solving problems on their own. For example, in Chapter 13, we discuss the fact that people with DS are very sensitive to others' feelings and emotions and this may be an excellent means to learning in certain situations. For example:

> *Jason, a young man with Down syndrome, worked in a grocery store. He had learned how to deal with a boss who was warm and personable. Unfortunately, this boss was transferred and an unfriendly boss took over. In the past, Jason had worked with teachers and others who were standoffish and had successfully dealt with them. Nevertheless, he was accustomed to his old boss and he tried on several occasions to shake his new boss's hand and to engage him in conversations, but the new boss did not reciprocate. Because of his reliance on concrete thinking, Jason could not use his previous experience with standoffish people to help him in this situation. Fortunately, after a number of unsuccessful attempts to engage the boss, Jason intuitively sensed that the boss was not interested in being his friend and Jason backed off. Despite his inability to use his past experience, his social sensitivity helped him to avoid the mistake of aggravating his boss with friendly overtures.*

Jason's experience notwithstanding, we usually find that most employers, teachers, etc. readily understand the connection between mental retardation and these types of memory problems and make accommodations for them. Strangely enough, it may be more difficult for people not familiar with Down syndrome to understand behavior that is linked to memory *strengths* that often go along with the syndrome. Several of these strengths were mentioned above and include the following:

◆ Visual memory;
◆ Recalling high-interest facts;
◆ Visual -spatial memory.

We explore these areas of strength in detail below.

AREAS OF STRENGTH

VISUAL MEMORY

One of the most important find-ings at the Center is that most people with Down syndrome, like Kristin in the above example, have an uncanny memory for people, places, and past events. We have found that this mem-ory is visual in nature, and may even be described as "photographic-like." People with Down syndrome may re-call past events in graphic detail, as if looking at a picture or a movie. Fami-lies are often astounded by the detail of recalled events. For example, recall of a family gathering may not only in-clude who came and what occurred, but such minutiae as the color and

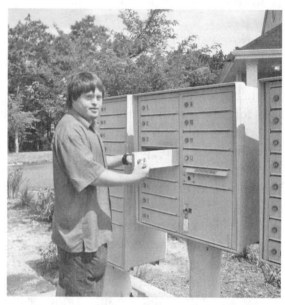

type of people's clothing, music played, etc. These recalled events may have occurred 20 or 30 years ago and still be crystal clear.

Families have given us clues as to how and why certain memories are recalled. It appears that present-day experiences often trigger recall of past people or events, particularly if there is a visual reminder. For example, many families tell us that their family member with Down syndrome points out places while riding in the car. These places may or may not be known to other family members. However, when these plac-es are investigated, they are invariably found to be a part of the person with Down syndrome's experience. For example:

> Anna and her mother went to the airport to pick up a beloved aunt, who had moved some time ago to a distant city. On the drive, Anna, who had some articulation limitations, pointed to a hot dog stand and tried repeatedly to say the name of this stand. When she persisted, her mother became irritated, commenting that Anna was being selfish, since she knew they had to pick up their aunt. Returning from the airport, Anna again

pointed at the hot dog stand, and her mother again told her they could not stop. After some time Anna's aunt smiled and then commented that she had not at first recognized the stand. She went on to explain to the mother that she and Anna had visited the stand on a number of occasions while she still lived in this town, much to the mother's surprise and the daughter's pleasure.

We have heard numerous other examples as well. For instance, pictures from old family albums not only elicit recognition of familiar events and people, but also more obscure people or events that others in the family barely remember.

MEMORY OF HIGH-INTEREST FACTS

We commonly hear that many people with Down syndrome have a remarkable memory for concrete bits of information (which are probably codified into visual form), such as the names and birth dates of others. This is especially true of things that are of interest. For example, many people remember statistics of favorite sports teams, as well as vast amounts of information on favorite music, movies, and television shows.

Many adolescents and adults with DS like to make lists of facts they are interested in, such as the names of Beatles songs or favorite movie characters. They may also make lists of things that are a part of their daily lives such as grocery items, activities planned for the month, the names of relatives, and even more mundane information such as items in their lunchbox or menu items of the week.

Writing and looking at lists may help people memorize the facts they are interested in. In many cases, the act of making the list may also be a relaxing or pleasurable task (as discussed in the Groove chapter), even if the facts are already memorized. However, this list making is not nearly as useful in helping people to remember facts that are not personally meaningful or of interest to them. This may include memorizing definitions of more abstract concepts encountered at school, or remembering events which do not directly affect them, such as politics or current events. This is one reason why mental status exams are not useful with people with DS and other disabilities. A mental status exam is a relatively brief assessment of a person's basic intellectual, social, and emotional functioning used by mental health professionals. Unfortunately, some of the key questions testing a person's cognitive function rely on knowledge of current events. This unfairly penalizes people with Down syndrome, who would not necessarily know or care to know this information.

VISUAL-SPATIAL MEMORY

Many people with Down syndrome are able to use their strong visual memory skills to remember locations of people, places, or things. For instance, they can often find their way, or direct others, back to places previously visited. Additionally, many people can use this memory skill to visually map their surroundings in order to acclimate and to orient themselves to an environment. For example, we have frequently heard from employers or teachers that the person with Down syndrome rarely gets lost, even in a maze-like high school or work setting.

People with Down syndrome may also use this skill to organize personal belongings. Interestingly, many people have extensive and meticulously maintained libraries of CDs, videotapes, or DVDs. Families are often amazed that the person with DS remembers exactly where a particular CD or tape is in his collection, even if he cannot read the titles on the CD or tape. Instead, he is remembering placement by visual memory. It is almost as if the person has a photograph of his room in his memory which he compares to the actual scene when he goes into his room after being away for some time.

ADVANTAGES OF A STRONG VISUAL MEMORY

There are many advantages to having good visual memory skills. For example, they can be very helpful in social situations because people with Down syndrome rarely forget a name or face. Family members tell us that they also benefit. They seldom have to worry about forgetting names in social situations as long as the person with Down

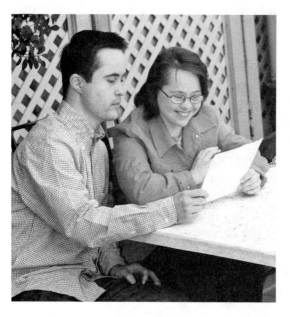

syndrome is present to remind them. Related to this, people with Down syndrome are often very thoughtful in remembering others' birthdays, anniversaries, etc. They may also use their memory of high-interest information to come up with something interesting to discuss in social situations, such as statistics about a favorite sports team, music, movies, celebrity facts, etc.

Visual memory skills can also greatly enhance independence in home and work settings. An adult who has a strong memory can memorize self-care or worksite tasks once he has had an opportunity to observe someone else doing the task. This is especially the case if the tasks are broken down and shown at a pace conducive to learning. Once they have learned a task, people with Down syndrome are able to repeat these tasks reliably in their daily routines. (See Chapter 9 for more on this.)

Finally, their visual memories may help people with DS relax when engaged in such activities as looking at photograph albums, especially of favorite holidays, vacations, family gatherings, etc. Watching movies is also a favorite past time for many people with DS, and many will replay the same video over and over. Additionally, we have found that visual memory may be paired with another favorite for people with DS, music. For example, we have found that music is often an essential part of a favorite movie or TV show. Many adults with Down syndrome enjoy musicals such as *Grease, Dirty Dancing, The Sound of Music,* and *Oklahoma.* Favorite TV shows may include "Barney" and many Disney shows that have strong musical scores. We have heard from many families that they hear certain songs or CDs as well as favorite musicals played over and over. While this is not exactly music to the ears of other family members (after hearing the same song 6000 times), still, for people with DS, there seems to be a great deal of comfort to seeing/hearing the same thing over and over.

DISADVANTAGES OF A STRONG VISUAL MEMORY

Despite the potential for great benefits, this type of memory recall can also lead to some significant problems. These are in addition to the problems that occur because teachers and employers often expect people with Down syndrome to use their weaker auditory memory skills without visual supports, and may become frustrated when spoken instructions are not followed or when the person seems to "tune them out." To help you understand the cause of these problems, we will discuss three key characteristics of memory recall for people with DS, then discuss the possibility for misinterpretation by others and the potential for posttraumatic stress resulting from memory recall. The three key characteristics of memory recall in people with DS include:

1. difficulty linking memories to time;
2. the tendency to relive past memories in the present; and
3. the tendency to repeat specific memories.

DIFFICULTIES LINKING MEMORIES TO TIME

Although people with Down syndrome have exceptional memory for past events, they often have little understanding of when these events occurred in time. This is due to their difficulty in comprehending more abstract notions of time (see Chapter 3). Many understand time in precise terms, such as dinner at 6:00, but have great difficulty grasping more abstract concepts of time and its passages, in past months or years. As a result, many people with Down syndrome do not have a good sense of recalled events as part of the past or as part of a historical sequence of events.

RELIVING PAST MEMORIES IN THE PRESENT

As discussed previously, people with Down syndrome often seem to think and recall events in picture or visual form. Combining this visual form of thinking with an absence of a sense of time results in a very interesting phenomenon. That is, many people with DS do not seem to remember a past event so much as to relive or re-experience it as if it is happening now, and quite often with the feelings and emotions experienced at the time of the original event.

This tendency may be good or bad, depending on the nature of the past event. For example, reliving positive experiences, such as holidays and vacations with family members, can be very pleasurable. On the other hand, re-experiencing negative experiences, such as a frightening thunderstorm or the funeral of a close family member, is not. Many people with DS may have trouble realizing that the event is not happening again, which may intensify the feelings associated with the re-experience of the event. This will be explained in greater detail below, in the section on post traumatic stress.

THE TENDENCY TO REPEAT MEMORIES

Many people with Down syndrome replay certain specific memories over and over. These repeated memories are often memories that elicit strong positive or negative emotions.

Understandably, people will want to re-experience positive events. For example, we frequently hear that people with DS love to look at pictures from photograph albums, especially of favorite holidays, vacations, etc. Given the intensity of their visual memory, they are able to transport themselves virtually back in time to relive these experiences. It is as if they are right there again, enjoying themselves with family and friends. Home videotapes are also very popular. People with DS often repeatedly view tapes of favorite or meaningful events.

Many people with DS also tend to replay negative experiences. This is probably a means for them to gain some sense of control over a negative experience—much as those of us without Down syndrome might have the same dream over and over until an issue is resolved. The person may feel compelled to repeat these experiences, as if he has little control over the process. This is particularly the case for people with DS who have a preexisting tendency for repetition and rumination, which is then increased with the presence of negative experiences (see Chapter 9).

One of the most commonly replayed types of negative memories is of situations in which the person with Down syndrome feels he was guilty of some wrongdoing. Sometimes the source of the guilt may be mystifying to caregivers. Often, the caregiver may experience the recalled event as trivial or may not even remember the event. (Irish guilt pales by comparison.) Ironically, others are often then put in the odd position of having to repeatedly receive apologies for events that occurred months or even years in the past and that they barely recall and have no negative feelings regarding. For example, one young man accidentally broke a plate at a dinner party given by friends of his parents. Although this accident occurred over six years ago, he continues to apologize to the parents of this family, whenever he sees them. Also, at times the need to repeat certain past events may be comical. We have heard many versions of the following example. At his first appointment at the ADSC, one young man with Down syndrome reported in a matter of fact way that his father tripped him. With humor his father explained that the event was an accident that had happened over seven years ago, and yet his son still needed to inform others about this infraction. To this, the father added, with a smile, "May God help you if you do anything bad, even by mistake, because it will never . . . and I mean never, be forgotten."

MEMORIES TRIGGERED BY EVENTS

In addition to choosing to replay memories, people with Down syndrome, like the rest of us, may have memories involuntarily triggered by occurrences in their daily lives. For example:

> After her father's death, Amanda, 33, was very upset whenever she went past her father's den and observed his pipe (which for her had a special association to him). Unfortunately, she had to go past the den frequently. As a result, she would become sad and preoccupied, which began to interfere in her daily activities. She was arriving late for work, had difficulty getting ready for bed, and was losing sleep. We were able to reduce the intensity of this preoccupation for her by simply having her family close the den door. Her family did open the door for a brief period in the evening. Amanda seemed to need this intense but limited exposure in order to grieve her father's loss. Nevertheless, she was still able to go about her daily business during other times of the day.

We have found that the intensity of emotionally charged events does not seem to diminish over time. For example, many older people with DS who have lost family members ten or more years ago still experience an intense sense of loss. Like Amanda, they too are transported back to the time of the loss. Fortunately, these past events are often experienced very intensely "in the moment." Then, most people are able to quickly move on to more positive thoughts or memories, especially if encouraged to do so by others. The difference, it seems, for those who become preoccupied with a loss, is the frequency of these "in the moment" experiences. For Amanda, we were able to limit the number of the most sensitive visual reminders of her father, which helped her to function at other times of her day. Caregivers and professionals who understand this type of "in the moment recall" can try to limit exposure to stimuli that trigger these memories, so that the adult with DS is not mired in it. Having pictures or even verbal reminders of positive events may also help to substitute positive memories for more painful or negative experiences.

Having said this, we have found that memories of emotionally charged experiences may be recalled with very little stimuli. In fact, what triggers a recalled experience may seem relatively insignificant or incongruous to an outside observer. In fact, we have found that small losses will often trigger the recall of a more serious loss. For instance:

> A nutritionist and school counselor were running an aerobics and nutrition awareness group for a group of eight well-adjusted young adults with Down syndrome. In the ensuing discussion, one young man

expressed sadness over the loss of his dog (actually a past event). This opened a floodgate of tears and emotions from other group participants, who had their own experiences of past losses. The two staff members were overwhelmed and at a loss to explain to the participants' families why the participants seemed so emotionally distraught after the group. Staff and family were relieved to find that the young adults returned to their normal emotional state fairly soon after the group.

Again, this group grief was due to the nature of the "in the moment" recall experience. At a subsequent meeting at the Adult Down Syndrome Center, we were also able to explain that this is a fairly common response by people with Down syndrome, even those who are well-adjusted individuals. It has been three years since this event, and there have been no long-lasting effects reported.

UNDERSTANDING WHY SPECIFIC MEMORIES ARE REPEATEDLY RECALLED

The repeated recall of memories may be a useful means of expression and communication if the listener understands the nature of the recall experience. At the Adult Down Syndrome Center, we have learned to listen carefully to family members or staff who share a common history with the person with Down syndrome. These individuals are often able to determine the correct time and context of the events discussed by the person. With this information, the caregivers hold the key to the translation of a potentially rich medium of experiences and emotions represented in the original event. Translating these events into meaning is enormously supportive to the person with Down syndrome and enormously informative to the caregiver and to us at the Adult Down Syndrome Center. This is especially important to people with Down syndrome who have limitations in verbal communication. For example:

Walter, 32, was brought to the Center by his mother and sister because he was uncharacteristically lethargic and unresponsive to family and friends. During the course of the meeting, he began to make comments which seemed to concern some type of accident. Eventually, they surmised that he was talking about an auto accident that his father had 15 years ago, when he himself was a teenager. His mother explained that this accident had created a great deal of stress for the family because the father was injured and out of work for several months. Apparently this was particularly difficult for Walter at the time, because he was very concerned for his father's welfare.

Having figured out what Walter was referring to, his mother and sister began to ask themselves what, if anything, this had to do with his present lethargic behavior. During the course of the meeting at the ADSC, several calls were made to his work and recreation sites to see if there was any explanation for Walter's comments. The answer came from his recreation site when we learned that one of the supervisors was convalescing from an auto accident. Not surprisingly, this was a supervisor Walter was very close to. With this knowledge, we deduced that this new accident had affected Walter much like his father's accident had affected him, so long ago. This insight helped to give his family and staff of the ADSC a strategy for helping Walter to deal with this problem. His family arranged for him to visit his supervisor regularly while he was recuperating. Assisting his supervisor was very therapeutic to Walter and his supervisor. An added benefit was that Walter was able to get accurate information about his supervisor's condition, which also helped to relieve his fears and concerns.

We often encourage caregivers from different settings (home, worksite, etc.,) to come to the evaluations at the Adult Down Syndrome Center. This increases the chance that someone can interpret events that the person with Down syndrome may refer to.

Sometimes the message expressed through a recalled event may be fairly simple and uncomplicated. For example, people often relate memories from a favorite holiday in anticipation of a future holiday. Many times families will try to repeat holiday traditions in an effort to be true to this memory. Other times, the message expressed in a recalled event may be more difficult to decipher. For example:

At an annual meeting to review his progress at his worksite, Eric, 30, commented that a bully harassed him. This created quite a stir, until his mother and a longtime supervisor explained that this had been a serious problem, but had actually occurred many years go. As they explained, the bully had not even been at the worksite for three years. In the ensuing discussion, an Adult Down Syndrome Center staff member, who was present at the meeting, was able to explain that the staffing may have triggered a replay of events that occurred at the time of the harassment.

Eric's mother reported that he did attend a staffing at the time of the harassment to deal with the problem. Most likely the present day meeting reminded him of the experience with the bully and triggered a reenactment in his mind. His comments about being harassed may have simply been a verbal confirmation of this. Staff and family also had noted that he was uncharacteristically anxious prior to and during the present day staffing. Both his comments about being harassed and his anxiety would indicate that he was re-experiencing many of the same emotions he had experienced when being harassed.

Interestingly, Eric's mother commented that he was still cautious when entering the workshop in the morning. He also seemed to be still on edge and worried despite the time lapsed since the harassment. Following this revelation, steps were taken to reassure him that he was safe at the workshop. For an extended period, Eric's favorite staff person met him at the door to reassure him that the bully would not return. Eric was also shown that another person occupied the bully's former locker and workstation. These steps were discontinued after several months, when his mother and staff observed that he no longer seemed worried or anxious. It has been four years since that time and he continues to function free of anxiety.

MISINTERPRETATION OF RECALLED EXPERIENCES

Unfortunately, this tendency to discuss (and relive) the past in present terms may be easily misinterpreted as a behavior problem or a mental illness by uninformed or inexperienced staff or professionals. It is easy to see how this happens. If there was no parent or experienced staff to explain the confusion of past and present events, Eric's statement about being bullied may have been viewed as an accusation or "lie," which defames or inflames others. His comments and his anxious behavior at the workshop may have also been viewed as an indication that he was out of touch with reality and in need of psychiatric treatment. In either case, such misinterpretations often result in medication or behavior measures that are unnecessary and may even be harmful.

Guidelines for recognizing and dealing with replayed memories include remembering that:

- Time concepts are difficult for people with Down syndrome to understand.
- Any statements by the person with DS about events, regardless of the tense used, may involve a past, present, or even a future event.
- Some people with DS may also confuse facts with events seen in movies or TV shows (see below on the mental replay of movies).
- To recognize the context of the discussed events, it is often necessary to be familiar with the person's history and with his day-to-day life and activities.
- If key caregivers in the person's current environments are not aware of a discussed event, chances are this event is from the past.
- Some event in the present is often the trigger which precipitates the replay of a past memory.
- One major clue that the event is replayed is that the person's emotions and behavior seem out of line with the current situation. For example, we have seen many people overreact to a seemingly insignificant loss (a pet hamster dies, or someone else has a loss, etc.) because it triggers memories of a real previous loss. For example, Eric's reactions to the present day meeting were a replay of a stressful bullying incident in the past.
- When dealing with replayed memories, it may be helpful to try to reassure the person that this event is not a current experience or threat. Verbal reassurances may not be enough if the adult has difficulty with time concepts. To get around this, try giving the person a visual time-

line based on photographs of himself at different ages. He may be able to see that the photograph of himself, at the time of the past event, is different from his current photograph, which may give him some sense of understanding and relief.

◆ Acknowledging that the person's feelings about the previous event are still very real is a must, particularly when he has the capacity to relive the experience. This may also offer the opportunity to resolve feelings left over from the previous event.

OTHER POTENTIALLY SERIOUS PROBLEMS

POSTTRAUMATIC STRESS DISORDER

People with Down syndrome who re-experience past events may be far more susceptible to posttraumatic stress disorder (PTSD). This is an anxiety condition that many people hear of during times of war, because it affects many soldiers who have been in combat. Affected soldiers have "flashbacks" which involve a dramatic re-experience of a traumatic event or events from combat, complete with the anxiety and fear experienced during the original event. For those with more severe PTSD, these flashbacks often last long after their return from war. In addition to combat veterans, this condition may also afflict anyone who has experienced a traumatic event, such as a violent crime or accident.

Two issues may complicate posttraumatic stress disorder for people with Down syndrome. First, people with Down syndrome may have more difficulty understanding that past events are in fact past. This may intensify the negative feelings they experience from a flashback. This may also be true for some people in the general population, but many have some understanding that the flashback is just a vivid memory. The person with Down syndrome, however, may actually feel he is reliving a nightmare all over again. Second, it is difficult enough for people in the general population to communicate the source of traumatic experiences in order to get assistance, but it may be even more difficult for people with Down syndrome. As a result, they may continue to be victimized by the previous experience.

Fortunately, we have been able to combine our understanding of memory recall in people with Down syndrome with the knowledge and experiences of caregivers to help identify people who experience traumatic flashbacks. For example:

Georgine, 35, lived in a foster home arrangement with a foster mother and another woman with Down syndrome. Georgine had lost both parents but she had strong support from her sister, Clare, who lived nearby. She also had a strong positive relationship with her foster mother. The strength of the relationship made the following behavior perplexing to her sister.

Apparently, every time Georgine visited her sister, she would refuse to get in the car to return to her foster family's home. This resulted in a daylong effort on Clare's part to talk Georgine into getting into the car for the ride to the foster home. Georgine's level of anxiety was quite high all day and during the forty-minute ride to the foster home. Interestingly, Georgine was noticeably relieved when she arrived at her foster home.

When discussing this situation at the Adult Down Syndrome Center, Clare commented that the problem may have been connected to a time 17 years ago when Georgine briefly lived in a group home. She and her parents had not felt Georgine was ready to move into a residence at that time, but they were worried that an opening in a residence might not come up again. The family had begun to suspect that Georgine was being victimized in the home, which was confirmed when they arrived one day and found her struggling to push a large male resident off of her. Her parents took her home that day and she never returned.

Clare related a history of difficulties with transitions much like Georgine's current resistance to return to her foster mother's home after a family visit. She would often get stuck when she was required to leave one place to go to another. In each case, she required a great deal of coaxing to finally leave. In discussing these issues with Clare, we mentioned our finding that many people seen at the Center have a potential for "flashbacks" and posttraumatic stress disorder because of their capacity for replaying experiences.

We concluded that Georgine might have had a flashback of her experience of returning to the previous group home every time she was to leave one place to go to another. The flashback may have been especially strong when she visited her sister because she was a part of the previous experience while living with her parents. Clare's attempts to tell Georgine where she was going did not seem to help. Even though she may have heard and understood what her sister was saying, the strength of the visual images seemed to have overpowered or canceled her sister's reassuring words.

To remedy the problem, Clare took numerous detailed pictures of the route she took when driving Georgine back to her foster home. This included pictures of each step as Georgine would experience them on the ride. The final two pictures showed the front of her foster mother's house and her foster mother. Looking at these photographs greatly helped to relieve Georgine's anxiety, as she was able to substitute the picture of the traumatic experience with positive pictures of the ride to her foster mother's house. We advised Georgine's sister and foster mother that other transitions would also be easier if they showed her some pictures of her destination. This again would help her to visualize the real destination in order to block the flashback of returning to her old group home.

Phobias

If we understand the tendency for people with DS to re-experience past memories, we may also understand one reason they may develop phobias. A phobia is a fear of a specific object or situation which, with exposure, often provokes intense anxiety and an avoidance response. It is easy to imagine how a strong negative experience would result in a visual replay from memory, complete with the same intense emotions and experiences of the original experience. Common phobias seen at the Center include fear of animals or of storms. Typically, each encounter or imagined encounter with a feared animal or storm results in a replay of the original experience. Many people also develop into what we call "weather watchers" who closely monitor the weather reports. In extreme situations, these fears may be debilitating if they interfere with other important activities in their lives.

We discuss phobias in more detail in Chapter 15.

Problems in Relating to Others

Most of us have had the experience of feeling as if we were treated shabbily by a friend or family member, and then having that experience color the way we look at that person for a short time. For instance, if a friend backs out on helping us with something he promised to do, we may feel like treating him relatively coldly the next time we see him. Usually, however, we don't let our hurt feelings affect our relationship very long, unless the other person did something really awful and won't make amends.

For people with Down syndrome, memories of real or imagined slights seem much more likely to affect how they respond to others. Again, this may be positive or negative depending on the nature of the event. For example:

> Brian, a 35-year-old man living in a group home, had support from a devoted brother and sister, who were both actively involved in his life. One weekend, Brian refused to go to his brother's home for a regularly scheduled visit. From this time forward, Brian refused to meet with his brother for any occasion.
>
> This had been going on for approximately six months when his sister brought him to the Center to discuss the problem. She had thought a great deal about the problem and she related Brian's refusal to meet with his brother to an incident just prior to his refusal. His brother had failed to come to the traditional family Christmas gathering at the sister's house because of a last-minute problem in his own family home. This event seemed to get stuck in Brian's memory. In addition, Brian had strong groove-like tendencies, which he expressed by ruminating on one issue. Unfortunately, the issue he got stuck on was his brother's absence and the hurt and anger that he felt as a result. He would not talk to or meet with his brother or listen to any explanations of why his brother could

not be at the Christmas gathering. His brother and sister were becoming increasingly alarmed and exasperated by Brian's behavior.

Our solution to this problem was to find a means to change the negative picture Brian had acquired of his brother back to the positive picture he had previously had. His sister did this by having Brian over to her house to look at pictures of enjoyable events he and his brother had participated in. His sister noticed a smile from Brian during this experience. Afterwards, he agreed to call his brother and had a positive meeting with him later that day.

Despite this breakthrough, we predicted that Brian might persist in avoiding his brother because of the strength and persistence of negative experiences for people with Down syndrome who have strong visual memories. Brian's sister continued to review pictures of positive experiences with him, which led to additional meetings with his brother. After each positive meeting with his brother, Brian's resistance to meet with him gradually dissipated. In time he no longer needed to review pictures of his brother to meet with him. In fact, his new experiences with his brother became the pictures that he would see when thinking of his brother rather than the negative pictures from the missed Christmas gathering.

On the plus side, we have used people's visual memory of close family members to help ease the pain of a loss. As discussed above, reviewing pictures of events with a loved one, especially if they were very positive, may make it possible for the person to feel as if they are with the person again.

Memory of Movies, TV Shows, and Music

We have found that many people with Down syndrome replay favorite movies and DVDs over and over. This should not be surprising. First, people with Down syndrome tend to have grooves and repeat activities. Second, as discussed in the previous section, the visual medium is very strong for people with DS. In addition, there is less of a boundary between fact and fantasy for most people with Down syndrome. Therefore, like children, adults with DS may experience a TV show or movie as more real than adults in the general population do. This may help to explain why so many people with DS reportedly talk to the screen during movies or TV shows. They may feel as if they are actually interacting with the characters in the show or movie.

We have also found that some people with Down syndrome are able to remember movies or TV shows in vivid detail. It is as if they are able to "videotape" the movie or TV show in their own memory and then replay it at will. What is interesting is that the memorized TV show or movie scenes may become like any other memory for the person with DS. As a result, people with DS may experience the replay as if is actually happening at that time.

We have found that the mental recording and replaying of movies or TV shows may have some very interesting results. Like any positive memory, a TV or movie replay from memory may be very entertaining during free time. It may also be comforting to replay "soft and fuzzy" movies or an uplifting show.

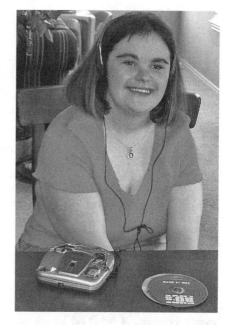

Unfortunately, the memory of a negative movie or show may result in traumatic experiences. Although many adolescents and adults with Down syndrome "love" scary or violent action movies, others are traumatized by these types of movies. For example, one young woman saw the movie *Nightmare on Elm Street* when she stayed overnight at a friend's house. She was so upset by the movie that she had difficulty sleeping and refused to go outside her house at night for almost a year. More recently, another patient was so upset by advertisements for a popular movie, *The Passion of the Christ,* depicting the crucifixion of Jesus Christ, that he also had difficulty sleeping at night. Fortunately, he was able to go to sleep when his family took our advice and had him look at family albums of favorite events before sleeping. This allowed him to substitute strong positive images of his past experiences for negative images from the movie ad.

We have found too that even when people are attracted to scary movies, they may be affected by them. For example:

> Meg, a young woman with Down syndrome, was brought to the Center by concerned staff because she was doing a great deal of agitated self-talk in her room. She would talk angrily or yell at people who were not present. This was happening later and later in the evening and it was affecting her sleep and her ability to function in the daytime. She also had other behaviors that were very odd and disturbing to staff and the other residents. These behaviors were very unusual for Meg, who was very capable in every other respect. She was very verbal, had excellent social skills, and was very conscientious and reliable at the office where she did computer and other clerical work. In addition, she had a strong network of support from family and friends.
>
> Staff were concerned that Meg was developing some type of psychosis. At the first meeting at the Center, we instructed staff to look for any possible problems or negative situations in Meg's life that she could be repeating through her agitated self-talk. Subsequently, a staff person

who was listening outside of Meg's room overheard self-talk that sounded somehow familiar to her. Eventually, she realized that Meg's self-talk was actually a scene-by-scene replay of one of the scary movies that Meg had recently watched. Staff continued to listen to her evening bouts of agitated self-talk, and, sure enough, she was replaying several scary movies that she had seen recently. In a follow-up appointment at the Center, Meg agreed to follow doctor's orders to stop playing scary movies. During the next several months, staff monitored her evening self-talk and noted a gradual reduction in the amount of agitated self-talk/movie replay she was doing. Equally important, she returned to a more normal pattern of sleep and daytime functioning. In a six-month follow-up, Meg and staff reported that she was only watching positive and not scary movies and that there were no additional problems.

Do's and Don'ts for Movie Viewing and the Mental Replay of Movies (MRM)

For the sake of brevity, in the following suggestions, "movies" may also mean TV shows.

Do's and Don'ts for Repeated Movie Viewing:

◆ Become familiar with the movies that the person with Down syndrome is watching. Most people with DS tend to have one or two favorites at any given time.

◆ Monitor the choice of movies if PTSD is a concern when the person views movies that may be too frightening or harmful in some way.

◆ Try to suggest alternate activities in order to limit the amount of movie watching (to an average of one hour per day) so that it does not interfere with beneficial social and recreational activities.

◆ Don't let movies be an excuse for not participating in social or recreation activities either inside or outside of the home.

Do's and Don'ts for the Mental Replay of Movies (MRM):

◆ Become familiar with the signs indicating that the person with DS is mentally replaying movies. This is usually apparent from gestures and comments that are recognizable from a favorite movie.

◆ Don't assume that people with limited verbal language do less MRM. They may actually do more. Recognition of MRM may just take a little more effort on the part of family members for people with limited verbal language. For example, the mental replay of *Star Wars* movies is often obvious from gestures indicating the flight and sound of fantasized space ships, etc.

◆ Don't try to eliminate or make the person feel bad for MRM. This is a normal and expected behavior in people with DS.

◆ Discuss MRM with the person with DS, especially if his MRM includes self-talk-like expressions and gestures when he enacts a scene. Let him know that, like self-talk, this is OK, but some people do not understand or are bothered by it, so not doing it in front of others is polite

◆ Do encourage appropriate (socially acceptable) places for MRM (such as when alone or when in one's room) and gently discourage inappropriate places (such as at work or school).

◆ As with self-talk, consider having a private signal to remind the adult if he is doing MRM inappropriately in public.

◆ Discuss MRM with others who come in contact with the person with DS (explain the normalcy).

Steps to Take When the Mental Replay of Movies Is Excessive:

1. If possible, don't expose the adolescent or adult with DS to boring or non-stimulating environments. In a competition between drab and monotonous school or work environments, a replay of favorite movies will win every time.

2. Include the person with DS in conversations. MRM is more likely when the conversation moves too fast or is over the person's head. (See Chapter 6 for more on this.)

3. Limit exposure to noisy, crowded, or over-stimulating environments. In these situations, the MRM may actually help people to tune out noise and static.

4. Expect a temporary increase in movie watching and MRM during times of loss or difficulty. Movies with positive messages and themes (for example, *The Sound of Music*) may actually be very soothing and inspiring during these times.

Steps to Take When MRM Is Both Excessive and Negative:

(This may be apparent if the person appears angry, agitated, or fearful when engaged in mentally replaying movies.)

1. Try to determine whether the person is replaying movies or if the behavior is actually agitated self-talk. It may be both. If agitated self-talk is present, see more on this in Chapter 8.

2. If MRM is observed, limit additional exposure to movies with negative or frightening themes or content.

3. Help the person fill his time with stimulating activities. Too much down time at work or less stimulating social or recreational activities may encourage negative MRM. The old maxim "an idle mind is the devil's workshop" is true, but in this case, the workshop is more of a movie house of horrors.

4. Similarly, try to limit alone time. People may be especially susceptible to negative MRM during quiet time in the evening. For example, it may be helpful to have the person watch TV with others rather than alone in his room, at least for a period of time.

5. Because the line between fact and fantasy is often blurred for people with DS, attempts to point out that movie images are not real may not be helpful or effective. Remember that verbal explanations and reassurances, even by a loved one, may not be strong enough to counteract the strength of negative visual images (see above case example of Georgine).

6. "Fight fire with fire" through the use of positive visual images. Verbal explanations and reassurances may have more power if augmented by pictures. This may include pictures of past positive events (see above example of *The Passion of the Christ*), but also pictures of what could be. For example, a number of adults with Down syndrome have fears about going to hell or of nothingness after they or loved ones die. These fears are often provoked by specific movies. Some families have learned to counteract this by showing the person artists' renditions of heaven and of life after death. This seems to help relieve fears.

CONCLUSION

Having a truly incredible visual memory is a wonderful characteristic of many people with Down syndrome. While there are many advantages to the strong memory, it can also be a source of concern. The characteristic strengths and weaknesses related to memory in people with Down syndrome must be carefully considered whenever an adolescent or adult with Down syndrome is being assessed for mental health issues.

Chapter 6

Communication
· · · · · · · · · · · · · · ·
Skills
· · · · · · ·

There is perhaps nothing so vital to us as human beings as our ability to communicate our thoughts and feelings effectively to others. We may take our communication ability for granted, but communication skills cannot be taken for granted for adults with Down syndrome. We have found that there are two key areas of communication that are difficult for people with DS and can lead to difficulties with mental health:

1. intelligibility of their spoken language, and
2. the expression of personal thoughts and feelings (McGuire & Chicoine, 1999).

INTELLIGIBILITY
· ·

Intelligibility is the degree to which one's speech is understood by others. Although people with Down syndrome have a wide range of intelligibility, from those who are highly verbal and intelligible to those who have no speech at all, most people fall in the middle: they use speech as their primary means of communication, but have difficulty being understood by others.

Fortunately, most caregivers who spend time with someone with DS on a day-to-day basis are able to understand her. Over time, most caregivers develop a keen

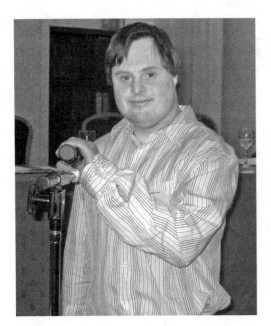

ear and fluency in understanding the person's particular articulation style. Sharing daily experiences also gives caregivers the context of the person's daily life and activities, which greatly helps with interpreting speech. Additionally, caregivers who share years of history with the person with DS are often in a better position to interpret the person's speech. This is because people with DS have exceptional memories and often talk about past events (see Chapter 5). Sometimes only listeners who have knowledge or personal experience with the particular event are able to understand what the person with DS is referring to.

We found convincing evidence of the importance of familiarity for understanding the speech of adolescents and adults with Down syndrome. (See the table below.) We did a survey of 579 of our patients with Down syndrome who were seen at the Center. We found that 75 percent of caregivers reported that they were able to understand the person with DS in their care "most of the time." Only 28 percent of the adults with DS were reported to have speech that was understood by strangers most of the time, while 40 percent of them could be understood by strangers some of the time, and 32 percent very little of the time.

How Understandable the Person with Down Syndrome Is to Familiar and Non-familiar Others (as Estimated by Caregivers, N = 579)

	Most of the time	Sometimes	Very little
Understood by familiar others:	75% (432)	12.7% (74)	12.3% (73)
Understood by strangers or unfamiliar others:	28% (161)	40% (233)	32% (185)

CAREGIVERS AS INTERPRETERS

Due in good part to their ability to understand the speech of the person with Down syndrome, caregivers play a critical role in the survival and success of most people with DS. These caregivers become what we call "interpreters." In this role they help the person with DS to get her message across to listeners who cannot understand her speech. Additionally, they help the person with DS to identify and meet basic wants and needs. They also advocate for her rights and needs in the community, such as by helping to locate the most advantageous programs and services.

It is difficult to understand how important interpreters are unless you have ever needed one. The closest we can come to explaining this experience is to describe what it means to be surrounded by people who speak a foreign language. The spouse of one of the authors is a native of Argentina. When the author visited this country for the first time, he attempted to visit stores and communicate with others on several occasions without his spouse, who was his interpreter. This gave him a sense of the tremendous frustration one can encounter when unable to get a point across to others. If this occurred to the author over the short period of several weeks, imagine what it is like to have this problem every day of your life.

OVER-DEPENDENCE ON INTERPRETERS

Despite the critical role caregivers have as interpreters, a number of problems may develop from this role. First, some people with DS become too dependent on their caregiver-interpreters. If this person leaves or is no longer present, the person with DS may feel lost and disoriented. For example, we have seen people who lose a special boss who had been taking the time to understand and communicate with them. In the absence of this person, they may flounder. This may also happen when close siblings leave for college, or in residential settings when close staff or other residents leave. Of course, the death of a family member such as a parent may be extremely difficult.

To avoid these types of problems, we recommend that families and other caregivers help develop as many interpreters in as many places as possible (home, school, work). This way, losing one interpreter may not be so devastating. Finding and cultivating people who may be able to serve in this capacity may require some time and effort. These should be people who are capable of being interpreters and show interest in, and genuine caring for, the person with Down syndrome. Once you have identified individuals who might serve as interpreters for your son or daughter, give them tips on understanding his or her particular articulation style and some key information that he or she may discuss more frequently, such as references to certain people and past events.

Additionally, we believe that anything that improves your child's ability to communicate with others, and especially unfamiliar others, is extremely important to her self-esteem and ability to get along in the world. This may include speech therapy to improve verbal language, but should also include efforts to improve comfort and fluency with nonverbal means of communicating, particularly because so many people with Down syndrome have intelligibility problems that persist despite speech therapy. We are not speech therapists and it is beyond the scope of this book to discuss the different nonverbal methods of communication. However, we have seen people successfully use a wide array of nonverbal means to communicate—from idiosyncratic hand gestures and pantomime, to picture books and more sophisticated devices such as talking computers. In our experience, anything (high or low tech) which improves communication and which the person is comfortable using should be considered.

NOT SPEAKING UP FOR THEMSELVES

As mentioned previously, caregivers are often called upon to speak on behalf of the adult with Down syndrome. Unfortunately, and with the best of intentions, caregivers may develop a habit of speaking too often for the person when she is able to speak for herself. This can occur for many reasons related to both the caregiver as listener and the person with DS as speaker.

When parents or other caregivers act as interpreters, over time a type of "shorthand" of understanding develops. Having seen the person with DS respond to different situations over many years, they are often able to anticipate how she will respond and what she may want and need in a given situation. This is just part of being a good "interpreter" and advocate. Still, there comes a time when they may make assumptions for the person that may not be correct. Additionally, as people age and mature, they want to have more of a say in decisions affecting their lives. Even if the caregiver is correct in assuming what the person wants, she may still want to speak for herself, just as we all do.

Another reason that "interpreters" may take over too much has to do with the difficulty that many people with DS have with the actual act of speaking. It takes a great deal of work and effort for many people with DS to conceptualize and then to successfully communicate their thoughts and opinions, even to familiar others. As a result, it may be easier for the person with DS to let the caregiver speak for her, even when, with time and effort, she could speak for herself. We see this frequently in our office. We ask the person with DS a direct question, and she looks at the caregiver and either says or clearly indicates that the caregiver should speak for her.

To better understand how and why this happens, it may be helpful, again, to compare the difficulty people with DS have in communicating with the author's difficulty with communicating in Spanish. What the author found is that, similar to people with Down syndrome, he was depending too much on his interpreter (his wife), even though he was often able to speak Spanish, if he took some time and effort. Again, the reason for this is the same as for people with DS—because the act of conceptualizing and speaking is extremely hard work. In order for the author to converse in Spanish, he has to translate back and forth between English and Spanish, then communicate clearly enough in Spanish to be understood by others. This is a daunting task, given the author's limited vocabulary and his tendency to pronounce certain letters or words differently than native language listeners are accustomed to, making comprehension far more difficult.

The person with Down syndrome has a number of similar hurdles to successfully converse with another. She has to understand the other's speech and formulate some thoughts or answers. This may take time because of a slower processing speed. After this, she must successfully communicate her thoughts, despite significant articulation limitations. This is often the part that is fraught with frustration and difficulty, even when others are familiar with her speech. Aside from having moderate to severe articulation limitations, many people with Down syndrome also stutter, or they get stuck repeating the first word or phrase. Many people also tend to speak at a low volume, or they speak too fast or too slow. Perhaps most importantly, the delay needed to process and respond to the other's speech may make them self-conscious or concerned that they may be trying the listener's patience.

Interestingly, self-consciousness is also a common problem for people speaking a foreign language. Both the person with DS and the person speaking a foreign language may be concerned with how they sound, or how long they need to formulate their ideas. This may make them hurry or force their speech, which may then interfere with the successful articulation of their thoughts. This, in turn, may make them less intelligible to the listener, making them feel even more apprehensive. Over time, an unproductive pattern may develop in which the person with DS, or the person trying to speak a foreign language, becomes more and more reluctant to speak to others. Often, they become increasingly dependent on one or a small number of interpreters, which then affects their ability to deal independently with the world, and, of course, their sense of pride and self-esteem.

The good news is that people with DS will speak for themselves if given the opportunity and strong encouragement from others. Returning again to the analogy of the foreign language speaker, recently the author was able to successfully communicate with a Spanish-speaking relative during a weeklong period when his wife (the interpreter) was out of town. This took a great deal of effort on the part of the author and the aunt. They struggled with many different words and expressions, but the feeling of accomplishment from successful communicating was very exhilarating and greatly reinforced the author's intention to speak for himself in Spanish.

We see a similar process when people with DS are encouraged to talk for themselves, only the stakes are much higher. This is their *only* means to verbalize their thoughts and feelings and not a second language. We have found that both the speaker and the listener must make a concerted effort for the person with DS to successfully speak for herself. Similar to nonnative language speakers, what is required for the person with DS to speak for herself is the following:.

1. If the listener starts the conversation, he needs to speak clearly and slowly enough for the person with Down syndrome to understand. He also needs to give the person with DS sufficient time to process the ideas communicated and to formulate an answer.
2. When the person with DS speaks, the listener has to be very patient.
3. As discussed previously, it helps to have an understanding of, or first-hand experience with, the person's life and activities to increase comprehension of her speech. On the other hand, the listener still must be very careful when making assumptions about what the person is trying to communicate.
4. Attempts to finish the person's sentences based on prior experiences may not be constructive. Some people may want the help, but for many others this tends to inhibit their efforts to speak.
5. Just as the listener needs to be patient and receptive, the person with DS must be willing to communicate without automatically looking for help from her "interpreter." We strongly encourage this at the Cen-

ter. When needed, we gently block parents or other caregivers from jumping in too quickly to speak for the person with DS. We may also need to coach the person with DS to speak for herself in the presence of parents. Once this process is set in motion, caregivers may simply need periodic reminders to back off and the person with DS may need encouragement to continue to speak for herself.

Again, the benefits of this approach are substantial, as there is perhaps nothing as important to self-esteem as to have your thoughts, feelings, and wishes listened to and understood. In our experience, most parents or other caregivers will try to change this pattern, given some time and encouragement. Of course, if this is a habitual pattern, it can be hard to break. Additionally, some caregivers strongly resist relinquishing control of this and other aspects of the adult's life. We have found that there are often reasons why this continues, even when people are aware of the negative consequences. For example:

> An elderly mother and her 35-year-old son, Daniel, came to the Center for the first time because the son had pneumonia and some other health concerns. Daniel did not talk and his mother made a point of telling staff that he was nonverbal. After a year and many visits to the Center, staff members were surprised to hear Daniel talk clearly for himself during a routine medical follow-up visit to the Center. The mother explained that she had been afraid that Center staff would "take him away" to live in a group home. She feared that this would leave her alone and without his help. Once she was assured that we would not do this, she let her son speak for himself.
>
> Interestingly, Daniel's mother later became concerned about what would happen to her son if anything happened to her. She had enough trust in the Center to ask for help in working with the appropriate agencies for residential placement. Fortunately, because of the mother's age, her son was a high priority for residential funding by the state. As per her wishes, a group home was located within a short distance from her home, which allowed him to visit her frequently.

In another family the problem was far more complex:

> In this family, all but Carlos, the youngest of five children, a young man with Down syndrome, had moved out and established their own lives and families. His parents brought Carlos to the Center when they were concerned about symptoms suggesting he was depressed. He refused to go to his workshop in the morning or to social and recreational activities in the evening. He had also developed a habit of whispering in a barely audible voice.
>
> On examination at the Center, the cause of the problem was found to be a long-standing conflict in his parents' marriage. After the last of

his siblings left home, the marital conflict intensified. His father spent more time away from the home involved in his work and his mother became over-involved in managing the young man's life and speaking for him. Carlos was very sensitive to the marital conflict and was sacrificing his own voice and life ambitions in order to reduce the conflict and tension in this relationship.

Our strategy was to try to refer his parents to counseling and to help this young man to move out of the middle of the parental conflict. The marital counseling was never started because the conflict was too entrenched. However, we were able to help Carlos move out of the conflict, and this in turn helped the parents to deal with their own issues. As part of the process, Carlos worked for months with Center staff and several key siblings to articulate his own thoughts and desires for his life. This was a slow process at first because he spoke so quietly and he was initially very hesitant to move out of his parents' home. Fortunately, he was a man of strong character and his siblings and Center staff appealed to his need for independence and growth.

The turning point came at an arranged meeting with his parents and siblings at the Center. His parents had difficulty at first letting him talk, but he persisted, even though he still talked very softly. In one particularly poignant exchange, he assertively stopped his parents from talking and told them very softly but emphatically that he was going to talk and they were going to listen. He went on to explain that he wanted to move on with his life and that he wanted to live in a group home. After this, he was able to spend extended periods of time in the homes of several nearby siblings. Fortunately, his siblings had started the process of applying for a group home some time before and a group home became available fairly quickly.

A fairly short time after Carlos moved into his group home, he began to speak at a more normal volume and to resume all normal activities, such as going to work and to all social and recreational activities. For their part, his parents were able to get a divorce and move on in their lives as well. After five years, Carlos continues to live successfully in his group home and he has visited with both of his parents in their separate residences without any additional problems.

COMMUNICATING IN GROUP SITUATIONS

There is one important speech and intelligibility issue that can affect the mental health of people with Down syndrome. We have found that the act of communicating in group situations tests the endurance and mental energy of people with DS (as well as of people speaking a foreign language in a group). For example, during a recent visit to Argen-

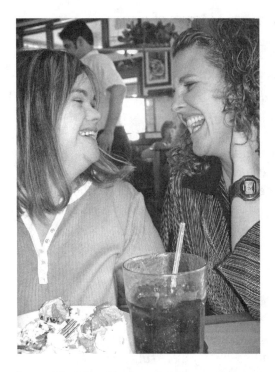

tina, the author and his brother-in-law, who spoke a little Spanish, attended an Easter brunch with his wife's large extended family. After several hours, the author went to an empty living room, where he encountered his brother-in-law, fast asleep on the couch. He, like the author, was exhausted and needed a break from the arduous task of trying to communicate with the family in Spanish. Additionally, both the author and his brother-in-law found that it was extremely difficult to maintain focus and respond to the conversation when in a group speaking Spanish to each other. They found that it was easy to drift off in their own thoughts and had difficulty not appearing rude and uninterested in the conversation.

With this in mind, it is interesting to hear from families that their family member with DS will often "make an appearance" at family gatherings but then retreat to the relative safety and quiet of her own room. Families want to know whether this is an indication of a problem, such as a symptom of a depressive withdrawal or antisocial personality. We usually find that this is normal. Like non-native language speakers, many people with DS simply cannot keep up with conversation because it moves too fast for them to process and to respond. The conversation may also revolve around adult topics they have little or no personal interest in, such as the cost of heating oil or traffic problems on the local highway. It is understandable then that the person with DS would want to leave the room.

Of course, there are some ways to make it easier for the person with Down syndrome to stay in a social situation. What the author found at social gatherings with others speaking in foreign tongues was that if his wife sat nearby and translated some of the conversation, this helped a great deal. This is certainly true for people with DS as well. It may not be necessary to translate everything verbatim, but paraphrases and summaries may help to keep the person with DS in the conversation. The interpreter should also assist the person with DS to articulate a response that allows her to participate and contribute to the conversation.

What Helps

Some do's and don'ts for family caregivers to help encourage participation by the person with DS in social conversations:

◆ Help to keep the person with DS in the conversation by sitting near her and quietly paraphrasing the topics of the discussion in understandable terms. This is not necessary with all topics of conversation but more so when the topics are more abstract.

♦ Encourage other people in social gatherings to be patient with the person with DS to allow her enough time to think, talk, ask questions, and articulate answers to questions.

♦ Make specific comments to help include the person with DS in the conversation. For example, say something like, "You know…Sharon had a similar experience once…. Sharon, do you remember when you…?" Any attempt to include the person with DS in talking about past events may also play to her memory strength.

♦ Encourage others to respond to the person with DS in a rewarding way and not just by saying "uh huh." The most effective way to do this is to simply repeat a part or all of what the person with DS has said, without making any interpretations or additional comments. This is often said with a slight inflection as if asking a question. "So …you went to the party?" This is called reflective listening and it is well known and widely practiced in the counseling profession (Rogers, 1951). It stimulates conversation by saying to the person with DS that you are listening and what she says is valued. This also allows you to facilitate and clarify the person's conversation without actually speaking for her or taking her voice.

If the adult's speech is difficult for others to understand, the above reflective listening technique may be very helpful. We also recommend these additional strategies:

♦ Help translate the person's comments, but only when needed. It is best to translate the person's actual statements without adding comments or interpretations which may distort or change what she is actually trying to say.

♦ Consider *briefly* stating or describing the context, topic, or background of what is said by the person with DS to improve others' understanding. We find this can help to orient the listener to the context of the conversation and make interpretation of the specifics much easier. For example, it may be helpful to say, "She is talking about… 'this party'… 'his job'… 'this movie,'" or "She is talking about the time when…."

♦ Get the permission of the person with DS before either translating or giving the context or background of her comments. This helps to maintain respect for the independence and integrity of her own thoughts and opinions. For the same reason, it is also important to ask the person with DS if your translation is correct, such as by saying, "What I heard you say is that you had a good time at the party. Is that correct?"

This brings up another important issue about the participation of adolescents and adults with Down syndrome in other types of group meetings. We have attended many meetings and staffings where the conversation moved too fast for the person with DS. How can she understand and respond to the proceedings, which may involve key decisions about her life, if it all sounds like a foreign language?

In these situations, it is imperative to translate the information so the adult with DS can understand it. It helps if, prior to the meeting, the person who will be acting as "interpreter" goes through the key points of the agenda with the person with Down syndrome. She would still require a translator/interpreter during the actual meeting to ensure that she understands the ongoing proceedings. The interpreter and the others attending the meeting must also allow the person to communicate verbally or nonverbally about the proceedings. This requires patience from others, but above all else, a belief that the person with DS has the ability to understand, to communicate for herself, and to contribute important thoughts.

In our experience, if someone is subjected to a meeting without a valid interpreter or means for understanding and communicating, she feels disenfranchised and devalued and thus subject to frustration, despair, and depression. Her situation is similar to that of someone who is being tried in a foreign court, where the language is not her own, and there is no attempt to keep her informed about proceedings or to solicit her opinion or feelings. Viewed from this perspective, it is easy to see how people with Down syndrome may begin to act "inappropriately" during such meetings. How can people help but drift off into their own thoughts and even to talk to themselves when they are so divorced from the process they are forced to attend? (See Chapter 8.)

SPECIAL ISSUES OF HIGHLY VERBAL AND NONVERBAL PEOPLE

As explained earlier, most people with DS are in the middle of the intelligibility spectrum and have moderate speech limitations. Although there are fewer people at either end of the spectrum (those who are highly verbal or nonverbal), these individuals have their own issues which merit special attention.

NONVERBAL ADULTS WITH DOWN SYNDROME

People who have significant speech limitations have to use nonverbal actions and behavior as their medium for communicating their thoughts, feelings, needs, and desires. We have found that most individuals with verbal limitations are able to find incredibly varied and creative means for communicating through facial expression, gestures, body language, signing, and such simple but effective tactics as pointing to get their point across.

For this type of nonverbal communication to be received, the listener-interpreter has to be attuned to all the subtle and idiosyncratic nuances of the behavior and actions of the adult with DS. Understanding nonverbal communication requires learning a unique language for each person. This obviously requires a listener who is a sensitive and patient observer. Not surprisingly, we have seen some of the most understanding and sensitive caregivers working with people with verbal limitations. These interpreters become very important to the adult with DS, and, therefore, their loss is often more devastating than for people with better expressive language skills. It is hard enough for a person with DS who has moderate verbal skills to lose an interpreter, but even more difficult for those who are nonverbal. Therefore, if you know a nonverbal adult with DS who has had a behavior change, consider whether she has lost an important interpreter lately. Additionally, whenever possible, make sure there are always several people in her life who can interpret for her.

Many people who are nonverbal use a variety of alternative and augmentative devices such as speaking devices or visual communication books to improve their abilities to communicate. This may greatly expand their communication potential. On the other hand, this still requires a caregiver who takes the time and effort to use the devices.

It is important to remember, too, that whether or not a person with Down syndrome has verbal skills, she often has excellent receptive language skills. Not surprisingly, caregivers who are good at interpreting nonverbal communication are often very much aware of this receptive skill. They will often use this to get the right interpretation by questioning the person with DS as to whether they are correct: "Is this what you mean?" Most interpreters are more often right than wrong in their interpretive guesses. However, we do need to repeat our warning regarding the interpretation of any communication made by people with DS. Caregiver-interpreters must be careful not to assume they already know what the person with DS is trying to communicate, especially when it comes to wants and needs. There may be a strong incentive for just deciding or choosing for the person with DS, especially if the process of getting her opinion is so much work. Still, there is nothing more important to one's self-esteem than having one's opinion and choices heard and acted upon. This may be even more important to people who do not have a history of responsiveness from others.

Finally, most successful interpreters capitalize on a rich variety of mediums which may be used for nonverbal communicators. As discussed previously, there are idiosyncratic gestures which are interpretable by observers who have lived with the person with DS. It is also important to ensure that the person learns to use some more standardized form of nonverbal communication, so she can voice her wants, needs, and choices to those who are less familiar with her communication methods.

WHEN COMMUNICATION PROBLEMS BECOME BEHAVIOR PROBLEMS

For nonverbal adults with Down syndrome, it may be extremely difficult to communicate more serious problems and issues. This may be especially true if the problem is something new or for which there is no prior history of communication to others. For example, one 29-year-old man with verbal language limitations was brought to the Center by his family when he began hitting himself very hard in the head. On examination, it was determined that he had a painful sinus infection. He had been very healthy for most of his adult years and had had little previous need to communicate physical pain to his family.

Sometimes people in the person's environment may fail to "hear" her communication. This may happen because no one is taking the time and effort to understand her nonverbal communication—for example, when a special caregiver-interpreter is absent or distracted by someone or something else. It may also happen if the person's skills and intelligence are underestimated, especially by inexperienced staff or professionals. These individuals may tend to discount or downplay the person's ability to understand and to communicate her thoughts, feelings, and needs to others.

Whatever the cause, we have found that when people are frustrated in trying to communicate a problem or need, they usually do one of two things:

1. they withdraw into depression and despair, or
2. they communicate their frustration and need through anger or aggressive behavior (toward property, self, or others).

In our experience, withdrawal into depression may be potentially more dangerous. This is because it may go undetected for some time and because it may be more difficult for caregivers and sensitive professionals to get to the cause. This is particularly the case if the person seems to have given up and makes no effort to try to communicate the source of the problem (see Chapter 14).

The other way to communicate a problem, through anger and aggressive behavior, is potentially more constructive, because the behavior often gives stronger clues as to the cause of the problem. For example, when the man mentioned above hit himself in the head, he communicated the source of the pain as his head. The other benefit is that it is often a more successful way to get help. In an insensitive environment, depression may be ignored, whereas aggression, particularly when directed at staff, often gets quick attention.

On the other hand, there is a danger that uninformed staff or professionals may misdiagnose aggressive behavior as a "behavior problem." While technically correct, this often means that there is a lack of understanding or interest in seeing the person's behavior as her primary means for communicating. Viewed from the "behavior problem" perspective, the treatment is often to chemically manage (sedate) the person rather than to try to uncover the source of the problem. Behavioral management techniques are also commonly used. These may be helpful, but also may be too restricting, especially if there is no attempt to uncover the cause of the person's angry behavior. Unfortunately, these techniques may end up suppressing the person's means for communicating and will often lead to more anger and despair. On the other hand, attempts to understand the person's behavior as communication can be very fruitful. (See Chapter 13.)

ABSENCE OF INTERPRETERS IN EARLY LIFE

There is one final issue related to people who are nonverbal. In our experience, most people with Down syndrome have family members and others who are willing and able to interpret for them when needed. Some adults, however, have not had this experience. Some of these individuals have grown up in larger facilities, or even in family homes were there was no attempt to encourage expressive language, whether verbal language or nonverbal, and there was also no speech therapy available to them.

Usually, we have found that the individuals growing up in these environments are nonverbal, even though many of them may have had the capacity to speak at some time in their lives. More importantly, even though many of these individuals have moved into more responsive environments, such as smaller group homes, most continue to be nonverbal or to have very limited expressive language skills. These individuals, like others who are nonverbal, may be more susceptible to depression because of the frustration and sense of hopelessness that may come from being unable to effectively communicate thoughts and feelings to others. Behavior problems are also more common because behavior may be the only means people have to communicate.

On the positive side, there are group and family living arrangements (in group homes, foster care situations, etc.) which can greatly reduce the effects of limited verbal language and thus also reduce the risk of depression and behavior problems. This happens when staff and other residents in these living arrangements become sensitive observers and responders to the nonverbal communication of the person with Down syndrome. Often this occurs in environments where residents and staff have lived and worked together for many years and thus have become like a supportive family. In these situations, the interpreters have the time and patience to understand and respond to the person even without verbal cues. We hear over and over from the family and staff that those who make the effort to interpret the communication of people who are nonverbal are greatly rewarded. The person's smile says to the interpreter that they "got it right."

HIGHLY ARTICULATE ADULTS WITH DOWN SYNDROME

On the other end of the intelligibility spectrum, people with Down syndrome who have excellent speech and language skills tend to have far more problems than would be expected. Unlike people who are nonverbal and whose skills are often underestimated, these individuals are often believed to be more capable than they are because of their language skills. There are a number of reasons this may happen. First, many people with DS are excellent observers and have exceptional memories. As a result, they may be able to memorize phrases that allow them to appear as if they understand more than they do. Second, many people want to fit in to conversations and social situations, like everyone else, and thus they may use certain remembered phrases or comments that help them appear to be part of the conversation. Third, they may be able to converse very fluently and capably about concrete situations and concepts, leading others to assume that they understand abstractions equally well.

In some situations, parents and other caregivers may also put intense pressure on the person with DS to be more capable. Caregivers may accentuate the person's expressive skills as evidence of her superior abilities or even of her "normalcy" compared to the others with DS who are "less capable." This is often part of a much larger problem of acceptance that is addressed in Chapter 7. But it may also be because teachers and other professionals have told families all along that the person with Down syndrome just needs to try harder or be more motivated to achieve more.

In fact, for many highly articulate people with Down syndrome, the real problem is that they are assumed to be more competent than they are because of their verbal skills. As a result, they may be allowed to manage aspects of their lives that are beyond their capability. This requires some explanation. As mentioned previously, we have been impressed with the fact that many people have uneven skills. They may have excellent speech and often can do many of their own self-care tasks reliably (see Chapter 9). This does not necessarily mean, however, that they are as capable in other important areas of their lives—for example, in knowing when to go to bed, what food to eat, or how to organize beneficial free-time activities (see "The Dennis Principle," Chapter 3).

Too often, we have seen people with DS blamed for their "failures" in jobs or living situations when in fact the failure is due to a misreading or misunderstanding of their skills by caregivers or staff.

Preventing Problems Related to Misinterpretation of Skills

If you have an adult child with Down syndrome who fits into this category, there are a number of things you can do to prevent or at least moderate these problems. First, it may be helpful to get a more complete picture of your child's strengths and weaknesses. There are many excellent assessment tools which look at a wide range of adaptive skills and not just verbal language. In fact, these measures were designed to measure the functional skills of people who may have limited verbal language. As such, they emphasize the person's behavior as observed and reported by caregivers and not verbal self-report. These measures include the *Vineland Adaptive Behavior Scales, The Scales of Independent Behavior-Revised* (SIB-R), the *AAMR Adaptive Behavior Scales* (ABS), and, to a lesser degree, the *Inventory for Client and Agency Planning* (ICAP). These assessments can not only help you understand your child's strengths and weaknesses, but also help you in advocating effectively for your child's real needs in work, residential, and other community settings. A standardized test administered by a professional can give your family an effective bargaining tool to help counteract inappropriate placements by well-meaning but misinformed staff in agencies and community programs.

Similarly, families may also ask professionals who have experience working with people with Down syndrome to consult with the agencies serving the needs of their sons and daughters. The purpose of this is to educate staff of the real strengths and weaknesses of the person with DS in order to avoid expectations that are either too high or too low. Interestingly, we often say the same things the family has been saying to these agencies, but as professionals, our opinion may carry more weight.

It may help to discuss examples of situations when expectations were too high for the person's skills and suggest some strategies to avoid this. For example, we have seen many people fail at jobs as cashiers in grocery stores. In these situations, the job placement agency failed to note that just because the adult with Down syndrome had good verbal skills did not mean she could manage money. This misplacement could have been avoided if the job placement agency had tested the person's ability to manage money before finding her a cashier's job. Had the staff of the ADSC been consulted, we would have also recommended a test of money management skill. This is because we have found that, regardless of skill level, most people with Down syndrome have difficulty managing money. Use of one of the Adaptive Skills Scales (discussed above) would have also identified this limitation.

Some people have also been given jobs as office receptionists because of their verbal skills. In a smaller office, some adults with Down syndrome are able to manage the job. For many others, however, handling a volume of calls, writing phone messages, and doing other complex office tasks were well beyond their ability. Again, job failure could have been avoided if the job placement agency had consulted with professionals or family caregivers who were aware of the person's limitations.

On the other hand, having a good understanding of a person's skills will allow a match of the right job with the right person. In these situations, everyone benefits: the person with DS, the employer, and the community. For example, we have found that many people with Down syndrome have exceptional memories and good organizational skills, which help them manage even the large number of stock items found in a grocery store. Similarly, we know many adults with DS who do exceptionally well in mail rooms or loading docks because of these skills. Additionally, if not under time pressure, such as receptionists or cashiers encounter, many people bring a degree of precision and reliability that is valued by many employers.

Residential settings can also be scenes of great success or great failure if expectations are too high, as described in some detail in Chapter 3. In these situations, people often failed when they are assumed to have more maturity for making appropriate decisions regarding sleeping and diet than they actually have.

One important way to keep overly high expectations from becoming a problem is for the person with DS to learn to advocate for her own needs. For example, people with DS can be taught to tell a person in authority when a job or job task is too difficult for them. This may not be as difficult as it sounds. We have found that most people with DS have a much better understanding and acceptance of their own limitations than they are often given credit for. For example, when we ask people if they are able to do certain tasks such as using the stove, most are quite honest and realistic in their answer. As discussed in Chapter 7, we have found that families who have a more realistic view of their child's strengths and weaknesses often have children who are also more accepting of their own abilities. This, of course, may be challenged somewhat during the adolescent drive for independence, but in general this holds true.

Finally, how can you get the right balance between tasks that are challenging but doable and tasks that are either too difficult or too easy, and thus demoralizing? Or, as one young man with Down syndrome put it, "why are you treating me like a baby?" How do we avoid either extreme? As discussed in Chapter 3, people need to be able to both fail and succeed in a task. Tasks should be neither too easy nor too hard that the person cannot learn to succeed, given some time, effort, and encouragement from others. Each task at each stage of development should be measured to meet and appropriately challenge the person's skills and abilities. This can usually be gauged from the tasks that she has already mastered.

THE EXPRESSION OF FEELINGS

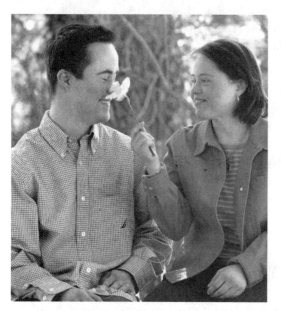

We have found that most people with Down syndrome cannot help but show their emotions nonverbally through facial expressions and body gestures. This includes negative feelings (disappointments, frustrations, anger, sadness) and positive feelings (happiness, elation, excitement). Nevertheless, quite a few people with Down syndrome have difficulty putting their feelings into words. As a result, it is not always possible for others to readily interpret the cause, source, or meaning of the person's expressed emotion.

Given some time and patience, many parents and other caregivers are able to discover the reason behind the person's feelings. Still, there may be situations where it is far more difficult to uncover the reason. Sometimes this occurs if changes or problems occurring in another setting are affecting a person's feelings. For example, parents may not know why their adult child is upset if something at work is affecting her. The intensity of the problem may also determine how difficult it is to verbalize feelings. As an example of how both intensity and location can complicate the situation:

> Staff in a small group home first noted that Bruce, 31, would not get out of bed to go to work in the morning. This was very unusual for him because he rarely missed work, even when ill. Staff became increasingly alarmed when he began to isolate himself in his room and when they observed a marked increase in agitation and self-talk, including frequent bouts of angry speech. Staff brought him to the Center on an emergency basis when he began to stay up all night and became so self-absorbed in his self-talk that he barely touched his meals. At the Center, a thorough physical and psychosocial evaluation showed the presence of hypothyroidism (see Chapter 2) but no other clear reasons for his change in behavior. While hypothyroidism may create some significant depression-like symptoms, it did not seem to explain the severity of his symptoms.

Fortunately, after we contacted staff in his workshop, they helped to solve the mystery. Bruce had been victimized by an aggressive bully who recently started at the workshop. Staff in his residence had begun to note a change in his behavior just after the bully began at the workshop. Shortly after this, the bully left for a more appropriate setting. At this point, we worked with Bruce and the staff from his residence and worksite to help him deal with his anxiety. Following our recommendations, Bruce was able to go back to work after much time and effort by all involved. For example, over a period of a week, residential staff members were able to get him up and out the door in the morning, but then he refused to go inside the workshop building once he arrived. Despite much reassurance, he seemed to be afraid that the bully was still at the workshop. Staff worked patiently with him and he began to go into the workshop and to his workstation very cautiously. In time, he went back to a normal schedule with no further problems or symptoms.

THE NONVERBAL EXPRESSION OF FEELINGS

One issue that is striking from the preceding example is that Bruce could not tell even close family and staff what was happening to him, even though his world was turned upside down by the bully. Fortunately, some extreme changes in his behavior drew his caregivers' immediate attention to the problem.

In our experience, Bruce's response is fairly common in people with Down syndrome who have experienced intense stress or emotional issues. That is, even if they are able to communicate with others about day-to-day issues, they may not be able to conceptualize and communicate more sensitive problems and issues. As a result, they may communicate these issues nonverbally through a change in behavior.

The problem with this type of nonverbal communication is that there must be a receptive "listener" or receiver of the message at the other end. Unfortunately, uninformed professionals or staff may too easily label nonverbal expressions of behavior and emotion as a "behavior problem" or a "mental health disorder." Such general labels tell us nothing about the possible causes or solutions to a problem. Moreover, these labels may actually point to solutions that maintain or worsen a problem. For example, what if we had not learned about the bully and had viewed Bruce's problem as a "behavior problem"? There is a good chance that we may have developed a "behavior plan" that forced him back to the workshop without eliminating the bully's threat. This would not have solved the problem and would most likely have intensified his fear and anxiety. Similarly, treating the problem as a "mental health disorder" with the use of psychotropic medications may have temporarily reduced some of his anxiety, but it also would not have eliminated the bully's threat. This too would have most likely resulted in a continuation and worsening of the problem.

When people with Down syndrome have to communicate their stress behaviorally, the causes are all too often misinterpreted. If professionals do not take the time and effort to look for all possible causes, however, the problem may continue. For example, we find many people who are treated for symptoms of depression (lethargy, loss of energy, etc.) with an antidepressant medication, when in fact the cause or a major source of the problem is hypothyroidism or sleep apnea. While antidepressant medications may temporarily reduce the symptoms, failure to treat the underlying medical condition may result in a continuation of the problem and the depressive symptoms. In short, one has to be careful not to assume that the behavior that is being used to communicate the presence of stress *is* the problem.

Even when parents or professionals are receptive listeners, the message may not always be received. Nonverbal messages are rarely clear. They often show the presence but not the source of the problem. To complicate matters, the problem may have more than one source. Thus, we have learned that we need to be very thorough when trying to track down all possible causes or stressors. For example, returning to the example of Bruce, he had a medical condition that may have aggravated his symptoms and behavior, even if the primary cause of the problem, the bully, had been dealt with effectively. Failing to treat this or other conditions or stressors may have delayed a resolution of the problem.

Numerous health conditions, sensory deficits, and environmental stressors may be associated with any given problem. Additionally, different people show stress in different ways, depending on their own characteristics and vulnerabilities. For example, many adolescents and adults with Down syndrome have compulsive tendencies or "grooves" (see Chapter 9) that are beneficial to them. They are able to follow through with routines and schedules that allow them to complete daily living tasks and worksite tasks very reliably. Unfortunately, under stress, they may become too rigid in completing tasks and this may begin to interfere in essential or beneficial activities. (This is further addressed in Chapters 9 and 16.)

Here are some guidelines to lessen the effects of the person's inability to verbalize her feelings:

- ◆ Consider teaching the person some skills to verbalize feelings. This may include having her work with a counselor to identify and label feelings or with a speech-language pathologist to learn ways to express her emotions. Or, teach the person with DS to look at pictures of expressions and indicate which one represents how she's feeling.
- ◆ Family members and other caregivers can help the person with DS identify her feelings during day-to-day activities. For example, if you witness a situation that obviously upsets the adult with DS, help her label her feelings, such as by saying something like, "Boy, I would feel really angry if that happened to me. Is that how you're feeling?"
- ◆ Family or long-time caregivers may need to teach less experienced staff (at school, work, or residential settings) to interpret the individual's expressive face and body language.
- ◆ Make sure that there is more than one person who is willing and able to interpret for the adult, as discussed above. The more people in more

settings who are able to understand and respond to her expressed needs, the more competent she will feel. Again, the more responsive caregivers there are, the less effect the loss of one will have on the person with DS.

◆ Family members should always continue to be active participants in meetings with work or residential staff in order to ensure the most advantageous or accurate interpretation of the adult's expressed needs.

CONCLUSION

Communication skills are vital to participating in society. Unfortunately, however, the expressive language problems of some people with Down syndrome create hurdles in daily life. Sometimes these problems can lead to misinterpretation of behavior or misdiagnosis of mental health problems. Sensitivity and patience on the part of family members and care providers improves mental health and improves the treatment of behavioral challenges.

Chapter 7

Self-Esteem
and
Self-Image

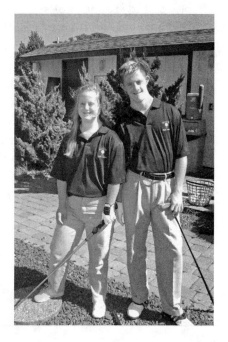

The Heritage Dictionary definition of esteem is "to regard with respect." Following from this, self-esteem is to regard oneself with pride and self-respect. The importance of self-esteem to one's health and wellbeing is well established: People with self-esteem are happier, live longer, are healthier, and have fewer mental health problems, to name some of the more important benefits (Seligman & Martin, 1998).

The promotion of self-esteem is any action which helps people regard themselves with pride and self-respect. This sounds simple enough, and yet, how do you promote self-esteem in people with Down syndrome when others stare at them because they think they look different? How do you encourage respect and pride when the world values speed, self-sufficiency, communication skills, and productivity? It will come as no surprise to anyone that people with DS move at their own pace, have far less independence and control in their lives, have limitations in communicating, and have far fewer job or career opportunities. Similar to other minorities, people with DS are often viewed and treated differently in our society.

Despite all this, the majority of people we have seen at the Adult Down Syndrome Center do have strong self-esteem and self-respect. How is this possible? Many seem to have an innate sense of self-respect, but much can also be attributed to families and

People with Down Syndrome as a Minority

For people with Down syndrome, being part of a minority actually has advantages and disadvantages. One of the most difficult challenges for people with DS and their families is the lack of understanding and acceptance by some others in the community. Despite efforts by parent groups and advocates to change stereotypes, people with DS are still viewed and treated differently in society. People with DS continue to be stared at, teased, and at times taken advantage of by the unscrupulous. Also, like other people who are in a minority, people with Down syndrome may lack positive role models who share their disability, or may have limited contact with others who have Down syndrome.

On the other hand, people with Down syndrome are recognizable as "belonging to a group." The same physical features that invite teasing from some members of the community signal more empathetic people of the possible need to take the disability into consideration when interacting with them (such as by being extra patient). This applies to adults as well as children. For example, a study found that school-age children were more accepting of peers with Down syndrome than of children with "invisible disabilities," such as learning disabilities (Siperstein and Bak, 1985). The authors of the study speculated that children with invisible disabilities may have looked like other children but there was something odd or different about them which may have confused or put the other children off. On the other hand, the distinctive physical features of the children with DS clearly identified them as disabled. This seemed to make it easier for others to accept them and their disability. In our own experience, we have found that people with DS are generally accepted in school and community settings. When staring, teasing, or discrimination occurs, it often involves a smaller number of people who are uninformed, bullies, or bigots.

Belonging to a group can also be an advantage by enabling people with Down syndrome and their families to connect with other people with Down syndrome and their families. Some families of people with intellectual disabilities that are not known to be secondary to a "syndrome" have shared with us that they do not have the same connection that families of people with Down syndrome have.

other care providers who have found ways to encourage and promote self-esteem. This chapter will describe some key issues around the promotion of self-esteem, including a discussion of the importance of accepting one's disability.

FAMILY ACCEPTANCE AND SELF-ESTEEM

Self-esteem starts with acceptance of who we are. For people with Down syndrome, that includes accepting that they have Down syndrome. They cannot be proud of themselves if they cannot accept that they have DS. Acceptance increases the use and development of their own skills and abilities and it encourages advocacy for their own rights and needs.

The development of pride and acceptance in the individual with DS often begins with the family's acceptance and willingness to discuss Down syndrome. This is not necessarily an easy or simple process. Anything that marks family members as different (race, creed, disability, etc.) may make a family susceptible to isolation due to real or perceived discrimination from others. For example, parents of a child with DS may feel as if some relatives are distant or unresponsive, which may make it difficult or uncomfortable to attend family gatherings. Many families report that these types of issues often extend well into the adult years.

Many families gain support and acceptance by joining parent organizations where they meet other families who have children or adults with DS. Finding families with similar experiences can be a powerful form of support, which promotes positive attitude and self-esteem in the family and the child with DS. Still, there are some families who continue to struggle with acceptance of their child's Down syndrome. There are also some families who had few, if any problems accepting Down syndrome while their child was young, 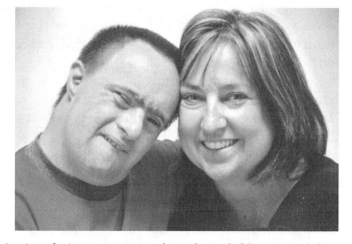 but who find themselves questioning their acceptance when their child enters adolescence or adulthood and fails to achieve some of the typical milestones associated with increasing independence.

It is beyond the scope of this book to explain in detail what families can do to accept Down syndrome. If your adult child with DS is struggling with self-esteem, however, it may be worthwhile to ask yourself whether you are having trouble with acceptance. Also be sure to read Chapter 3 on the role that families play in supporting adults with DS.

SELF-ESTEEM IN PEOPLE WITH DOWN SYNDROME

The development of pride and acceptance in the individual with DS is a complex and often creative process, involving the person's own attitude and abilities and the environment he lives in. In our experience, acceptance appears to be a four-step process involving:

1. awareness,
2. development of a sense of competence,
3. development of one's own unique talents or gifts, and
4. feeling loved and accepted by family and friends.

DEVELOPING AWARENESS

Awareness of any type of disability or difference in oneself may result in feelings of anger, loss, and sadness. For children with Down syndrome, awareness of differences in skills and opportunities compared to typically developing peers and siblings will invariably increase as these children are included in regular classrooms and community settings. As the children grow into adolescents and adults, many become even more aware of discrepancies in skills and opportunity. For example, a young child with DS may play on the same block, go to the same neighborhood school, and be in the same classroom as all the other children from the neighborhood. Later, the type and frequency of activities shared with peers without disabilities often decreases. This may occur as early as grade school, but the difference is particularly noticeable when others learn to drive, date, go to college, get married, and have careers. Some people with DS do have these opportunities, but we have seen a number who feel left behind.

Even people who attend self-contained programs throughout their school years are still in the community enough to experience the stares and the different treatment given them by others. Remember, people with DS are often very sensitive to the reactions of others.

When they compare themselves to others, people with Down syndrome are invariably forced to consider their own identities (of who and what they are). This is not unique to people with DS. We all have to figure out who we are. Furthermore, comparisons between people with DS and the general population are probably no less disappointing or humbling than the comparisons the rest of us make. After all, we may all dream of being what we are not, such as larger or smaller, more attractive, or more successful. Many of us may even dream of being rock stars, sports legends, etc.

As for all of us, the process of "coming to terms with one's identity" for people with DS often starts early in childhood and continues into adulthood. We have heard of many creative ways that families of children and adults with DS have discussed and promoted a positive view of Down syndrome. This may include dealing with the inappropriate or unkind actions of others and the self-blame that sometimes occurs in response to these actions (a common experience of minority members). Over time, the result of this process of awareness and acceptance leads to the development of a more honest, realistic, and positive view of self.

Sheila Hebein, the Executive Director of the National Association for Down Syndrome (NADS), has described an important event in her son Chris's development of acceptance and self-esteem:

> *On a visit to the park when Chris was 9, two young girls curiously asked him whether he was "retarded." He quickly answered "No." When they persisted, he was irritated but he continued to play. Later that day at home, Chris asked his mother if he was "retarded." His mother had already explained that he had Down syndrome and that he may be slower than others in doing some things. Now she told Chris that she and Chris's father did not use the word "retarded" to describe someone who learns slowly, but that some people did. She then sat down with Chris and together they made a list of what Chris could do and things that were hard for him to do. After making the list, Chris concluded that he could do far more than he couldn't do and that "having Down syndrome wasn't bad at all."*

It may be instructive to look at some of the steps in this successful process. First, Sheila did not intervene in the park incident. After careful observation, she determined that the girls' questions were based on normal curiosity and offered a wonderful learning opportunity for Chris. Second, Sheila respectfully waited for Chris to initiate a discussion of the incident. She knew that he needed time to think through the issues and she trusted that Chris would come to discuss the issue when ready. Third, her explanation of "Down syndrome" was direct and honest and yet also extremely encouraging and respectful of his skills and abilities. On the one hand, she did not gloss over the fact that DS was a disability that may make him "slower than others." On the other hand, she conveyed great confidence in his ability to deal with this issue on his own terms and at his own speed by waiting for him to initiate the discussion and by asking him to talk about things he could do. Finally, the sense of pride and acceptance Chris experienced came from a natural event in the community. This incident, in turn, was the result of a family decision to let Chris explore and experience the world.

Clearly, for Chris, the message from this experience was that he had the right and capability to be in the community regardless of his limitations. No doubt, the confidence and pride he experienced from this incident has carried over to subsequent incidents in his life. Chris is a now an adult working successfully in a community setting, and, despite the challenges he has faced, he has maintained a strong positive view of himself and of Down syndrome.

BREAKING THE NEWS

At this point it may be helpful to discuss what to do if you have an adolescent or an adult with DS in the family who has not discussed the fact that he has Down syndrome or who has not discussed this issue for some time. The following are frequently asked questions regarding this:

Why do adolescents and adults with DS need to know they have DS?

As we discussed earlier, it is difficult to develop your own talents and skills and to advocate for yourself if you cannot accept DS. This is true whether the person is a younger child or an adult.

Is the person with DS ever too old to learn about DS?

We do not think so. If anything, there is a greater need with increasing age, because most people already know they are different than others. By adolescence, and certainly by early adulthood, most people have been stared at or treated differently literally hundreds of times. Regardless of how sensitive or insensitive you think the person is to these issues, it would be very difficult for him to miss the fact that he is different unless he lives in a vacuum. At this later stage of life, the question then is not *whether* they are different but how and why?

If we discussed these issues when he was younger is it important to discuss them again now that he is older?

Yes, because the discrepancy in skills between people with DS and peers in the general population is more apparent in adolescence and adulthood, so people's awareness of this difference is also greater at this time. Your son or daughter needs to discuss their DS in order to develop a positive and realistic view of themselves as teens or adults.

What response should we expect from our son or daughter to this discussion?

We have found that some people have difficulty accepting the message, but most experience some sense of relief after learning that they have Down syndrome. The discussion will often confirm and validate feelings and observations they have about being different. There is a name for what they have been experiencing (Down syndrome). They have something that helps to explain what has been happening to them all these years.

Should we wait for the person to initiate a conversation about his Down syndrome?

Certainly, if he brings up the subject it is very important to respond to the topic. On the other hand, if he does not bring it up, it is not always advantageous to wait. Many people are very aware and sensitive to the world around them but they may have difficulty articulating their feelings and thoughts to others. Taking the responsibility to discuss these issues may allow them to voice issues and concerns they have and have been unable to express. Additionally, people with DS are often sensitive to cues from others. If this topic is broached, they may feel free to discuss it; otherwise, they may not be sure that this is what the parent wants.

How do you talk about Down syndrome?

We recommend simple and honest statements similar to what Sheila told Chris in the above example. People need to know the name (Down syndrome) of what they have. This makes it a concrete reality. They need to know that there are some significant differences compared to most others, and what they are. For example, they may need more time to do certain tasks and are more dependent on others for assistance with finances, travel, or whatever the case may be.

One way to discuss Down syndrome is to discuss the person's strengths and weaknesses. As shown in the above example, it is important to praise and encourage the person for what he can do. It is also important to mention his special talents and gifts. On the other hand, being forthright about the person's limitations is also essential. Anything less than honesty about these issues and you run the risk of undermining your credibility, and, more importantly, of denigrating and patronizing the person with DS. Most people with DS are very perceptive about the veracity and authenticity of another's comments. If the person with DS thinks you are less than honest about his weaknesses, he will probably not trust your comments about his strengths.

Are there ways of promoting and broadening a more positive image of DS?

It may be helpful to point to other people of different ages and levels of skill in the community who are good role models of Down syndrome. Additionally, celebrities like actor Chris Burke offer excellent role models of people who are successful and have good self-esteem (see peers discussion on pages 132-36).

Are there ways of normalizing DS?

There are ways to help the person with DS to see that while his DS may be unique, many of his issues and concerns are not. For example it may be helpful to discuss the fact that we all have strengths and weaknesses. We too have dreams of being rock stars, sports figures, or more successful in work or in love, and we too all have to live with what we were born with.

Additionally, it may help to discuss the fact that not all of their differences are related to Down syndrome. For example, an older sister may be able to have a cell phone because she has reached a certain age and not because she does not have DS.

When do you broach the subject?

There are many different types of situations when the subject may be broached:

- ◆ You might broach the subject when your son or daughter is confronted with comments from others (as happened with Chris in the above example). We have heard of many examples from adolescents and adults of being stared at, teased, or even being made the victim of unintentionally hurtful comments. These situations often demand some type of response and discussion by family members to help the person with DS to learn from and deal effectively with these issues.
- ◆ Another opportunity might be when the person with DS compares himself unfavorably with others without disabilities. This may happen when others have major life experiences that the person with DS will probably not experience, such as getting married, going to college, etc. It may also include more day to-day-issues, such as the person with DS needing an escort to go into the community when his younger sibling is free to go alone.

◆ Parents may also broach the subject at a time when there are no negative issues or concerns related to the person's Down syndrome. This
may allow you to discuss the issue under less stressful circumstances.
This has some advantages and disadvantages. Someone may be more
intensely interested in the subject when he is in the midst of problem
situations, such as described immediately above. On the other hand,
when there are no problems, you can gradually introduce the issues.
You can then discuss them over an extended period of time, allowing
the person to more easily process the information. There may be many
ways to bring up the subject of DS—for example, if you see someone in
the community or on television who has DS.

DEVELOPING A SENSE OF COMPETENCE

Following awareness, the essential next step for positive acceptance is to emphasize the person's own strengths and skills. Over time, and with encouragement from
family and friends, the person needs

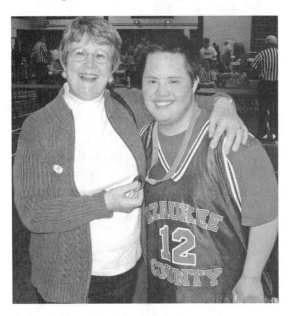

to change his perspective from "what
cannot be done" because of his disability to "what can be done." Psychologists call this process the development
of competence. Competence is the term
used to describe every-man's need "to
do for self" as a means to gain some
sense of control and mastery over the
world. The promotion of competence
begins at home at the earliest age and
continues throughout life as a day-to-
day process of growth and learning.
Over time, competence with daily living tasks leads to a greater sense of
independence and to enhanced pride
and self-esteem.

Developmental psychologists believe that the best way for parents to promote
competence is by "good enough" parenting. This means that the parent is available
for love, support, and guidance when needed, but the child is also allowed to experience manageable amounts of frustration and failure as an incentive to learn and
develop independence.

At the ADSC, we have found that families of adults with DS who are most successful with promoting competence and self-pride follow this "good enough" formula.
Parents are aware of their adult child's limitations but are also aware of his potential
for independence. Parents are there to guide and aid him as needed while also encouraging him to "do for self" whenever possible—doing daily living tasks at home, as

well as tasks at school, work, and other community settings. The process of trial and error and of learning from one's mistakes is the same for people with DS as for other children; just the starting point and the level of skill attained is different.

Families who have more difficulty promoting competence may expect either too much or too little from the person with Down syndrome. When parental expectations are too high, the person may give up in frustration and failure. We have seen this occur in adults who become depressed and despondent when, despite family expectations, they could not achieve the same goals in sports, school, job, career, marriage, etc. as "normal" brothers, sisters or same age peers.

On the other hand, frustration and underachievement may result if families expect too little from the person with DS and do not allow him to do self-care tasks that would increase his independence. As a result, when opportunities for independence occur, he may simply not have the experience or confidence to know how to respond effectively. Equally important, when people do not get experience in dealing with day-to-day challenges, they may develop a sense of helplessness and despair in the face of more serious problems and issues. This has been aptly described in the literature as "learned helplessness" and puts people at far greater risk for depression and a host of other health and mental health problems (Seligman, 1967).

Whether people expect too much or too little of the person with DS, the pride that comes from the development of independence skills goes unrealized. This occurs if the person is pushed to be something he is not or cannot be or if his talents and skills are grossly underestimated. These topics are further addressed in Chapter 3.

Do's and Don'ts in Promoting Competence at Home

- ◆ Encourage the person with DS to do new tasks that he is physically and developmentally capable of doing. If the task is too far beyond him, this may demoralize him rather than create competence.
- ◆ If the task is too difficult, it may still be possible to break it into manageable and doable steps.
- ◆ Tasks that are most important to the person with DS are an added incentive.
- ◆ Don't be too quick to "take over" when the person is trying a new task.
- ◆ Above all else, encourage the person to accept mistakes and a lack of success as a necessary part of the learning process. How else can people learn if they cannot learn from their mistakes and failures?

Competence in School

Families who support competence and self-esteem at school are careful not to confuse their own wishes and ambitions with those of the person with DS. These families are most likely to honestly and realistically appraise the person's skills and interests in order to find the right environment for his needs. They also encourage school staff to build on existing strengths and positive experiences to increase confidence and motivation.

Again, families who overestimate or underestimate their child's skills and abilities may fail to find school settings that promote pride and self-esteem. True,

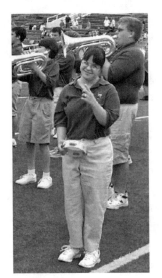

in the United States, inclusion in the schools is every student's right. However, the child's needs and abilities should determine the curriculum. Academic programs which are over the student's head or which simply serve as a babysitting service do nothing to promote independence, pride, or competence in dealing with the world. Also, when students are included in classes geared to college-bound students, they often are not taught the practical job skills, money handling, reading, food preparation, self-travel, and other tasks needed to live as independently as possible. Additionally, including a student in a setting where there is exposure to few if any other students with DS or other disabilities may have a negative effect on the student's social and emotional development.

In the upper grades, education should focus on the realities of life after school. It is fine to continue to take academic classes, especially in subjects such as reading, writing, and math that adults need for independent living. However, most older students with DS also need to learn social and work skills needed to succeed in jobs and to live independently in the community. Moreover, job experience is essential to any successful school program. Research has clearly shown that the greater one's job experience while still in school, the greater

The Importance of Having Friends with Intellectual Disabilities

Why is it important for people with Down syndrome to have friends who have DS and other intellectual disabilities? If you think about your friends, they probably tend to be people who are the same intellectual level as you. We seek out these people. They are the ones who are most likely to understand what we are trying to say, to share our interests, and to experience the world the same as we do. They serve as a type of mirror and validation for who and what we are.

The same applies for people with DS. They also need others who are most likely to experience the world as they do. They may not always be able to talk to these others because of expressive language limitations, but this may not be necessary. As mentioned in Chapter 4, people with DS are very aware of and sensitive to others in their environment. In observing how others experience and deal with the world, they come to feel that they are not alone in their perceptions and experiences. They validate who and what they are, which offers a strong sense of support and identity.

one's chance of being successful at finding and keeping a job once they age out of school (Weyman et al., 1988). In our experience, exposure to different types of jobs is also valuable so people can choose an area of interest to them. Parents who do not understand the importance of job experience in school often find out too late that these experiences are critical to success in the job sphere.

Equally important, success in job experiences usually requires a competent job coordinator and job coach. Successful programs will emphasize the skills and talents needed to succeed on the job, such as patience and persistence on job tasks, a strong work ethic, and taking care of one's appearance. In addition, the job coach will help to teach appropriate social skills in the worksite (see job section below for more on this).

A good outcome is usually the result of a program that is both appropriate for the person's skills and addresses the life skills necessary after graduation. A nationally recognized school district in the Chicago area discovered these challenges. The focus of this district is on college preparation, since a very high percentage of the graduates go on to college. The approach was not altered for students with intellectual disabilities, many of whom became frustrated and graduated without appropriate job skills. The school district then modified its approach and developed a transition program. This program emphasizes skills for living and working in the community and provides ample opportunity for supervised job experiences in a host of settings. The students are now having a much more positive experience and are much better prepared for occupations after graduation.

POSTSECONDARY PROGRAMS

We have heard from a number of young adults with Down syndrome who attend postsecondary programs at colleges or community colleges. Most of these individuals commute to programs at local community colleges and take one or two courses outside of their normal work and social schedule. Typically, these local programs make courses available to people with cognitive disabilities, but offer little else in the way of support or organized social activities. Still, people with DS attending these programs enjoy their courses and they often describe their participation in them with pride. Many seem to feel they are experiencing something that is fairly rare for persons with disabilities. As one student described his courses, "I can go to college just like my brothers and sisters." It is not clear how much substantive learning occurs in these courses, but this may be beside the point. For participants, the experience seems to be invaluable in and of itself.

There are also specialized community college programs which do have supports and counselors available for students with developmental disabilities. Some even have social activities available, ranging from drop-in centers on campus to dances or other social outings and events. The most successful and popular of these programs have courses which emphasize independent functioning in the community, as well as job training and adaptive skills in the workplace. The network of support with other students in these programs is also of great importance.

These types of programs take up where secondary schools leave off and they may be very beneficial in offering support and training for people in the community. Unfortunately, there are not many of these programs because they do not appear to be a high priority for state educators.

There are a number of more intensive programs, usually located on college campuses, in which participating students usually live in dorms. There are two different types of campus programs: 1) those that are adapted for students with learning disabilities, but which sometimes also admit students with Down syndrome, and 2) those which are specifically designed to serve the needs of people with DS and other disabilities. We have found that the former are not always optimal environments for people with DS. Many of the students who do not have DS have learning problems, but most have average or low average intelligence. Because of the emphasis on these students, the courses are often too difficult for most students with DS. Perhaps more importantly, there is also more of an emphasis on academic rather than on work and community skills, so they may not be appropriate to the needs of adults with DS. Additionally, supervision in the dorms may be inadequate. This follows from the expectation in these programs that most of the students have the cognitive ability to manage their own lives and schedules. As discussed in Chapter 3, adults with DS may be technically proficient with their own self-care, grooming, etc., but still be immature with such decisions as when to go to bed, what to eat, when to attend beneficial recreation activities, etc. We have heard of a few students who have done well in this type of environment, but most have not.

Given the problems associated with these programs, why would people with Down syndrome attend them? Many parents may hope that their son or daughter with DS may learn from and even rise to the level of the others in the program. While this may be possible to a limited degree, the demands on the student and the lack of adequate support and supervision make this a bad fit for most people with DS. Most students with DS are simply overwhelmed.

The second type of campus program is more specifically designed for people with Down syndrome and other intellectual disabilities. The stated goals of most of these programs are to help people develop self-esteem and the skills for living independently in the community. Most of these programs are relatively new and have had to learn through trial and error how to best meet these goals. The most successful programs emphasize adaptive living skills in the dorm, worksite, and community more than they emphasize traditional lecture-style coursework. Additionally, more successful programs have an understanding of the needs and limits of people with DS. For example, they are more active in helping students to structure schedules and routines for them to follow. The most successful schools also continue providing supports to students who have graduated and are living in the community.

Left to their own, young adults with Down syndrome may flounder, but with the right amount of help and guidance, many have matured and prospered in these environments.

COMPETENCE AT WORK

There is perhaps nothing as important to an adult's sense of competence and self-esteem as his work. We have found that most people with DS are very motivated and conscientious about their work. We have heard high praise from employers regarding the work ethic and performance of people with DS. Employers report that people with DS are not necessarily fast but they are quite often thorough, persistent, and reliable (see Chapter 9). Many are also reluctant to take time off and are rarely tardy. Some employers actively recruit people with DS because of the positive experience they have had with this group. For example, one camera company hires a large number of people with DS for assembly of cameras and related items. The precision and care people bring to the job is valued by this and other employers.

Success in community jobs depends on a number of factors, including:
1. exposure to different work sites;
2. adequate training in work tasks, ability to communicate with supervisors and others, social skills; and
3. ongoing support.

There has been much progress in the area of community jobs, particularly in the past ten years. The most common jobs held by adults with DS are in grocery stores, janitorial and cleaning positions in offices, or fast food restaurants. We also frequently hear about jobs in offices, mail rooms, nursing homes, day care centers, and factories.

Exposure to Different Jobs. Exposure to a wide variety of different types of work is a key component of any successful school or post-school job training or placement program. This allows people with DS to try out different types of work and find out what fits their wants, needs, skills, and resources. Job trainers are able to see them perform in different work sites to assess strengths and areas that need additional training. When people are not given this type of exposure, they may be placed in jobs that are not appropriate to their skills or interests. For example:

> One man's family found the "perfect job" for him as a greeter in a large discount department store. Unfortunately, no one checked to see if he thought the job was perfect. His family found out fairly quickly that this was not what he wanted when he refused to get up and greet people. Fortunately, his family worked together with the manager so that he was able to try different work tasks in the store. After several different job tasks did not work out, he found the right job in the stock room doing merchandise preparation.

> Dominic, another adult with DS, had been assigned a "prized job" in a grocery store by a job placement agency. After approximately six months on the job, he began to send carts out into the middle of a busy street that ran along the side of the store. He told his family that he tried to do the job

because he knew he was lucky to have gotten it, but that he just could not take the job anymore. Dominic now works in a greenhouse, which seems to be much better suited to his needs and interests.

There are two additional examples of adults with Down syndrome failing at poorly suited jobs described in Chapter 9. All of these failures might have been prevented if there had been some exposure to different job environments in order to determine what the individuals were capable of and interested in doing.

Adequate Job Training. Training to do the tasks required in the job is also essential. Job training usually works best if it is done at the job site and if tasks are broken down and taught in manageable units by a patient job coach or trainer. We have found that it is also helpful if people with DS are encouraged to capitalize on their excellent visual memories to memorize and repeat the steps required to do the task.

Unfortunately, we have also seen people have problems and failures in jobs because they did not have adequate job task training and supervision. For example:

When Marion, 24, started her job at a large discount department store, the only preparation her supervisor gave her was to hand her a rag and to tell her, "Dust the store." The assignment was overwhelming, and, needless to say, this did not work. Marion seemed to be paralyzed in one spot.

A similar problem occurred with Meg, a 32-year-old woman working on a janitorial crew. She was given the job of vacuuming a large ballroom. Although she knew how to vacuum and she enjoyed this job, she was also paralyzed in one spot with the enormity of the job. When the supervisor came back three hours later, Meg had managed to vacuum only a twenty-square-foot section. Fortunately, the solution to Meg's problem was rather simple. Her supervisor and job coach partitioned the ballroom into more manageable sections and Meg was able to continue doing her job as effectively as ever.

For Marion, whose job was to dust the entire department store, the outcome was not positive; she lost her job. This should not have happened. A job coach should have been present to break the job down into more manageable tasks. The store supervisor also demonstrated a lack of tolerance or patience for adapting the job to Marion's needs. Despite this, Marion actually had the last laugh in this situation. She was able to find a job in a nearby competitor's store, and, with a little bit of direction from a good job coach, she has been a model employee who is much valued by her employer.

Social Skills Training. Besides training people in job tasks, perhaps the most important role of job trainers is teaching appropriate social skills and "job etiquette" at the worksite. Researchers have consistently found that what creates problems on the job for adults with developmental disabilities is social skill deficits, not a lack of job skills (Greenspan and Shouts, 1981; Hill and Weyman, 1981, Weyman et al, 1988).

Social competence on the job includes knowing how to deal with the boss, other employees, and customers or the public. Social competence with the boss is especially important. Difficulties in this area is one of the primary reasons for job dismissal. For example, one boss told a new employee with DS to "come and see me anytime." He was quite surprised when this young man repeatedly took him up on this offer.

Some adults may not understand that others besides their job coach or immediate supervisor may be in charge. For example, one young man in a grocery store was almost fired when he told the store manager that he only took orders from his immediate supervisor. Still others may be too easily swayed to do anything they are told to do by coworkers who are not in charge. For example:

> In the midst of a bitter battle between union and management in a grocery store, Samantha was manipulated by angry employees to write down complaints she had about her boss. Some of her complaints were appropriate, such as about her boss's disorganization around weekly scheduling. On the other hand, some complaints were true but should not have been expressed. For example, she described her boss as "grumpy," "yelling sometimes," etc. Unfortunately, Samantha showed a lack of common sense by delivering this list of complaints directly to her boss, much to the horror of her family and the employees who had put her up to this.
>
> Fortunately, Samantha's boss had a sense of humor and knew how others had manipulated her. Additionally, the boss had enough concern and knowledge of Samantha's needs that he called a meeting with the family, the job coach agency representative, and ADSC staff. Interestingly, the job coach agency representative explained that Samantha did not have regular meetings with her job coach because she already knew her job. The agency representative steadfastly refused to accept responsibility for Samantha's social competence on the job. On hearing this and with encouragement from ADSC staff, the family agreed to contract with a new job coach agency. The new job coach met with Samantha regularly to help her work on social skills and there have not been any additional problems since that time. Samantha continues to do her job as competently as ever.

People with Down syndrome may also have some difficulty dealing with customers or people encountered while on the job. For example, a close friend of one of the authors was buying some items at a grocery store for a breakfast meeting. She was in a hurry, and, without thinking, reached over to try to help a woman with Down syndrome bag her groceries. The young woman responded immediately in a tone of frustration and disgust that "you people are all the same . . . you are always in a hurry." In retelling the incident, the woman smiled and commented that the woman with DS was correct (see "The Pace" in Chapter 16).

Unfortunately, many customers may not be so understanding. There are many mean-spirited and angry people who may see the worker with DS as an easy target. For example, one man with DS almost lost his job in a restaurant because he "talked back" to a woman who chided him for being too slow in bussing the table she was waiting for. (He actually said, "I am going as fast as I can.") She complained to the administrative office of the restaurant chain, which directed the restaurant manager to put him on probation. Fortunately, this young man had a good job coach and was also well liked by the restaurant manager and the other employees. The job coach and restaurant staff took a great deal of time and effort to teach him how to control his comments and anger in these types of situations. As a result, he learned a valuable lesson, and has stayed in his job for many years without any further complaints from customers.

Ongoing Support. A different type of social issue we have found is that many people with Down syndrome who have jobs in the community appear to be alone and isolated. For example:

> *Ellen, 30, was diagnosed at the Center with depression. She had had recent losses in her life but we also found she had no friends or confidants in her job. She worked doing cleanup in a fast food restaurant where there were few repeat customers and there was much turnover in the employees and management. Many of the other employees spoke primarily Spanish and they had difficulty understanding or talking to Ellen. We started Ellen on an antidepressant medication, which reduced her symptoms, but we also strongly recommended that she work in a more supportive work environment. This follows from our belief that gains made from medication will be limited or not sustained if the person's environment does not change. Soon afterwards, Ellen moved to a different restaurant employing a number of people with disabilities, including a close friend of hers. She continued to make steady progress after this job change, and, after three years, she has had no new bouts of depression.*

We have seen many people with Down syndrome who do especially well in what are called "enclaves," where they work at a jobsite with several other employees with disabilities, as well as employees without disabilities. This is an excellent means to reduce the problem of isolation and also to make the most productive use of a job coach's time.

Some people with Down syndrome may find the most supportive work environment to be a sheltered workshop. These workshops have been developed since the 1950s-60s, and later by parent groups and others to give people with disabilities access to training and work in a segregated (sheltered) setting. These centers usually have different levels to meet the needs of workers with differing degrees of adaptive skills. The lower levels emphasize training of work and daily living skills, whereas the higher levels have work consisting of basic factory-like assembly work. Although the "gold standard" is community employment, we have found that sheltered workshops have great potential. This may be especially true for people in their 40s who missed out on the job training that is more widely available today. Yes, there are still workshops consisting of loud cavernous rooms with repetitious busy work. On the other hand, we have also seen a growing number that compete with any community job site in terms of meaningful work. In addition, people with DS are often able to connect to peers in these settings.

Workshops generally have piece work and assembly tasks as the primary type of paid work. Better workshops often have a variety of different assembly jobs, as well as other types of work such as janitorial and shipping jobs. These workshops also try very hard to recruit more work and a variety of jobs to keep people busy and interested in their work. They try to pay based on piece rate, just like any factory. People who are most productive should be able to earn more money. Although this may never be a livable wage, it should still be a fair rate of compensation for a day's work. We have found that most people with Down syndrome are proud of their paychecks even if they do not completely understand the value of the money.

Many of the better workshops have social, recreational, and exercise programs available to employees during and after work. Aerobics exercise programs are becoming more frequent and not just during "down time" but as a regular part of the daily work routine. Additionally, we have seen arts and crafts programs in workshops. Some are simply glorified busy work, but there are a growing number of exceptional programs taught by professionals. These programs are beneficial to all participants in building pride and the joy of self-expression.

Some people with DS benefit from a combination of community work and time in a workshop setting. This allows the pride and excitement of a community job while also allowing access to friends and supports at the workshop.

Of course, we do not mean to suggest that all adults with DS need to work with "their own kind." Some adults with Down syndrome do quite well as the only employee with a disability. However, if you know an adult with DS who seems unhappy and withdrawn while at work, it may be worth having him try another job where he would have more coworkers with disabilities.

COMPETENCE AT HOME

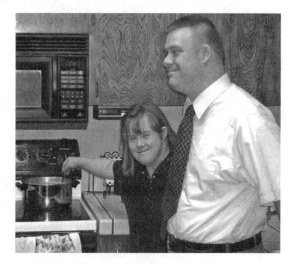

Residential environments should promote independence, pride, and self-esteem. Parents, caregivers in group homes, or others providing supervision need to follow a "good enough" model of direction and supervision. Adults with Down syndrome need to be given autonomy to do what they are able to, yet also receive help and guidance when needed.

Problems develop when people with DS are given either too little or too much independence. In our experience, too much independence is far more common. This may result from a disturbing tendency to judge a person's need for supervision on his ability to do self-care tasks rather on his level of maturity around certain key issues. For example, many people can independently do routine grooming, hygiene, and housekeeping tasks. However, they may make decisions about nutrition, sleeping, and free-time activities that are harmful to their health, well-being, and self-esteem. For example:

> *Three women from the same apartment were referred to the Center for depression and an apparent loss of skills. Symptoms included a lack of interest or participation in social or recreation activities that they previously enjoyed; significant weight gain; a loss of energy, fatigue, and a tendency to nap or to be "out of it" during daytime hours, which affected their work activities. In fact, one of the women was close to losing a job she loved at an animal shelter and another was earning a third of what she had previously earned at her workshop job. At the first appointment, neither the women themselves nor their case managers were able to shed light on what caused their depression and fatigue. Their case managers were actually surprised by the symptoms because the women had been very capable and social, and productive in their jobs.*
>
> *Fortunately, an explanation was found when their second appointments were scheduled in the late afternoon. This time, the evening staff person accompanied them to the appointment. This staff person explained that, as per agency policy, the women in the apartment were independent enough to be left alone at night. She would make certain that lights were out and the women were in bed when she left at 11:00 p.m. Recently, while driving away from the apartment at night, she had observed that all the lights were being turned back on in the apartment. The women admitted sheepishly, when questioned, that they got out of bed after staff left for the night, and watched their favorite TV shows and movies until early in the morning. Compounding the problem, they often ate many snacks while up watching their shows. This pattern had been going on for at least three months; thus, the cumulative effect of the sleep deprivation had begun to take an increasingly negative toll on their functioning.*
>
> *To resolve this problem, a number of meetings were held with the women, their parents, and caregivers, as well as many key staff and administrators from the agency. After some discussion about the limits of patient rights, the agency agreed to give the women 24-hour supervision to resolve the problem. In time and with a more normal pattern of sleep, they were back on track.*

We have also found that many people in less supervised community settings may not have the skill or initiative to attend beneficial social or recreational programs if they are responsible for organizing these activities. This may be true even for individuals who have the capability to manage all other self-care tasks successfully. As a result, they may become isolated and therefore at great risk for depression or other health or mental health problems (see "The Dennis Principle" in Chapter 3). For example:

> Peter, 31, moved from a fifteen-bed group home to a three-person residence in a more residential neighborhood. His level of skills warranted a move to a more independent living situation. After a year in the new residence, his sister and case manager brought him to the Center because he was becoming increasingly withdrawn and lethargic. He had also gained a considerable amount of weight due to inactivity. Peter had been active in social and recreation programs while living in the larger group home, but in his new residence he was responsible for scheduling and getting to recreation activities on his own. Although he had the training and the skill, he seemed to lack the motivation or initiative to go to activities. As a result, he spent most of his free time sitting on the couch watching television. Furthermore, Peter was alone most of the time in his new apartment because his two roommates were involved in their own activities. Peter's sister scheduled an appointment at the ADSC when he refused to visit her at her house, which was something he had always treasured.
>
> At the first meeting, it became clear to ADSC staff that Peter was depressed because of his social situation. After this, a second meeting at the Center was scheduled to include administrative staff from the group home. In this meeting, the administrative staff initially stated that Peter had a "right" to choose whether he would attend social activities. In response, the ADSC staff reported that his health and wellbeing were greatly affected by his inability to organize social activities. In the ensuing discussion, agency administrators developed an understanding that not only Peter, but a number of other individuals living in less supervised settings were also at risk for depression.
>
> By the conclusion of the meeting, a program was developed to provide Peter and others with more choices of social activities. For this plan, staff would work with Peter and the others to schedule and transport them to a full calendar of social and recreational events. For Peter, the "social plan" included riding to events in vans with others who lived in nearby apartments. Peter made some new friends among these people and reestablished friendships with the many people he had met over the years who attended the social activities. After he began his new social schedule, he began to lose weight and regained his positive mood and spirit. Within nine months, his sister reported that Peter was back to his old self.

For both Peter and the women noted above, the good news is that competence and self-esteem will return when appropriate help and guidance are provided. Interestingly, it is often not people with DS or their families who need to be convinced of the need for such help, but rather residential service providers, who are often strapped with limited budgets and inadequate staffing levels.

Challenging Agencies to Provide Adequate Support

We have discovered that the pattern of inadequate supervision shown in the above case examples is a problem affecting many people in community group homes. Agencies have limited finances for staff, but it may also be a little too convenient to attribute inadequate supervision to a "rights issue." We have found that families are often reluctant to challenge agencies to provide more supervision for fear of losing the residential placement. However, an interested third party such as a case management, social service, or healthcare provider may be able to join with the family to advocate for the needs of the person with Down syndrome. With this strategy, the family often feels that there is less risk of jeopardizing the placement with this strategy.

At the Adult Down Syndrome Center, we are able to challenge agencies when they misuse the "rights issue" and persuade them to provide more supervision and education, particularly when this is a threat to the person's health and wellbeing. If needed, we will even write doctor's orders specifying what is required to assist the person. Again, the areas of concern often include more serious problems with sleeping and eating, as well as a failure to participate in beneficial social and recreation activities. These activities are of critical importance to the person's wellbeing. By staying active and avoiding a sedentary lifestyle, people are more able to stay fit and healthy. This is particularly important for people with DS, who need regular exercise and activity because of slower metabolism. Regular attendance at social and recreation programs is also essential to avoid social isolation, as discussed below.

Adequate social supports are not just a problem in residential settings; they can also be less than optimal when an adult with Down syndrome is living with parents or other family members. In our experience, some teens and adults living at home have little opportunity for social or recreation activities. Sometimes this is due to a lack of transportation to these programs, such as when parents are working or unable to drive. There may be different ways to solve this problem. For example, most communities have some form of transportation available for people who are elderly or disabled, such as a cab, van, or bus service. It may also be possible to get rides from the families of other program participants. Case managers of agencies serving the needs of persons with disabilities and some staff in the recreational programs are often knowledgeable about such services. Families who spend the time and effort to locate a means for transport are usually rewarded. For the person with DS, time and effort is also well worth the effort.

Another problem families sometimes face is lack of appropriate social activities. These families may do well to band together and organize social activities. For example, parents in the Chicago area reported a successful "pizza and movie" activity (*NADS News*, January 2004). This began as a get together for two or three young women with DS at one of the participant's family homes and it has expanded to include eight to ten people who meet at different participants' houses at least every other Friday night. There are now at least two of these groups going in different parts of the Chicago area. The beauty of this activity is that there is no plan. No one has to conform to any rules or minimum requirements for participation other than to show up at a specified time and place. People simply get together for the pizza and the movie. For people with DS, who are often told what to do for most of their day, this is quite a welcome change. What is surprising to the families is how the groups have evolved and participants have grown together. Over time, participants have felt free to share their personal feelings with each other, and a closeness and genuine friendship has developed between members. Participation is voluntary, but most people rarely miss pizza night.

Although there are special recreation programs available in most Chicago communities, these pizza and movie groups serve a special purpose for the participants. This type of group activity may be even more beneficial in communities where there are relatively few social programs available, such as more rural areas or communities in which people live in unincorporated areas near cities (which are without a government structure and tax base to pay for programs). Parents in these less densely populated locales may need to travel some distance between households to have these meetings, but again, this may be well worth the effort.

There may also be other resources available in communities for organizing these types of groups. For instance, social groups have been formed by graduate students from the special education departments of universities. We have also been impressed with programs which pair teens or adults with DS with peers in the general population. Many high schools have such programs, which are called different names by the different schools, such as Peer Buddies. These programs often pair one teen peer as a special associate of the teen with DS, but they also have group activities with all participants in the program. These programs often help to integrate people with DS into the mainstream of the school, and especially the extracurricular programs, which is where so much of the socializing occurs among students in high schools.

There are similar programs for college age students which bring together students with teens and adults with DS and other disabilities. Unlike with the high school programs, the people with Down syndrome rarely attend the colleges from which the students come. These programs go by different names at different universities and colleges, such as "Best Buddies" and "Natural Ties." We have heard many comments from families and people with Down syndrome themselves about the benefits of these programs. Interestingly, those who report the greatest benefit are often the college or the high school students. Their comments are often similar to those made by families regarding the affection and sensitivity of people with DS, but they also comment on the lessons on life learned from them, such as to slow down and appreciate things here and now. We have also heard that many people continue their friendships long after they leave college, which is an indication of the strength of these relationships.

If you are creative and persistent, you can probably think of many other options. For example, perhaps you could join with other families to hire a special education teacher or professional to organize a social calendar for these adults.

"The Right to Choose" versus "The Need to Make Healthy Choices"

Whenever possible, adults with Down syndrome should be allowed to make their own choices and to learn from their mistakes. But what happens when they continually make choices that are harmful to themselves? When and how should a family step in to protect the adult from the consequences of bad choices? The answer to this question will often depend on three key areas of concern:1) safety; 2) people with influence; and 3) legal issues.

First, we believe that safety is the paramount concern. We think that families should step in when the person consistently makes choices which put him at risk for physical or emotional harm. We have discussed some of the most common reasons this can occur, such as more serious problems with sleeping, diet, and social isolation. More immediate dangers can involve risks from being unaccompanied in the community or left alone in a home, exposing him to such risks as fire, unsavory people, etc.

The second consideration is whether there are differences of opinion as to the amount of independence the person with Down syndrome can handle. Parents, grown siblings, teachers in a school, staff in a group home or worksite, or other people with influence over the adult with DS may all have differing agendas or philosophies which may compete for influence on the person's choices. This puts the person with DS in the middle, which may be very stressful. It may also be counterproductive if one of the parties encourages a degree of independence which the person cannot handle and thus puts him at risk for harm (as shown in the above examples of Peter and the women in the apartment). In these situations, families may be well advised to work with a third party who may be able to negotiate a more positive solution (see discussion on page 123). Again, agencies that have experience and authority to work with people with DS may be good candidates for this role.

The third issue has to do with whether the family members are legal guardians or whether the adult with Down syndrome is his own guardian. Guardianship issues may affect how easily parents and service providers resolve differences of opinion over levels of supervision. Parents who are guardians have the legal right to challenge a service provider to provide appropriate supervision. If they fear losing the placement, they may work in conjunction with a third party (see above). On the other hand, if the adult with DS is his own guardian, an agency or service provider may correctly say that he has the right to make up his own mind, even if his decision is harmful. See the section on Legal Guardianship in Chapter 13 for more information about the pros and cons of appointing a guardian.

DEVELOPING UNIQUE TALENTS AND CHARACTERISTICS

In addition to a sense of awareness and a sense of competence in essential tasks at home, school, and work, there is one more area that is essential to the self-esteem of adults with Down syndrome. That is the identification and development of the individual's unique talents and gifts.

Some people with Down syndrome have conventional talents that others readily recognize—whether it be writing poetry, public speaking, playing a musical instrument, creating art, acting, swimming, or something else. Others are truly gifted in people skills, such as being able to read others' emotions or bring out the best in others, although communication skills may make their talents difficult to appreciate at times. Still other people with Down syndrome may not have talents that are readily appreciated by outsiders, but instead have relative strengths that family members and others are aware of and appreciate.

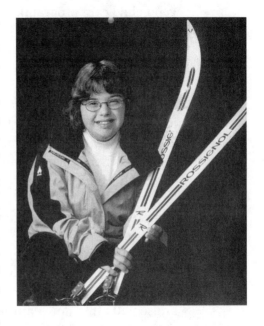

Whether or not an adult is a "superstar" in the Down syndrome universe, he needs to feel encouraged and proud of developing his unique talents and skills. For people with Down syndrome, who are often judged more by what they do not have or are not able to do, this is a way to say that "I am more than that."

Just as for any person who is part of a minority group, people with DS want to be seen as both a part of the group and yet possessing their own unique talents. In effect, these talents define the person as much or more than the DS, and as such, they need to be identified and nurtured. Most families know how important this is. So often we hear family members make statements like this: *"Sure, he has limitations, like others with Down Syndrome, **but did you know that he. . .** is an artist . . . can do this job better than anyone . . . has changed our family . . . is especially sensitive to others' feelings and needs . . . has an exceptional memory,"* etc. The pride and respect expressed in these statements is so important to the person with Down syndrome. It says to the person that he has something special and unique to contribute to the family and the world. He may have limitations in some areas, but strengths and talents in other areas, and this is who and what he is.

Do's and Don'ts for Nurturing Gifts and Talents

Here are some do's and don'ts for helping an adult with Down syndrome to identify and appreciate his own unique talents and characteristics (with examples from different talent areas):

◆ Assume the person with DS has talents and gifts of some kind.

◆ Expose him to a wide variety of different activities to help identify these talents and gifts.

◆ Don't assume he doesn't have skills in certain areas. Try everything.

◆ Encourage talents that the person with DS shows real interest in. If it comes from the person himself there will be true interest and pride from the talent.

◆ Look for ways to successfully develop the talent he is interested in developing. For example, if talented in art or music, it may help to have instruction from an appropriate teacher. If sensitive to others, find an avenue to express this (such as volunteering in a nursing home, or a good child care program). For athletes, find different sports and recreation venues.

◆ Find ways to encourage talents at home. For example, for artists or musicians, have a place to work or practice with the appropriate instrument or art materials. For those sensitive to others, encourage them to use this talent with family and friends. For athletes, take time to play or to organize neighborhood sports activities.

◆ Encourage but be careful not to over-pressure. Nothing dampens the spirit and energy like too much pressure from others.

◆ Take time to observe or acknowledge the person's talent. For example, look at his art, listen to his music, observe him volunteer at a nursing home, attend his sports activities, etc.

◆ Offer sincere praise but don't overdo it. People with DS will usually know when praise is not genuine.

◆ Excessive praise may increase the person's interest in doing the talent to please others rather than enhance his own self-esteem.

◆ Praise will often flow naturally from others in the community when the person with DS puts his heart into his talent. (See the example of Emily, immediately below.) Sports, artistic endeavors, and other types of activities will also generate praise from others, including peers (which is a valued form of praise).

◆ Finally, praise should emphasize self-pride rather than pleasing others. For example, say, "you should be very proud of yourself" rather than, "I'm so proud of you!"

One mother was concerned about how her 29-year-old daughter, Emily, would respond to her grandmother's deterioration from dementia and her move to a nursing home. After delaying a visit to the nursing home for some time, Emily's mother finally took her to visit her grandmother. Her mother was amazed and immensely proud to find that Emily was not only unusually sensitive and caring toward her grandmother, but she also responded sensitively to a host of others in the nursing home, particularly those who were lonely and in greatest need of care. Emily's mother let her know how proud she was, but the elderly residents who benefited from her caring interest also expressed their profound thanks through their words and facial expressions. Emily returned to the nursing home many times before and after her grandmother's death. Eventually, the administrator of the nursing home asked her to continue as a volunteer, which she has done with much benefit to all, including herself.

LOVE, FRIENDSHIP, AND SELF-ESTEEM

As discussed in the preceding sections, three key factors in the development of self-esteem are: 1) the acceptance of one's identity, 2) the development of competence, and 3) an understanding of one's own talents and gifts. A fourth, equally essential key to self-esteem is the feeling that one is loved and lovable.

So much of counseling for *all* people revolves around their perceptions of being unloved and unlovable, and, alternatively, on how to find ways and means for obtaining love in their life.

While some people with DS clearly have some difficulty finding the love they need, we have found that many are quite adept in this area. In any event, most people with DS are very sensitive to, and aware of, expressions of love. Most are also keenly aware when these expression are absent in their lives. In many cases they are so good at eliciting love that they are often able to change the amount and intensity of love expressed in the family. Like all skills, this may have enormous benefits, but it may also have some negative consequences, which we will discuss in this section.

EXPRESSING LOVE AND AFFECTION

The feeling of being loved is essential for all of us, but for people with Down syndrome, there are also some unique issues. Before we discuss this, first let us explain that we have consistently heard two stereotypes regarding people with DS. The first is that they are stubborn. We discuss this in Chapter 9. The second stereotype is the notion that people with DS are unusually loving and affectionate. For the most part, we find that this stereotype is true. Many families assert that their son or daughter with DS has been a strong positive influence by increasing the amount of love and affection family members express toward each other. We experience this affection firsthand at the Center. Our patients with DS are poked, prodded, and worst of all, bored by questions, and yet we still receive more hugs than most professionals on planet Earth. We enjoy these hugs just as much as we know families do.

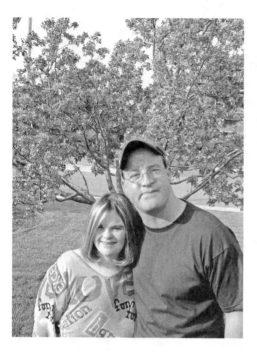

As you might expect, there is a down side to the expression of love and affection. There are important social skill issues related to when, where, and with whom the person with DS expresses his love and affection. Parents, teachers, and caregivers often spend much time and effort teaching about the appropriate expression of affection. For example, people with DS learn that affection with family and friends is fine but not necessarily in public settings. Similarly affection with a "girl or boyfriend" may also be appropriate in private spaces, but not at work or in community settings. Of course, not all people with DS are naturally outgoing and affectionate, and some actively resist being touched by others, especially strangers. Some families actually spend more time teaching others that they would prefer their child be greeted with a "high five" or a handshake than they do teaching their child how to greet others.

When an adolescent or adult with Down syndrome *is* physically demonstrative, the biggest concern is with expression of affection toward strangers or people who are not family or close friends. This makes sense. There are unscrupulous people who may take advantage of people with DS, just as there are people who take advantage of children. Families' concern for the safety and wellbeing of their sons and daughters with DS is justified, and the openness and affection shown by many people with DS no doubt intensify it.

Recently, there has been more concern with safety issues in the general population and in the field of disabilities. We believe this may be contributing to a different problem that we have encountered. The problem seems to occur most often when adults with DS move from their family home to group homes. In their family home, people with Down syndrome are usually free to give and receive love and affection. In group homes, however, staff are strongly discouraged from showing physical affection to people in their care due to growing concerns with sexual abuse.

We believe that many adults feel a great sense of loss when they move from their family home to a more sterile or affectionless environment. The adult with Down syndrome may or may not understand why staff are not allowed to show him physical affection. He may think, "This is my house and this is a person I care about and who cares for me. But he (she) never hugs me." The problem may be exacerbated if the adult takes longer to connect to people because of expressive language limitations. The lack of physical contact and expressive limitation may be major reasons why people have difficulties adapting to a group home. They may also be the reasons why coping with turnover of certain staff members is so difficult.

Do's and Don'ts for Safe Expression of Affection

The needs to express and receive physical affection and to protect people with Down syndrome from sexual abuse and sexual predators are both very important. There is not an easy solution to address both needs.

Some guidelines to help ensure safety for adults with DS include:

- ◆ If possible, enroll the adult in a program designed to teach people with developmental disabilities to be street-savvy and security conscious. These types of programs are typically offered by a local ARC or by an agency serving the needs of people with intellectual disabilities. These programs may be successful, particularly if what is learned in the program becomes a part of the adult's regular routine. For example, one man who was sometimes left alone in his house was instructed not to open the door to anyone. His parents were relieved to find that he was steadfast in maintaining this rule even when it was just a neighbor borrowing sugar. In a similar vein, one woman refused a ride from a neighbor because she was not a family member, even though it was raining.

- ◆ Teach the person with Down syndrome which physical demonstrations of affection are appropriate. Remember that people with DS are visual learners and learn best from seeing the appropriate behavior.

- ◆ Bear in mind that although adults with Down syndrome often have a general understanding of appropriate physical touch, many situations may be confusing and seemingly contradictory. For example: Why is it OK to hug people at a wedding reception but not at a mall? Why is it OK to show affection to parents and not to staff in one's group home, especially when these people behave much like parents? Similarly, at the Down Syndrome Center we allow our patients to hug us, but what happens when they try to hug other doctors? Because of these types of contradictory expectations, people with DS may need more specific guidelines on who, when, and where it is appropriate to show affection. They may need to specifically identify each person who they can show physical affection to and not just a class of all people, such as all doctors, all caregivers, etc.

Some guidelines to ensure that adults with DS are able to safely give and receive physical affection include:

- ◆ If and when they move out of the family home, try to ensure that they still see family members regularly, and that those family members give them ample, appropriate opportunities to hug, etc.

- ◆ Encourage the adult with Down syndrome to attend dances with friends where physical contact is part of the activity.

- ◆ Ensure that the adult has the support, opportunities, and privacy needed to show affection with a date, or at some type of get-together with a boy or girl friend. We find that such get-togethers rarely involve sexual intimacy and the hand holding and other forms of affection are very enriching.

◆ Pets may also be a safe and wonderful way for people with DS to give and receive affection. In addition taking responsibility for the care of the animal adds another important dimension.

◆ Do not forget that giving care to those in need may be a beneficial way for people with DS to share their caring and affectionate nature. Caregivers may need to determine that the person receiving care is appropriate and not taking advantage of the person with DS. However, when this is the case both the person receiving the care and the person with DS may benefit greatly from this experience. By giving of themselves, people receive affection and thanks in return, and also acquire a sense of accomplishment and pride from helping others.

While continued efforts to maintain safety are encouraged, the solution cannot be the complete loss of physical contact. A hug, a pat on the shoulder, and other non-sexual acts of physical contact are very important. Continued efforts, monitoring, and working with compassionate, caring care providers are essential to maximizing emotional support and safety.

PEER RELATIONS

Peer friendships are critical to everyone's health and wellbeing. Peer friendships are different from parent or teacher relationships, but they serve an equally important

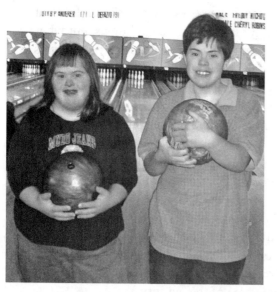

role in the development of self and self-esteem. Like a parent-child relationship, a peer relationship involves the expression of positive feelings and support, but it also provides the all-important feeling of fitting in with one's peer group. Peers share common interests, they struggle with similar developmental tasks and issues, and they serve an important mirroring role in the formation of one's identity. Peers with similar disabilities play an even greater role in showing the way to pride and self-respect despite whatever limitations the disability causes. Similarly, peers with a disability who are in the public eye, such as actors Chris Burke and Andrea Friedman or many of the artists and musicians who display their talents at Down syndrome conventions, play an equally important role. They project a positive image about DS that people can take pride in and aspire to.

And yet, some families and researchers call into question the quality of peer friendships between people with Down syndrome and other disabilities. These individuals point to difficulties people with Down syndrome have with initiating and maintaining conversations, and with reported difficulties in showing interest in and taking another's perspective. On the other hand, many families report that even when there is an apparent lack of interactional skills, peer relationships are usually strong, longstanding, and critically important. Typically, these peer relationships develop over much time and familiarity, such as when people are in the same job or school program over many years. Although these friendships may take more time to develop, once established, they are an essential source of support and self-esteem.

Families who have some difficulty accepting Down syndrome may discourage the development of relationships with peers who have disabilities. Other families may inadvertently discourage these relationships if they are so intent on "inclusion" of their child with DS at school and in community activities that he rarely if ever encounters someone else with Down syndrome. This is not to say that friendships with peers without disabilities are not possible or that they are not extremely beneficial. However, these relationships are not as common as parents may hope and when they do develop it may be difficult to maintain over the long term because these peers often move on in their lives.

Discouraging friendships with peers with disabilities is unwise. Some of the saddest people we have encountered at the Center are people who do not want to associate with peers who have Down syndrome (or other disabilities). These individuals are caught between two worlds and have difficulty maintaining a positive self-image. On the one hand, they are not always readily accepted by typically developing peers, or they lose touch with them over time. On the other hand, they voluntarily cut themselves off from peers with disabilities who could be their friends and who often stay behind when nondisabled peers leave for college or other typical adult pursuits.

Some of our patients live in what we describe as an "Existential Hell." They have found that their high school friends without disabilities have moved on to other aspects of their lives. And yet, they believe that it is inappropriate to associate with people with disabilities. Furthermore, they are struggling with their own identity because of their inability to accept or "deal with" having Down syndrome. They find themselves isolated between two worlds. They feel they are by themselves, but unfortunately, they aren't even comfortable with themselves. The approaches discussed in this chapter are much better used as prevention strategies to avoid this occurrence. However, if it does occur, we start back at the concepts discussed at the beginning of this chapter and work on reestablishing self-esteem.

Do's and Don'ts in Encouraging Peer Friendships

In the meantime, there are some things families can do to encourage the person with Down syndrome to interact with, rather than to avoid, others with disabilities:

- ◆ Encourage participation in Special Olympics and other recreation activities for people with disabilities. This is important even when the person resists participating in these activities. We find that people will often get caught up in the team effort, which helps to create a rapport and positive experience with other teammates (even though they have disabilities).

◆ Try to find situations where the avoider has to help another person with a disability. For example, have him teach a coworker how to do a job task or a housemate how to do a chore. This strategy does three things:

1. The incentive to show that he can do a good job at the task will often get the avoider past his initial reluctance to interact with another with a disability. In setting this up, it may be helpful to appeal to the helper's skill in doing the job.

2. Taking on the role of helper will often change the avoider's attitude and demeanor from negative or apathetic to positive and helpful.

3. This in turn will usually change the attitude and response of the person who is being helped. This is important because many people with DS are aware when they are not liked or appreciated by others and they usually avoid these others or respond negatively to them.

The result of this is the potential for a positive experience between the avoider and the person he is avoiding. This may change the avoider's attitude and subsequent behavior toward others with disabilities. After a number of these positive experiences, he may develop a more permanent positive attitude toward others with disabilities.

◆ We have found that some people who tend to avoid others with DS may be more open to interacting with someone who has a different type of disability, such as a physical handicap. For example, some people with DS enjoy helping others in wheelchairs get from one place to another. You can then capitalize on this to praise the person for his sensitivity. Then you may be able to point out that the person with DS simply has a different type of disability than the person with a physical disability, which may help him to be more accepting of his own disability. (See Chapter 13 on counseling persons with acceptance issues for more on this.)

◆ See if the adult is less resistant to assisting younger people, such as children in day care settings. Many times the children they help look up to them as heroes and role models. This may not only help them view themselves and their Down syndrome more positively, but also benefit the children.

◆ Arrange for the adult to attend Down syndrome conferences and conventions. At these conferences, he will be surrounded by people and programs which are supportive and positive about DS. Perhaps more importantly, he may be influenced positively by leaders and self-advocates with DS who have found acceptance and self-pride despite their own disability.

◆ Keep a careful eye on your own and other caregivers' attitudes and behaviors toward individuals with disabilities. Your attitudes will strongly influence the person with DS in your care. Even if you feel you are hiding your attitude, any negativity will often be detected by your family member with DS. If you feel you do not have a positive attitude toward people with disabilities, you need to talk to someone who can help or go to support groups for parents who have similar problems.

ENCOURAGING FRIENDSHIPS FOR ADULTS WHO ARE SHY OR LACK EXPERIENCE

Sometimes adolescents and adults with DS avoid others because they are shy or have little experience socializing—not necessarily because they are resistant to interacting with people with disabilities. These are some successful strategies used by families who attend the ADCS:

◆ Encourage participation in Special Olympics and similar recreation activities. Participating in structured activities is far easier than participating in more unstructured social events. Over time, people often develop more comfort with interacting with others, especially when caught up in team activities which build rapport.

◆ Dances may be a surprisingly good way for shy adults to get together with others. Many people with DS love to dance, whether or not they are with someone. In these situations everyone seems to dance and to have a good time and there does not seem to be the same type of social pressure that accompanies dances for teens or young adults in the general population.

◆ Some people may find that participating in programs for teens and adults at DS conferences and conventions is a good way to connect with peers. These programs often allow people to comfortably interact with peers while engaged in the program activities and may include activities specifically designed for building confidence in social situations. Additionally, experienced self-advocates in attendance are often able to inspire and influence positive attitude and self-pride. This can translate into more confidence in social situations with peers.

◆ Volunteering or working at programs serving young people or children with Down syndrome may help to build more confidence in social situations. Again, if the younger people look up to the older person who is helping, it helps to build pride and self-confidence.

◆ Participation in Buddy Walks or other programs may help instill confidence, particularly when there is strong support from those attending for people with DS. There is also exposure to people with DS who have strong pride and self-esteem.

◆ Try to develop casual get-togethers for peers with DS such as the pizza and movie night described above. This is the type of planned activity that people often feel more comfortable attending, especially when it occurs in a comfortable home environment. Also, having different participants host the get-together allows them to develop confidence in taking care of others in a social situation. As an added incentive, people are often able to show off their music and other hobbies and interests, which can build interest and rapport with others.

Summary

Families who are most successful at promoting self-esteem:

◆ Develop an understanding and acceptance of DS and encourage the same in their child with DS.

◆ Are aware of their child's limitations as well as his potential for developing independent living skills and more unique talents and abilities.

◆ Promote self-esteem and independence through competence with self-care tasks and day-to-day challenges encountered in the home and community.

◆ Encourage expressive language skills and social relationships with peers.

◆ Encourage productive "grooves"; especially those that assist the person in reliably completing self-care and job tasks.

◆ Encourage participation in social and recreational activities.

◆ Try to find the right school, work, or residential program to meet their son's or daughter's needs and abilities. They also encourage staff to build on their child's existing strengths and positive experiences to increase confidence and motivation in these environments.

Finally, families who promote independence understand their child's ability to teach valuable lessons on slowing down and on experiencing the here and now.

Chapter 8

Self-Talk,

Imaginary Friends,

and

Fantasy Life

In examining and evaluating our patients at the Adult Down Syndrome Center we have heard repeatedly that adults with Down syndrome talk to themselves. Sometimes the reports from parents and caregivers reflect deep concern that this behavior is "not normal" and symptomatic of severe psychological problems.

Preventing misinterpretation of self-talk as a sign of psychosis in people with Down syndrome was a major motivation in our investigating self-talk in our patients. We believe that too often these conversations with self or imaginary companions have been equated with "hearing of voices" and treated with anti-psychotic medications (such as Haldol or Risperdal). Since it is extremely difficult to evaluate the thought processes of adolescents and adults with cognitive impairments and limited verbal skills, we urge a very cautious approach in interpreting and treating what seems to be a common and sometimes very helpful coping behavior for adults with Down syndrome.

Since the Center opened in 1992, we have been asking our patients, their families, and caregivers about self-talk. Our records indicate that 83 percent of our patients engage in conversations with themselves or imaginary companions (McGuire and Chicoine, 2002). This includes people with Down syndrome with an age range from 12 to 83. This high prevalence of self-talk does not seem to be widely known. For some parents and caregivers, learning this fact is reassuring. But the contents of these conversations, their frequency, tone, and context can be important in determining whether treatment is warranted.

Intertwined with the issue of self-talk is the tendency of people with Down syndrome to have rich fantasy lives. Some people with Down syndrome converse with imaginary friends or act out scenes from their imagination for entertainment. Again, it is important to understand how and why this may be "normal" for someone with Down syndrome, and not a sign of psychosis.

HELPFUL SELF-TALK

Many "normal" people talk to themselves at times. Self-talk is very common in typically developing young children, and not unheard of in otherwise "normal" adults. In general, people talk to themselves for four reasons:

1. to direct their own behavior (for instance, someone knitting a sweater might mutter "knit two, purl two" to herself);
2. to think out loud (for example, to ponder a question or to review the events that occurred in the course of one's day);
3. to let off steam in the midst of strong emotions (for example, many people swear out loud or criticize themselves with comments like, "Boy, was that stupid");
4. to entertain themselves (for instance, on long, boring car trips, some of us sing or talk to ourselves or talk to the radio even though we know the radio can't hear us).

Most often when people with Down syndrome talk to themselves, it is for one of these same normal purposes. They are often less likely to censor themselves in front of others, however, and therefore are caught talking to themselves much more often.

USING SELF-TALK TO DIRECT BEHAVIOR

Families and caregivers should understand that self-talk is not only "normal" but also useful. Self-talk plays an essential role in the cognitive development of all children up until the age of about seven, although this may be as late as nine in some children (Diaz and Berk, 1991; Vygotsky, 1991). Self-talk helps children coordinate their actions and thoughts. It also seems to be an important tool for learning new skills and higher level thinking. For example, three-year-old Suzy says to herself,

"This red piece goes in the round hole." Then Suzy puts the red piece into the round hole of the puzzle.

We suspect that self-talk serves the same useful purpose of directing behavior for many adolescents and adults with Down syndrome. Consider twenty-two-year-old Nick. His mother reported the following scene. She asked Nick to attend a family function on a Sunday afternoon even though Nick's regular routine was to go to the movies on Sunday afternoons. Nick told his mother he would not go with the family. Then his mother asked Nick to think it over. Nick stormed off to his room and slammed the door. His mother overheard this dialogue (Nick's is the only voice being heard):

"You should go with your family, Nick."

"But I want to go to the movies."

"Listen to your Mom!"

"But Sunday is my movie day."

"You can go next Sunday."

Nick's mother said he went to the family function, with the proviso that he could go to the movies the next Sunday. Nick may have been talking to an imaginary person or arguing with himself, but Nick clearly managed to cope with a situation not to his liking. He used "self-talk" to sort through the issue.

Children without identified learning problems progressively internalize self-talk with age. Moreover, children with higher intellectual abilities seem to internalize their self-talk earlier. As self-talk is transformed into higher level thinking, it becomes abbreviated and the child begins to *think rather than say* the directions for his or her behavior. Thus, the intellectual and speech difficulties of adults with Down syndrome may contribute to the high prevalence of audible self-talk reported to us at the Center. We consider the behavior to be "developmentally appropriate," given the intellectual and adaptive limitations of most adults with Down syndrome.

In general, the functions of self-talk among adults who do not have an intellectual disability are not well researched or understood. There is, however, a growing body of evidence suggesting that a high percentage of athletes use self-talk to motivate themselves and enhance performance. One study even found that a high percentage of people who exercise use self-talk, at least fairly often (Gamage et. al., 2001). Common experience suggests that adults who are not participating in sports or exercise programs may also talk out loud to themselves when they are alone and confronting new or difficult tasks. Though the occurrence may be less frequent, the uses of an adult's self-talk seem consistent with the findings about children. Adults talk to themselves to direct their behavior and learn new skills. Adults are more sensitive to social context and therefore this self-talk is observed less frequently because they may not want others to overhear these private conversations.

In the general population, self-talk among older persons is frequently noted, and, usually, easily accepted, just as it is with children. Social isolation and the increasing difficulty of some tasks of daily living may explain this greater frequency of self-talk in the elderly. For adults with Down syndrome, these explanations also make sense. Adults with Down syndrome are at greater risk for social isolation and the challenges of daily living can be daunting.

Using Self-talk to Think Out Loud and to Vent Emotions

Additionally, we have found that many adults with Down syndrome rely on self-talk to vent feelings such as sadness or frustration. They *think out loud* in order to process daily life events. This may be because their speech or cognitive impairments inhibit communication. In fact, caregivers frequently note that the amount and intensity of the self-talk reflects the number and emotional intensity of the daily life events experienced by the person with Down syndrome. They also note that the person's speech is often clearer when talking to herself than when carrying on a conversation. This may be because there is less social pressure when the person is speaking to herself.

Using Self-talk for Entertainment

For adults with Down syndrome, self-talk may be the only, or preferred, entertainment available when they are alone for long periods of time. For example, a mother reported that her daughter Debbie, a 23-year-old woman with Down syndrome, spent hours in her room talking to her "fantasy friends" after they moved to a new neighborhood. Once Debbie became more involved in social and work activities in her new neighborhood, she did not have the time or the need to talk to her imaginary friends as often.

Many people with Down syndrome seem to enjoy retelling favorite stories or movies to themselves during down time, or when bored with what is going on around them. The section on "Imagination and Fantasy" below delves more into the role of imagination in self-talk and other aspects of life for people with Down syndrome.

Appropriateness of Self-talk

Adults with Down syndrome show some sensitivity about the private nature of their self-talk. Like Nick in the example above, parents and caregivers report that self-talk often occurs behind closed doors or in settings where the adults think they are alone. Having trouble judging what is supposed to be private and what is considered "socially appropriate" may contribute to the high prevalence of self-talk among adults with Down syndrome we have seen.

When to Worry

The distinction between helpful and worrisome self-talk is not easy to cast in stone. In some cases, even very loud and threatening self-talk can be harmless. This use for self-talk by an adult with Down syndrome may not be that different from someone

Self-talk Do's and Don'ts

- ◆ Don't make the person with Down syndrome feel bad because she uses self-talk.
- ◆ Don't try to eliminate self-talk.
- ◆ Discuss self-talk with the person: self-talk is OK but some people don't understand or are bothered by it, so not doing it in front of others is polite.
- ◆ Do encourage appropriate (socially acceptable) places for self-talk and gently discourage inappropriate places (such as at work or school).
- ◆ Consider having a private signal to remind the person if she is doing self-talk in public.
- ◆ Discuss self-talk with others who come in contact with the person with Down syndrome (explain the normalcy).

who rarely swears but screams out a four-letter word after hitting her thumb with a hammer. Such outbursts may simply be an immediate, almost reflexive outlet for some of life's frustrations.

Our best advice about when to worry is to listen carefully for changes in the frequency and context of the self-talk. If self-talk becomes dominated by self-disparagement and self-devaluation, intervention may be warranted. For example, it may be quite harmless when Jenny yells, "I am a dummy," once, right after her failure to bake a cake from scratch. However, if Jenny begins to tell herself over and over, "I am a dummy and can't do anything right," it may be time to worry and possibly to take her for a psychological evaluation.

A marked increase in the frequency and a change in tone of the self-talk also may signal a developing problem. For example, Irving began to talk to himself more frequently and not just in his room at the group home. He seemed to lose interest in his housemates and spent more time in these conversations with himself. Irving talked to himself, sometimes loudly and in a threatening manner, at the bus stop, at the workshop, and at the group home. Irving was diagnosed as experiencing a severe form of depression. Over an extended period of time, he began to respond to an antidepressant medication and to group counseling.

In another case, Ray (like Irving) showed a dramatic increase in self-talk. Ray refused to go to his job and to participate in the social activities that he once enjoyed. It turned out that Ray's change in behavior was not due to depression. Instead, Ray's family and staff at his worksite discovered that he was being intimidated and harassed by a new coworker. After the bully was removed from his workshop, Ray gradually regained his sense of trust in the safety of the workshop. His self-talk and interest in participating in activities returned to earlier levels.

Further study of the content, context, tone, and frequency of the self-talk of adults with Down syndrome may provide more insight into their private inner worlds. What we have observed and heard from family and caregivers suggests that self-talk is an im-

Warning Signs That Self-talk May Signal a Problem

- ◆ Self-talk markedly increases in frequency.
- ◆ Self-talk becomes increasingly self-critical.
- ◆ Self-talk becomes loud or threatening.
- ◆ Self-talk becomes agitated.
- ◆ The person uses self-talk in public places (when previously he or she only used it in private places).

What to do if these changes are noticed:
- ◆ Ask the person with Down syndrome if something is bothering her.
- ◆ Listen to the self-talk for clues as to the problem.
- ◆ Check with teachers, employers, other family members, etc. to see if there may be a new stress.
- ◆ Watch for signs of physical illness and obtain a medical examination.
- ◆ If the above steps do not result in the identification of a cause (and a solution), obtain a psychological evaluation.

portant coping tool and only rarely should it be considered a symptom of severe mental illness or psychosis. A dramatic change in self-talk may indicate a mental health or situational problem. Despite the odd or disturbing nature of the self-talk, our experience at the Center indicates that self-talk allows adults with Down syndrome to problem-solve, to vent their feelings, to entertain themselves, and to process the events of their daily lives.

IMAGINATION AND FANTASY

We have found that people with Down syndrome often have a rich and creative imagination and fantasy life. They easily create fantasies from their rich and fertile bank of visual memories and from favorite movies and TV shows which are also saved in memory (see Chapter 5 for more on memory). Common examples involve people imagining themselves to be police- or firemen, pro wrestling or other sports figures, princesses, heroes and superheroes, and, of course, movie and music stars. Interestingly, the most popular music stars are not always present-day celebrities but include "oldies" stars such as the Beatles, the Beach boys, and Elvis (who lives on in the world of Down syndrome). Similarly, movie and TV stars live on through videotapes and TV reruns, and, as a result, are also very popular with this group. Musicals such as *Grease* and *Cats* are often particular favorites.

We have also heard more fanciful tales of marriages, babies delivered, relationships with stars, and accomplishments by the person or significant others that are gross exaggerations or fantasies. Parents, caregivers, and professionals frequently express concerns that such behavior is "inappropriate" for an adult with Down syndrome. In most cases, we do not agree. When evaluating the appropriateness of such stories and fantasies, it is important to consider developmental, rather than chronological, age. For example, an individual with a chronological age of 27 years may actually have the developmental age of a 5- or 6-year-old in terms of abstract thinking, maturity of decision-making, etc.

Similarly, the line between fact and fantasy is blurred for many people with DS, just as it is for typically developing children up to about the age of 6 or later for some children. For example, some 7-year-olds and even some children who are older still believe in Santa Claus. As a result, fantasized events and characters from movies and cartoons may be easily confused with real-life people and events. With this in mind, creating and believing in fantasies is quite normal and appropriate for most people with Down syndrome.

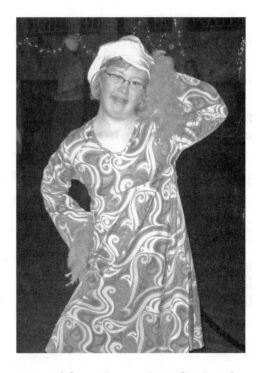

Another concern is whether made-up stories and fantasies are just "lies" and or even a symptom of psychosis. While we have seen some people with Down syndrome who lie or have psychotic symptoms, generally we have found that instances of fantasy creation are most often simply an indication of an active and creative imagination.

Positive Consequences of Fantasies

If we take the younger developmental age for most people with Down syndrome, and combine this with a rich fantasy life, fueled by vivid visual memories from movies and life experiences, then there is a potential for the development of some very interesting stories and fantasies. The results of this fantasizing may be both positive and negative. On the plus side, we have seen that this can fuel brilliance in such creative endeavors as painting, music, and dancing. As mentioned previously, imaginative play may also be a wonderful way to fill free-time activity. People may replay memories of movies or past events or they may have props, such as pictures from favorite hobby magazines (e.g., wrestling, sports, celebrity, etc). They may also incorporate toys or collectibles (such as dolls, Matchbox cars, etc.) into their fantasy play.

Additionally, we can make a strong case that fantasy is a necessary part of a healthy life for all of us. In fact, creative fantasies serve an important function that has been described by Daniel Levinson as "the dream." A dream may include all our hopes and aspirations for a successful career, marriage, and family life, but also such fantasies as being a rock star, sports celebrity, etc. The truth is, we are rarely able to completely fulfill our dreams, and yet, this is still an essential part of our development as human beings. We need to have something to aspire to even if that something is not attainable.

It is interesting to note that the dreams and fantasies of people with Down syndrome are quite often to simply have the same life and activities that their siblings and parents have (such as marriage, career, children, etc.). Like all of us, they may not achieve their dreams, but this is usually not a problem. For example, for the past ten years that one man has been coming to the Center, he has promised that he will get married in five years. Obviously, if this doesn't happen, his world won't come to an end, but he still needs to dream, as we all do.

NEGATIVE CONSEQUENCES OF FANTASIES

On the other hand, this rich reservoir of memory and fantasy may compete with what is going on in an adult's real life. It is easy to see how this could happen, especially if the "here and now" happens to be a noisy, boring, or stressful environment and the fantasized life is full of fun, entertaining, soothing, or exciting things. Unfortunately, when someone lavishes too much attention on her fantasy life, particularly in public situations, this may be misinterpreted as a symptom of a behavior problem or a mental illness. For example:

> Dr. McGuire was asked to consult with a school district regarding Tim, a 15-year-old with Down syndrome who was reportedly displaying odd behavior in class. When Dr. McGuire arrived at the school, he found Tim underneath a table making noises with his mouth, gesturing with his arms, and talking loudly to himself. In a subsequent meeting with family and school authorities, his teachers reported that he was exhibiting this and other odd behavior in a number of his classes. The school was concerned that Tim was showing signs of a psychosis.
>
> In looking closer at the situation, it became very obvious that this young man was trying to communicate extreme boredom. What he was doing under the table was playing "Star Wars" and other imaginative fantasy play to fill the hours of boredom. His mother described him as extremely imaginative and creative in his play. It turned out that the classes where he exhibited the most self-talk and fantasy play were academic classes that were not suited to his skills or interests. On the other hand, he showed little of the self-talk or fantasy play in either his art class, where he excelled, or his vocational programs, which consisted primarily of on-the-job training. Based on our recommendation, he was moved out of the academic classes into more suitable vocational classes and the problem was all but solved.

Another example from the other end of the age cycle can be seen in Phil:

> Phil was a pleasant 52-year-old man with DS who lived with his brother and sister-in-law. He had been doing janitorial work at a local workshop. Phil had an incredibly rich and complex imaginary family consisting of family members from his real life (many of whom were deceased) and

characters from classic TV shows ("All in the Family" and "I Love Lucy" were his favorites). Although his brother reported that Phil had always had a rich fantasy life, it appeared that he was spending more and more time with his imaginary world. This was especially the case at his workshop where he had been able to reliably and meticulously clean three large bathrooms for many years. Unfortunately, he was now spending so much time in conversation with his imaginary family that he could barely finish one bathroom by the end of the day. Staff in the workshop were concerned that he was psychotic or demented, because he appeared forgetful and confused at times.

Fortunately, Phil's behavior changed when he was moved from his cleaning job, where he was alone most of the day, to a workshop with 15 other participants and a supervisor. After the move, staff members were amazed to find that he was very social with others in the group and he no longer seemed to need to talk with his imaginary family. Additionally, his work activities became focused and there were no more incidents of confusion or forgetfulness. What caused the positive change? We believe he may have simply needed the social stimulation of the group and a change in job duties. Just like Tim, Phil may have been trying to communicate the need for something (a social group) that would be more engaging than his rich fantasy life.

We have encountered some people with Down syndrome who not only imagine themselves to be one of their favorite movie or TV characters, but who go a step farther and assume the role of the character in their own life. For example, one man became the Disney movie character "Inspector Gadget," with all the detective paraphernalia from the movie. Everyone in his life also became a character from the movie. This was a little irritating to these people but fortunately, it did not interfere with his ability to go about his normal home and work activities.

We have also seen a number of adults with Down syndrome who become firemen or police officers, complete with uniform shirts, badge, radio, and other paraphernalia. Some become sports figures or movie or music stars. Sometimes this type of role taking may become too extreme (or "over the top" as described by one father). For example:

One man assumed the leather-jacket-clad persona of Fonzie from the "Happy Days" TV show. This was "cute" for a while. Unfortunately, his role playing almost cost him his job when he called his female boss a "babe." He was also almost expelled from his group home when he called female staff "chicks" and slapped several across their backsides. This problem was resolved fairly quickly when an emergency meeting was called and all key caregivers, including family and residential and worksite staff, made it clear to him that there would be serious consequences if he kept up the Fonzie role.

In another situation, a therapeutic intervention was required to solve the problem. This involved a 28-year-old man with Down syndrome, Jack:

Jack had developed a relationship with a female companion in his life based on romanticized love relationships from his favorite TV show and movie, "The Partridge Family." He had experienced considerable stress and loss in his own life and the movie gave him a means to escape to a more perfect world. Unfortunately, the reality of his relationship was not like the movies. At first he tried to get the woman to change. When this did not work, he became more and more preoccupied with reenacting the movie in his own imagination, to the detriment of his work and social life.

After this had gone on for some time, Jack was brought to the Adult Down Syndrome Center, where he was treated for depression with obsessive compulsive features. He responded to the medications, as well as to the staff at his worksite supporting him and redirecting him back into his daily activities. In time, he was able to get back to his normal activities.

Do's and Don'ts in Dealing with Fantasy

◆ Do try to limit a fantasy if it is interfering with work or school or peer relationships.

◆ If the involvement is interfering with the person's life, redirect her toward other activities.

◆ When redirecting the person, it may or may not be helpful to tell her that the object of the person's fantasy is not real (e.g., "Rocky is only a character on TV. The man you see in the movie is just an actor pretending to be Rocky.") Often, however, this is not comprehended or accepted. If so, it is not necessary or generally helpful to continue insisting that the character is not real.

◆ When redirecting the person away from the fantasy (such as by limiting access to videos, DVDs, games, etc. that the person is obsessed with), do so in a positive fashion so that you are directing the person *toward* something else rather than *away* from these objects.

CONCLUSION

Far from being signs of mental illness, self-talk and imaginary friends are usually quite "normal" in adolescents and adults with Down syndrome. For most people with Down syndrome, talking aloud to themselves or to imaginary friends can serve many possible useful purposes. Intervention is generally only necessary if there are other symptoms that are consistent with mental illness and/or the behavior interferes significantly with participation in other activities.

Chapter 9

The Groove

and

Flexibility

Don would wake each work day at the same time and invariably follow the same routine. First he would have his toast and juice, then shave, shower, and dress in the same meticulous way. His parents and boss could count on him to be clean and well groomed for work. Likewise, his boss could count on him to be punctual and reliable with his work activities. After work he would have a snack, do his chores (take out the garbage, set the table), and make sure everything in his room was put away. Each Tuesday he would wash his clothes; Wednesdays he would pick up and vacuum the house. After dinner he would relax in his room with his favorite movie or music while writing in his notebook or doing word search puzzles. Saturdays he would get up at the same time to eat breakfast, then on to shave, shower, dress, and off to bowling and later to a social club. His family grew to expect this regularity of Don and he was very reliable with his routines.

At the Adult Down Syndrome Center, we have discovered that an unusually high number of people with Down syndrome, like Don, need sameness, repetition, and order in their lives. We call this tendency "The Groove" because people's behavior tends to follow fairly well-worn paths or grooves. We have found these groove-like tendencies to be so common in people with DS that the absence of this tendency is notable for its rarity. We will summarize ideas on different types of grooves and the advantages and disadvantages of grooves. Following this we will discuss means for identifying and resolving problems arising from "stuck grooves."

WHAT IS A GROOVE?

A simple definition of a groove is a set pattern or routine in one's actions or thoughts. We all have grooves in our daily lives or absolutely nothing would get done. For example, if every morning we had to rethink when or how to take a shower, brush our teeth, put on socks, tie our shoes, and make toast, we would never leave home in the morning. Multiply this by all the other automatic and routine tasks we do every day at home, at work, and in the community and it is easy to see that a world without grooves would grind to a halt.

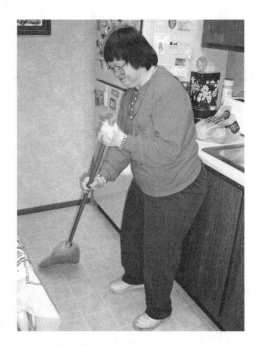

People with Down syndrome are particularly good at this business of having and following grooves in their daily lives. Many follow grooves with a degree of precision that would impress a fussy accountant. Examples of grooves we have seen include:

- ◆ Having a set order and timing to daily routines, to include set morning, evening, and work routines, as well as routines for activities that are relaxing. For example, many people with Down syndrome draw or copy words or letters during their time at home.
- ◆ Being quite meticulous in the care of their appearance and grooming, as well as of their rooms and possessions. People with DS often have a set place for furniture and other personal items in their rooms or living spaces. Items that are moved or disturbed by others are usually returned to the original location in short order.
- ◆ Developing grooves around less frequent activities, such as a set method for packing clothes, for ordering in restaurants, or for celebrating weddings, birthdays, holidays, etc.
- ◆ Having grooves which center on personal preferences for such things as music, sports teams, social and recreation activities, or celebrities,

as well as for more personal issues such as a favorite relative or a love interest. These preferences help to define who the person is by what he likes to do and who he likes to do it with.

ADVANTAGES OF GROOVES

There are numerous advantages to these grooves. Grooves give an important sense of order and structure to people's daily lives. Grooves are of great benefit in increasing independence. Once an activity is learned and becomes a part of a daily routine, these tasks will be completed faithfully. Independence and performance may also be enhanced in the work environment. Employers are often impressed with how reliable workers with Down syndrome are in completing routine work tasks and in following time schedules.

USING GROOVES TO RELAX

Groove activities may also offer a refuge from the stresses and strains of daily life in the home or on the job. These activities often involve repeating a specific enjoyable activity in a quiet or private space, sometimes as part of the daily routine. At home, the person's private space will often be his bedroom or bathroom. Some of the most common activities people with DS enjoy repeating include reading, writing or drawing, listening to music, watching TV or videos, looking at family pictures, or doing such crafts and hobbies as needlework or arranging collected items. In fact, some of the most common activities may appear rather unusual, such as copying letters or words onto paper or a notebook or cleaning or organizing their rooms. However, there is no question that this is relaxing to the person. In the bathroom, relaxing activities include cleaning or grooming tasks, as well as just sitting and relaxing.

On the job, repeating a relaxing activity may give adults with Down syndrome a brief but valuable respite from interacting with others, from the noise and hassle of the workplace, and from the tedium of work. At work, the chosen space is quite often the bathroom because this is frequently the only place where there is some quiet or privacy. As at home, relaxing grooves may include doing some grooming tasks or just sitting and relaxing in one of the stalls. Debra, 32, an office assistant, frequently relaxes during breaks by listening to music on her headphones or by doing "word searches" at her desk.

GROOVES RELATED TO APPEARANCE AND POSSESSIONS

Also of great benefit to people with DS are grooves involving the meticulous care of their own appearance, room, and personal items. Careful grooming and dressing conveys an image of pride, self-respect, and dignity to others and may increase one's own pride and self-respect. This may be especially important for people with Down syndrome, who have distinctive physical features that clearly mark them as different.

This difference makes them susceptible to discrimination, which may occur with any minority group. The self-pride that comes from attention to dress and grooming may go a long way to reduce the stigmatizing effect of being different.

ORDERING GROOVES

Ordering grooves are also very important to many people with Down syndrome. Ordering involves being neat and tidy with one's room, furniture, clothing, and other personal items, such as videos, pictures, CD's, etc. When ordering and arranging, many people feel a need to close doors and cabinets and turn off lights. Many people are very careful with folding and putting away clothing in drawers and on hangers in their closets. If taken to an extreme, these ordering tendencies can be difficult for families to live with, as detailed in the section on "Disadvantages" below.

GROOVES RELATED TO PERSONAL PREFERENCES

Finally, and most importantly, the groove is a powerful means of expression and communication. This is especially true for people with Down syndrome who have a limited ability to express themselves verbally. Each groove is a clear and unambiguous statement of a personal choice or preference. For example, daily grooves and routines express how someone chooses to organize and manage such things as his own grooming, appearance, and personal items; his participation in social, recreational, and work activities; and his personal preferences in music, hobbies, and artistic endeavors. Each person's choices will, in turn, help to shape and define his own unique style and personality.

For some, grooves may even take on a life-saving role. For example:

> *Cassie, 28, has Down syndrome as well as a genetic disease that causes progressive and irreversible muscle deterioration that will eventually lead to an untimely death. This horrible disease has already taken the life of all but one sibling. Cassie is well aware of her condition and yet she continues to maintain a strong positive attitude about life and about the people in her life. In fact, when we first met Cassie, one of the most difficult aspects of her disease was not the pain and discomfort it caused but the fact that she frequently missed seeing her friends at work or at social activities because she was too tired or ill to go out.*
>
> *We discovered that the primary reason Cassie is able to maintain her positive attitude is that she has developed a number of routines that are not only extremely relaxing but also allow her to connect to others. True to the nature of grooves, these routines often occur at a set time and in a set order. For example, she often starts with a favorite activity, which is to make one of her endless lists of things on her computer. She frequently follows this with a period of thoughtful letter writing to friends and to*

extended family members. Finally, she carefully and meticulously writes personal thoughts in her diary.

Despite Cassie's illness and many losses in her life, these routines give her free time a shape and form which serves at least three important purposes. First, she is able to avoid despair because she is simply too busy for self-pity. Second, her letters allow her to connect with family and friends, even if not in person. Thanks to her exceptional visual memory, she feels almost as if she is conversing with them while writing. She is even able to write to her deceased family members "in heaven," which gives her a great deal of comfort. Third, through her letters and diary, she is able to express her feelings—including positive feelings as well as her fears and concerns about her illness and her great sense of loss for her family. As grooves, these activities are repeated reliably every day, ensuring that she continues to get the benefits of these activities.

DISADVANTAGES OF GROOVES

Although there are many benefits and advantages to grooves, there may also be problems and disadvantages. Some of the problems are not serious or need not be serious if handled appropriately by others. For example, an adult with Down syndrome may be interested in a particular issue, such as a favorite sports team, and bring it up repeatedly with family and friends. This may be a minor irritant to his friends, but it is not necessarily a problem that interferes with important spheres of the adult's life.

There are also grooves that may be useful if done at the appropriate time or place but a problem if done at the wrong time or place. For example, a groove related to cleaning the bathroom may be greatly appreciated by family members unless it is done in the morning when everyone needs to get ready for work. A better plan would be to schedule this task into an afternoon routine. Similarly, a restaurant manager may be pleased with how clean an employee with Down syndrome keeps the bathrooms unless patrons have to wait for long periods while he does a meticulous job. A better plan may be for the employee to do this job when there are fewer patrons or before the restaurant opens.

It is not uncommon for ordering grooves to become problematic to a greater or lesser degree. For example, some people are described as "having their own sense of order." They arrange things in their room "just so" but not necessarily in a way that others would consider tidy or even practical. Books, clothing, videos, paper, etc. may be arranged in piles in different spots on the floor, which may be inconvenient and make it difficult to walk through the room or clean it.

Some adults with Down syndrome have a habit of folding and putting away even worn clothing. Some may spend an excessive amount of time ordering belongings or rearranging folded or hung up clothing "just so," which may delay an outing or interfere with other activities. These adults may "over-arrange" everything from everyday clothing or furniture items to special magazines or memorabilia, to unique or unusual items such as cut-up paper, bottle caps, etc.

Saving items such as these unique or nonsensical things, as well as pictures, magazines, memorabilia, pens, CDs, etc. is another fairly common groove. Many people with DS take saved or special items "on the road, " carefully packing special items in bags or backpacks and bringing them everywhere they go. The behavior becomes less adaptive, or hoarding, when it includes resistance to giving up items, when backpacks become excessively heavy, or when hoarded items include garbage or refuse items. (See hoarding in Chapter 16.)

Less adaptive ordering may also involve inflexible insistence on always doing things the same way, such as sitting in the same chair or in the same fixed spot for meals, using the same cup, having food arranged "just so" on one's plate, etc.

The pace of completing routines is also an area of inflexibility for some people with Down syndrome. For example, attempts to move people along at a faster pace may only result in them slowing down further. Sometimes when adults with DS are pushed too far, they respond by shutting down (what some families call a "meltdown"). They may even start the sequence of a routine all over again. We often hear of this happening during morning routines when there is a limited amount of time to get up and out the door. This may also happen when there are unexpected last-minute changes to the daily schedule. On the other hand, shutting down may also happen in response to a more significant change in an adult's life. For example:

> Susan, 39, often refused to go out in the evening for recreation activities with the five other residents in her group home. This refusal had created growing resentment among the other residents, who enjoyed regular outings. It turns out that Susan had recently moved from a residence with fifteen older women who had a more sedentary lifestyle and far fewer outings.
>
> In an attempt to solve the problem, staff became increasing more forceful with Susan because they believed her reason for staying home— so she wouldn't miss her nightly 7:00 bath—was an absurd excuse. Predictably, she met their attempts to push her with even more resistance. At first, she slowed her pace when getting ready, which then delayed the outing. With increasing pressure, she not only slowed her pace to a crawl but also became more meticulous about her dressing and grooming and would start the routine all over again if not "just so."
>
> A meeting at the Center with all parties resulted in a recommendation that Susan move to a new home with older residents, which was believed to be better suited to her needs. Before this plan could be carried out, a second option became available. It was proposed that residents from several nearby group homes could go on joint outings, freeing up one staff person who could stay home with Susan. This latter plan was adopted as the best option for Susan. Interestingly, as Susan became more comfortable

with her group home, she began to go out more often on planned outings. This significantly improved her relationship with other residents and also helped her with weight management.

We obviously hear about routines in our clinical work, but we have also developed a healthy respect for the routines of the interns and employees with Down syndrome at the Adult Down Syndrome Center. In most instances, we have found ways of making routines work for people, so that they are able to do assigned office tasks reliably. However, sometimes routines do create minor problems. For example, one man had a set lunchtime at 12:00 and he could not adjust his work routine to eat lunch at 12:30 with others in the office. We were able to let him have his own lunch schedule, but this meant missing out on a beneficial social period with other employees. Fortunately, after several weeks of gentle encouragement, he agreed to lunch with the other employees. In some cases, we have simply learned to stay out of people's way when they do their routines. For example, we have learned to try not to interrupt people with DS who are doing a copying job, in order to quickly make "just one copy." This is just too disruptive.

MORE SERIOUS PROBLEMS

Sometimes a groove may become a more serious problem, and, occasionally, may even meet the criteria of an obsessive-compulsive disorder (OCD). The groove may become OCD when it includes repetitive thoughts (obsessions) or repetitive behaviors (compulsions) that interfere significantly in normal and essential activities of life. For example, a groove is significantly problematic when morning or evening routines become so elaborate that someone consistently misses work or beneficial social activities. Obsessive-compulsive disorder is addressed in Chapter 16.

RISK OF MALADAPTIVE GROOVES

People with Down syndrome are more susceptible to maladaptive grooves than other people are. After depression, maladaptive grooves are the second most common mental health problem diagnosed at the Adult Down Syndrome Center. On the positive side, maladaptive grooves, especially in the form of a more severe OCD, are not inevitable in adults with Down syndrome. Grooves clearly seem to be built into the chemistry of most people with DS (as described below), but we have found that grooves have different degrees of strength in people with DS.

One way to look at grooves is to compare them to the concept of temperament (Carey and McDevitt, 1995). Temperament is an accepted psychological term for our own innate personality traits or characteristics which govern our moods and emotional nature. Any parent with more than one child will testify to the differences in temperament that each child displays from birth. This is not to say that families or outside forces do not have a strong influence on temperament—just that a strong biological component plays a major role in any aspect of one's emotions and moods. Grooves also appear to have an inherent biological basis, but, as with temperament, there appears to be a wide variation in the strength of this tendency. In other words, some people have an inherent tendency for more intensity or rigidity in their grooves than others. We have found that this may affect how susceptible people are to the development of maladaptive grooves. In addition, in our experience, people with better adaptive skills overall are often more flexible and less susceptible to more severe grooves or OCD.

THE BIOCHEMICAL BASIS OF GROOVES

In order to understand the tendency toward maladaptive grooves in some people with Down syndrome, it may be helpful to understand the underlying chemical process in the brain. Researchers have known for some time that human behavior is the result of nerve activity in the brain. The brain's system of nerve pathways function much like an electrical system, but with gaps at junction points. These junction points are bridged by chemical substances (neurotransmitters), which allow the nerve system to work properly.

More recently, researchers have used sophisticated brain scans to actually locate specific nerve pathways and regions of the brain that are associated with specific types of human behavior (Saxena et al., 1998; Schwartz, Stoessel, Baxter et al., 1996; Breiter, Rauch, Kwong, et al., 1996). For example, grooves (obsessions and compulsions) are associated with the nerve systems located in and between the frontal lobe and the basal ganglia of the brain. Researchers also found that deficiencies in the chemical substance serotonin, bridging specific nerve synapses, may result in maladaptive behavior. In other words, specific nerve activity is associated with adaptive grooves and routines but may also result in less functional or maladaptive grooves when serotonin deficiencies exist at the nerve synapses. See Chapter 13 for more information about brain chemicals.

THE GROOVE CONTINUUM

The fact that all grooves, whether adaptive or maladaptive, are connected to the same biochemical process may help to explain how maladaptive grooves develop in people with Down syndrome. In order to understand this, it may be helpful to conceptualize grooves on a continuum from most to least adaptive:

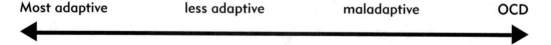

| Most adaptive | less adaptive | maladaptive | OCD |

The left end of the continuum represents adaptive grooves, which we believe are essential to the day-to-day survival and functioning of everybody, including people with DS. Grooves allow people to reliably complete daily self-care and job tasks. We could take this one step further and state that grooves are the basis of our own survival and serve as a foundation and structure of civilized society.

Closer to the center of the continuum, a groove may become less adaptive and less functional. This occurs when people adhere too rigidly to the groove, or when the groove has no useful purpose. Families usually preface their descriptions of these types of grooves with "I don't know why he/she does this, but..." For example, some people with Down syndrome are driven to repeat the same question over and over when they already know the answer. Other common examples include a need to arrange furniture or personal items in a room "just so," to turn lights on and off, or to close doors repeatedly before leaving a room or house. Grooves may also include repetitious thoughts or activities that have no real functional purpose even when a part of the activity *is* functional. For example, eating is necessary, but there is no need to arrange one's chair "just so" or sit in the exact same spot every time to eat dinner. Also, there is no need to arrange food on plates so as to avoid contact between different food items.

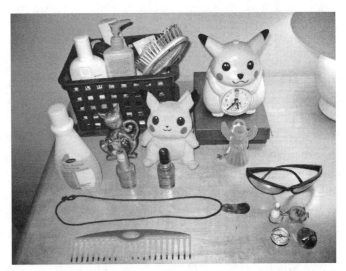

Example of ordering items on a dresser by a teenaged girl with Down syndrome.

Even in the case of people whose grooves are overwhelmingly adaptive, there are invariably a few areas where there are nonsensical or unexplainable repetitious thoughts or behaviors. The truth is, most of us have some nonsensical repetitious thoughts or behaviors such as counting to ourselves, checking the stove numerous times, cleaning meticulously, or arranging things "just so." What is going on here? We have to consider again that the chemical process resulting in grooves may fluctuate or sometimes result in chemical deficiencies for most of us, which result in some "nonsensical" behaviors.

When do we then say that a groove is pathological? Actually, no matter how illogical, odd, or nonsensical the repetitious behavior, it may not be maladaptive or meet the criteria for an obsessive-compulsive disorder unless it interferes with functioning in the key social, home, or work spheres of life. For example, arranging your chair or food "just so" at meals is odd but not a problem unless this activity keeps you from eating the meal in a timely fashion. Similarly, repeating questions or comments about a favorite star, sports team, or holiday may drive other people a little crazy, but it is not a real problem unless the preoccupation interferes with work or social activities.

Moving further to the right on the continuum, there is a point at which the groove begins to interfere with life activities and becomes increasingly more maladaptive. Once the repetitious thought or behavior interferes significantly in normal life activities, then the criteria of an obsessive-compulsive disorder are met. It is important to note that we have found a difference in how OCD is presented in the general population and in adolescents and adults with Down syndrome. In the general population, the hallmark of this disorder is odd or disturbing thoughts which intrude on people's thinking. This in turn results in the classic and debilitating rituals and repetitious behaviors that people do to try to stave off or manage these disturbing thoughts. For example, illogical fears of dirt or infection can result in repeated washing rituals. What makes this a treatable problem is not necessarily the odd thoughts but the resulting change in behavior which interferes with people's lives.

On the other hand, people with Down syndrome are far less likely to report disturbing thoughts associated with compulsions. This may be due in part to expressive language limitations that may make it difficult to conceptualize and communicate such thoughts, or it may be that most people with DS do not have these disturbing thoughts—at least not consciously. However, there are instances when we may infer that disturbing thoughts are present. For instance, we have treated a few people who spent an excessive amount of time showering or doing cleaning tasks, which seemed to indicate fears about contamination from dirt, germs, or other harmful substances. Irrational fears may also be inferred from rituals that consistently result in avoidance of some specific activity, such as outings in the community or a ride in a car. Even in instances where such contamination or safety fears seem obvious, people with DS are rarely able to verbalize fears and anxieties, even if asked by a trusted confidant. Regardless, the presence or absence of a disturbing thought may not matter so much as the presence of a repetitious behavior that interferes with their lives.

The intensity of maladaptive grooves may be reduced if stress is reduced and if the groove can be diverted to more productive ends, such as completing self-care tasks or work activities. However, when grooves continue to interfere in essential life functions, the person may benefit from the use of an antidepressant medication to normalize the biochemical imbalance. This is discussed in more detail in Chapter 16.

HOW STRESS AFFECTS GROOVES

Up to this point, we have described the chemical process underlying grooves and discussed what constitutes a truly maladaptive groove versus just odd or nonsensical behavior. We now need to discuss some of the other causes or stressors which result in maladaptive grooves. To this end, we need to consider one simple but important notion, and that is that people with Down syndrome have a strong propensity to repeat thoughts or behaviors once begun. Unfortunately, this may include thoughts or behaviors that are not always appropriate and may even be a serious threat to their health and wellbeing, and, thus maladaptive. For example, many families complain that the adult with DS acquires "bad habits" by first mimicking and then repeating others' behavior, such as hand flapping, hitting, picking at skin, and even faking seizures. People with Down syndrome may also develop maladaptive routines when they make poor decisions about behavior, and it then becomes a habitual pattern. For example, they may "get in the habit" of staying up too late to watch movies or TV while also consuming unhealthy foods or soft drinks.

We need to also consider that this propensity for grooves may lead to the development of maladaptive grooves when someone experiences too much stress. This happens because grooves represent preexisting tendencies or pathways, which then become natural conduits for expressing stress. In other words, a groove is similar to any type of physical predisposition. For example, people may have predispositions for headaches or for stomach or bowel problems, which become activated during periods of stress. These areas seem to be the "weak areas" for those individuals and are the location of physical symptoms secondary to stress. Similarly, the tendency of people with Down syndrome to develop routines and grooves may result in grooves that become "stuck" and unproductive with stress.

The specific process for developing a problem groove may be explained if we consider again the association of grooves to the chemical process in an obsessive-compulsive disorder. Under stress, the chemical needed to bridge the gap between nerve endings may become deficient and thus more like the chemical deficiencies seen in OCD. As a result, the groove may become more rigid and maladaptive. For example, when under stress, someone who is ordinarily somewhat flexible may rigidly adhere to a routine such as taking a bath at 7:00 in the evening, even if it prevents him from doing a previously desirable activity such as going to the movies. Another common example is to become so preoccupied by a favorite star or a love interest (real or imagined) that this then begins to interfere with home or work activities.

In short, people with Down syndrome often have a tendency for repeating thoughts and behaviors that may be extremely beneficial but also a formula for major problems. Ironically, maladaptive grooves may be very useful as a communication method. Just as adaptive grooves are a powerful means for expressing people's choices and preferences, so too a stuck groove may be a powerful means to express the presence of health, sensory, social, or emotional stress. This is similar to the notion of physical pain, which may be the only clue that a health problem exists. A stuck groove may express stress related to any area of functioning, such as health problems, a sensory impairment, or an environmental stress at work or at home.

INTERPRETING "STUCK" GROOVES

We have found that stuck grooves may express a general warning that an individual with Down syndrome is experiencing stress. In addition, they may communicate a more specific message about a problem.

INDICATIONS OF PAIN OR PHYSICAL PROBLEMS

Returning to the analogy of a headache, a headache may be a general warning of a health problem, while also pointing more specifically to a problem in the region of the head, such as a sinus infection. Similarly, a stuck groove, such as repeated trips to the bathroom, may sound a general warning of a problem, but may also point to a specific health problem, such as a bladder or kidney infection. In some instances, people with Down syndrome who have had ritualistic-like actions involving touching or poking their face or ears have been found to have serious sinus or ear infections. Similar actions may alert caregivers to the presence of a hearing or vision impairment.

We believe that physical problems result in an increased sensitivity to the affected area of the body, which then triggers an accompanying repetitious pattern or behavior. When an adult with DS has a stuck groove, it is always important to take him to a medical doctor in addition to a mental health professional, particularly if he is exhibiting a groove that has some association to the body or a bodily function.

> Henry repeatedly pushed his hand up his own rectum. He was diagnosed in our Center with a painful and uncomfortable bladder problem, which did not allow him to urinate. His actions brought some relief by stimulating his bladder to urinate. His actions, although unorthodox and alarming, were also successful at warning caregivers of a serious health problem and pointed to the specific area of the problem. As you may imagine, this also resulted in immediate help from staff, especially since Henry was not careful to wash his hands and would smear feces on the walls in his group home and bathroom. Successful treatment of the bladder condition did eventually eliminate the problem. However, it took several months after the physical problem had resolved for him to unlearn the groove.

SENSORY ISSUES AND GROOVES

Sensory issues, such as touch, taste, smell, and sight, may also create stuck grooves. These types of grooves will often sound a general warning but may also point to a specific sensory problem. For example, touch or tactile sensitivity is probably one of the major reasons underlying the unusual preferences some adults with DS have related to their clothing. For example, we have seen many people who will only wear soft and loose clothing, such as sweatpants, due to an apparent sensitivity to certain types of fabrics. Quite a few people also refuse to wear new jeans and some will not wear any type of new clothing. Some people will even try to wear the same clothing every day or the same "uniform" consisting of the same broken-in shirts and pants.

Family members often come up with creative solutions and adaptations to deal with these idiosyncrasies. For example, if an adult will only wear one outfit no matter what the occasion (wedding, meeting the President, etc.), there is the nightly washing routine while the person sleeps. Other families wash new clothing 20 times before it is worn or seek out special pre-worn jeans or carefully selected secondhand clothing.

Fortunately, we have seen that these issues often wax and wane based on the degree of stress an adult is experiencing, maturity, or other factors. As a result, people are at times more able to try different solutions to these problems. For example, an adult may be more willing to try something other than sweats, such as soft cotton shorts in warmer weather, or softer cotton pants, which may look better at more formal occasions. Fortunately, too, many people who tend to wear one outfit, or only one uniform, periodically change to something different. Still, if the problem gets out of control and begins to interfere in essential home or work activities, we have been able to help people become a little more flexible by using behavior strategies, and, if needed, medications (serotonin reuptake inhibitors). See the OCD chapter for more on this.

Many people with Down syndrome also have food-related rituals that may turn into maladaptive grooves. One of the many possible causes is an aversion to certain textures and tastes in the mouth. People with this problem are often described as picky eaters because they often avoid certain foods. Sometimes people may also refuse certain types of foods, based on past experience with the food prepared in a way that is aversive for them (crispy, soft, etc.) Over time and through trial and error, most families find enough foods and enough ways to prepare the foods so that they are acceptable to the person. A few adults with DS develop more extreme aversion to food and may refuse to eat. Fortunately, this problem is not common or a long-lasting problem, and those with this problem generally respond to medication and behavior treatments. See more on treatment in Chapter 18.

Another common sensory issue in adults with Down syndrome is a type of depth perception or related visual problem which makes it difficult for them to climb up stairs or to cross uneven surfaces. This problem often seems to worsen with age, although some people have this problem even as children. Usually, this is not an unmanageable problem. Most people continue to walk across uneven surfaces (even wet or snowy surfaces) or to go up and down stairs, just very slowly and carefully. However, a number of people develop grooves and rituals around this difficulty that may cause problems in certain situations. For example, we have found that many people with DS have difficulty negotiating stairs in an auditorium, movie theater, or sports stadium, particularly if the facility is dark or very crowded.

Many people try to deal with the problem by moving very slowly and methodically, which may not always be practical when they are at large venue events. However, families can usually deal with this problem by being early for the event and by waiting until most people have left before they leave. Still, some people with Down syndrome flatly refuse to go to these types of settings, probably because of a previous negative experience. This may become a more severe problem if it also affects the person's ability to negotiate stairs that are present in unavoidable settings such as shopping centers, schools, or work sites. These problems usually involve an anxiety disorder as well as a more severe maladaptive groove (OCD). See the chapters on anxiety and OCD for more on these problems.

Many other types of sensory issues may also result in stuck grooves. This may appear as repetitive hand or body movements, including mild self-injurious behavior such as picking at sores, chewing fingers, etc. The cause of these behaviors is varied and may include anxiety or even tics, which may be outside of the individual's conscious control. However, these types of repetitive behaviors may also be linked to sensory issues, including the aforementioned touch, taste, vision, hearing, smell, but also less well-known areas such as proprioception and the vestibular system (which has to do with movement and orientation of the body in space). These problems may be best evaluated by an occupational therapist (OT) who specializes in sensory integration issues. OTs have made great progress over the past 25-plus years in identifying and resolving problems that arise from a malfunction of the complex sensory system.

Indications of Environmental Stress

A stuck groove may also point to the presence of some kind of environmental stress. One of the most common messages expressed by a stuck groove is one of avoidance. Often, a stuck groove that is used to avoid something develops from a groove originally used to relax. For example, as described previously, people with DS often relax by repeating an enjoyable activity in a quiet or private space. As tensions or conflicts in an environment increase, they may spend more and more time in their private space doing their own relaxing or self-absorbing activity. Some adults with DS move more slowly and become even more meticulous in completing their morning routines as a way to avoid a school or worksite problem. If they are slow enough, they may miss the bus and avoid the conflict altogether.

There are many different situations or conflicts that people may try to avoid, such as physical or verbal aggression, or an overprotective or intrusive care provider. On the job, adults with DS may try to avoid serious conflicts or tensions with others as well as the noise and tedium of the work, perhaps by staying in a quiet place such as a bathroom stall.

Other Reasons

Sometimes the message of a stuck groove is a clear expression of a relatively harmless or benign issue. For example, people may get stuck in grooming tasks as they enter the self-conscious teen stage of development. (Remember, this often begins later for adults with DS compared to the general population; see Chapter 10.) For instance, they may brush or comb their hair excessively, or repeatedly put on and take off different outfits in the morning in an attempt to find the most becoming one.

Odd or out-of-character behavior, such as repetitious talk or drawings with sexual or violent content, may alert others to the possibility of sexual or physical abuse. For instance, after Gary suddenly started repeatedly drawing sexually explicit drawings, careful investigation led to the discovery that he was being sexually abused. Appropriate treatment and removal from the abusive situation led to a reduction in the repetitive behavior.

How Others Can Affect the Development of Healthy Grooves

Parents, siblings, coworkers, friends, roommates, and support people can all have an important effect on an adult's grooves. Indeed, how well they understand, accept, and respond to grooves can determine whether the person's grooves become adaptive and useful or maladaptive and problematic. The primary ways that families and others in the adult's environment can affect the development of grooves are:

1. How they interpret behavior related to the groove (for instance, whether they see it as deliberate oppositional behavior or something the person needs to do);
2. Whether they set and enforce rules that interfere with healthy grooves;
3. Whether they provide the right level of supervision to prevent bad habits that can turn into maladaptive grooves;
4. How well they encourage flexibility.

Interpreting Behavior

It is relatively easy to misinterpret someone's need to complete routines or grooves as oppositional behavior. For example, most people with Down syndrome will try to finish a routine before starting a newly assigned task. Unfortunately, if the person who has assigned the task believes the motivation for delaying the assigned task is to resist authority, then an escalating conflict may ensue. Further pressure by the parent, teacher, or supervisor may cause further entrenchment by the person with DS. Is this oppositional behavior, or is this a behavior that is not completely under the person's control, involving a type of biological imperative? If you believe it is willful and oppositional behavior, then you will probably continue to force the issue, which will no doubt create more entrenchment in the person's behavior.

What may confuse the issue is that most people feel a push for independence and a normal urge to rebel in any situation where they are told what to do. However, biology is probably a stronger force here, and biology (like Mother Nature) is not to be trifled with or ignored or you pay a price. An analogy can be found in the tumultuous behavior and moods of teenagers who are in the midst of the hormonal changes of this developmental period. Parents who are successful with teenage sons and daughters have a healthy respect for the way hormonal changes affect mood and temperament. They learn to respond very carefully and patiently to the teenager's moods and have learned that reacting too strongly only makes things worse. An analogy may also be seen in people who have problems with low blood sugar, and who may become moody and unreasonable when the blood sugar is low. Family members often learn to encourage the person to eat before discussing any important issues. Similarly, for a person with DS, pushing hard to force the issue will backfire, as the person will become more mired in the "problem behavior."

In our experience it is always important to look for reasons behind a person's behavior, including behavior such as an annoying or nonsensical groove, before concluding that the person is just being stubborn and oppositional. As discussed throughout this book, it is important to consider that people with DS are not always capable of articulating or communicating issues or concerns verbally and therefore may need to express them behaviorally. The fact that grooves are a natural part of these individuals' lives may make it a logical vehicle for communicating stress. Whenever possible, identifying and reducing stress in people's lives may also reduce problematic or annoying grooves.

Having said this, there *are* situations where people are not just compulsive, but also oppositional. We are usually able to determine whether this is the case by noting the number and intensity of situations where the behavior occurs. For example, if someone's intention is to be oppositional, he may act this way whenever he is asked to do things by authority figures. If he is just trying to complete a groove in a given situation, then this should not affect other areas where he has adequate time. Another clue is how the person responds to attempts to solve the problem. If he is given more time and he persists with a negative attitude, then the purpose of his behavior may not be to gain more time but to oppose the person of authority. This person may very well need more freedom and independence, but this is a different type of problem than merely adjusting time to adapt to someone's grooves.

ENFORCING SENSIBLE RULES

Problems may also occur if adults in charge set rules that interfere with the completion of grooves or that show a lack of understanding or allowance for grooves. For example:

> Lynne, 42, was brought to the Adult Down Syndrome Center for assessment of behavior challenges that included yelling at the staff and other residents in her group home, as well as occasionally striking the person who was sweeping the floor. The rules of her house included sharing the chores. On Monday, Lynne swept the floor; Tuesday, she cleared the table; Wednesday, she took out the trash, etc. Each day she did a different chore and each of the women took turns with each chore. However, Lynne really liked to sweep and she was very good at it. She became upset when she had to do a different chore. Upon further questioning, we discovered that the other women did not care whether they swept the floor. The staff person who accompanied Lynne asked if this was an example of obsessive-compulsive disorder. It is an example of OCD, but not in Lynne. The rules were too compulsive for the situation and were creating unnecessary conflict. We encouraged a change in house policy, and when Lynne was able to sweep daily, the floor sparkled and "peace reigned."

We have most often encountered these types of problems with rules in work or residential settings when staff or administrators have had little experience with people with Down syndrome. They may also occur in the person's home if his family does not fully understand groove-like issues. For example:

> *The Baker family continually had difficulty with their teenage son, Greg, who was chronically late getting ready for school in the morning. With the best of intentions, Greg's parents had made the same rules for him and his two brothers, because they wanted Greg to be like everyone else. In many areas, he was just like others, but he definitely did not move as fast in the morning. Like many people with Down syndrome, he was slow, precise, and methodical in bathing, grooming, and dressing. As a result, he looked very neat and handsome, but still he was late.*
>
> *The Bakers came to the Center when the conflict and tensions in the morning reached a boiling point. In the parents' words, they had begun to "encourage" him to move faster. In his words, they were rushing and babying him. The harder they tried, the more he resisted. Finally a shouting match erupted. Greg even began to refuse to go to school, which was very unusual for him. At the Center, all agreed that what had been attempted had not worked and that a new strategy was in order. Greg's parents patiently listened to our explanations about the groove. They recognized that he had many groove-like tendencies and that they were generally beneficial for him. They had not considered that this was behind his morning slowness. All agreed that Greg would be better off with more time to get ready. He took the initiative to set his own alarm clock, and from this time forward there were no further problems around this issue.*

We have also encountered situations similar to Greg's in school or work settings. For example, staff at work sites have complained that employees with DS were chronically late getting back to their work after their lunch break. As it turned out, the break was only half an hour, which was not enough time for the adults to eat and to return to work, given their slower pace. In negotiating a solution to these kinds of problems, it is often possible to discuss the benefits of the groove. Employers will often readily admit that the person's reliability and attention to detail makes him excellent at their job tasks. When it is explained to them that the adult's pace is related to his precision with his work, they will often agree to whatever extra time is needed (usually just five to ten minutes).

Similarly, we have heard that students with Down syndrome are often late after physical education (PE) class because they need extra time to shower and dress. When we have worked with the schools, we have often discovered that the parents have already tried to communicate the need for more time. The schools often downplay this explanation because they feel the parents are biased or overprotective of their child. Staff from the Center, however, are viewed by the school as less biased and more professional, and thus school staff are often more willing to listen to us, even if we state the same things the family already stated. We have found that what the students with DS need is often just a matter of a few extra minutes. Once this is understood, the problems are solved fairly easily.

Sometimes it may not be possible or in the person's best interest for him to take as much time as he would really like. For instance, extended time bathing may aggravate dry skin problems. We have had some success using timers. Whenever possible, however, we put the person with Down syndrome in charge of the timer.

We need to balance the person's needs and abilities against the needs of the family, school, etc. If the individual is physically incapable of moving fast enough to follow the rules, then this is unfair to him. If, on the other hand, the person is taking a long time as a delaying tactic, it often indicates a more serious problem. For instance, the person with Down syndrome does not want to be there for whatever reason.

We believe that this type of misinterpretation of the groove is one of the reasons people with Down syndrome have a reputation for being "stubborn." Understanding this tendency and modifying your approach to setting and enforcing rules based on this understanding can avoid many problems.

PROVIDING THE RIGHT LEVEL OF SUPERVISION

Adults in authority also play a role in allowing or preventing the development of "bad habits" that could become maladaptive grooves. For instance, in a previous example, several roommates with Down syndrome got in the habit of staying up late to watch movies or TV. This obviously involved a poor decision on the part of the adults with DS, but we also think there was a lack of supervision appropriate to the developmental age and maturity of these adults.

As discussed in Chapter 4, developmental age can be different than the individual's chronological age. For example, a man with Down syndrome who is 30 years old may have many strong daily living skills, but his ability to make judgments may lag far behind. If others assume that his problem solving skills are in line with his cleaning, cooking, and grooming skills, he may not receive the supervision or support he needs in other areas. In group living situations, inadequate support may be due to funding and staffing restrictions that may be rationalized on misguided or disingenuous notions of treating people in an "age appropriate manner."

Secondly, a lack of understanding or recognition of the power and persistence of grooves often compounds these situations. Caregivers may not understand that there is a natural tendency to repeat a behavior once started. Unfortunately, once someone gets a taste of late shows and midnight snacks, he or she may soon develop a bad habit of staying up too late. Not surprisingly, this can create major problems with sleep deprivation, daytime fatigue and lethargy, truancy, tardiness, and unproductiveness at work, as well as an increased risk for depression, weight gain, and a long list of associated health problems.

Recommendations for Discouraging Maladaptive Grooves:

◆ *Remember that people with Down syndrome tend to do what people do and not what they say (rather than the classic maxim of "Do what I do and not what I say").*

Many people with DS are visual learners (discussed in detail in Chapter 5). They learn from observing those around them. If you do not want the person to develop bad habits, then limit exposure to people who have them. People with DS who are exposed to people who eat, sleep, and exercise right generally follow these same practices.

◆ *Provide people with DS with "good enough" parenting and supervision.*

Described in more detail in Chapter 7, this is the practice of allowing people to have as much freedom as they are capable of handling, while still maintaining their health and wellbeing. Too much supervision may be stifling, but too little may encourage the development of poor sleeping or eating habits.

◆ *Limit exposure to situations with a higher degree of risk.*

Most parents know that a number of different situations can put the person with DS at risk for developing maladaptive grooves. Exposing him to these situations would be like putting several boxes of chocolate in front of a "chocoholic." Chances are very good that the chocolate will be eaten in short order. Likewise, some people with Down syndrome may be easily addicted to TV or movie watching. Allowing them to decide how long to engage in these activities will no doubt result in too much of this and too little of more beneficial activities such as social or recreational activities. Fortunately, grooves may work both ways. Once adolescents and adults with DS have a schedule that includes a more reasonable pattern of TV or movie watching, they will generally follow it.

◆ *Take time to talk about it.*

Our habits and patterns of behavior are not just what we are exposed to and not just what we want or desire. We can reason and respond to others' influence. People with DS may have some difficulty with abstract reasoning, but they are still very sensitive to the feelings and opinions of others. Taking the time to talk to them about why they should do productive activities may be very helpful and respectful. Even if they do not completely comprehend why a reasonable diet or social and recreation activities are beneficial, the fact that this matters to those who are close to them is very important. Additionally, it may help to take time to explain the issue in more concrete terms. For example, try explaining that a reasonable diet and exercise may help them to fit into their pants, to have more energy, feel better, etc.

ENCOURAGING FLEXIBILITY

While we certainly recommend respecting a person's groove, we also acknowledge that too much groove can be a problem. We therefore recommend encouraging the individual to develop some flexibility. This is an ongoing process done on a day-to-day basis. It involves respect for the groove while at the same time gently encouraging and directing the person to see other options.

Do's and don'ts of encouraging flexibility with behavior that has become groove-like:

- ◆ Pick a behavior that is possible to change. A task that is too difficult will lead to demoralization and more rigidity.
- ◆ Pick a time to encourage flexibility when you have the time to be patient.
- ◆ Explain clearly and patiently what behaviors would constitute flexible options to the current behavior.
- ◆ Break the activity down into manageable steps to facilitate learning.
- ◆ Use visual cues: pictures, a calendar, a demonstration of an alternative behavior, or some other type of cue to facilitate learning and comprehension.
- ◆ Don't try to change a groove when the person with DS is under extra stress.
- ◆ Don't be judgmental or critical. (Nothing will encourage rigidity quite like saying something along the lines of, "It drives me crazy when you ____.")
- ◆ Explain with enough time for the person to prepare for the change but not so long to encourage obsessing about the change.
- ◆ It may be helpful to deliberately teach the word "flexible" by pointing out and praising instances when the person with DS is being flexible (see example below).

A wonderful example of flexibility is seen in the following story:

> *William, 34, came home from work and found his mother and his aunt, who was visiting from Europe, talking at the kitchen table. His mother invited William to go to a movie with them that evening. William indicated that it was Tuesday night and that on Tuesday nights he always did one hour of exercise to his favorite exercise video. His mother suggested that he could change his usual schedule and go with them to the movie, and, perhaps, make up the session later in the week.*
>
> *William went to his room and his mother overheard him talking to himself regarding this issue. He returned to the kitchen and said to his mother, "I want to talk about the 'F' word." His mother braced for the embarrassment of this (never-before-had) conversation in front of his aunt. William went on, "I want to talk about flexibility. I will go to the*

movie tonight with you and Aunt Jenny." Years of gently encouraging
William to look at alternatives to his grooves when appropriate ended in a
successful and enjoyable evening.

CONCLUSION

We have reviewed many ways that grooves are displayed. Each of them can have a beneficial function. Unfortunately, we have also seen patients with each of these grooves
that have shifted to the right on the continuum to the point where they become significant challenges. These behaviors may become maladaptive grooves or may even
become problematic enough to meet the criteria for obsessive-compulsive disorder. If
the person is simply unable to be more flexible after a great deal of gentle prodding
from others and his grooves are causing lots of conflicts or problems, then it may be
time to consider an assessment for OCD or a trial of medication. Assessment and treatment options are explained in more detail in Chapter 16.

Although many adults with Down syndrome have difficulty being flexible with
routines, most of the time these routines do not interfere significantly in their lives.
Most people with Down syndrome are able to adapt to change, given some time and
encouragement from others. Even in situations such as Susan's, on page 152, when
rigid routines create problems, these problems may be resolved if others help them to
develop new, more productive routines or find environments that are more accepting
and accommodating of their routines.

Grooves are clearly a common characteristic of people with Down syndrome.
Complete elimination of grooves is not only unlikely to be successful, but can be detrimental. Using grooves in a healthy way can often be very advantageous. We recommend continued efforts to respect a person's grooves, while at the same time striking
a balance between the groove and flexibility.

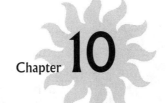

Chapter 10

Life Span
• • • • • • • •
Issues
• • • • • • • •

"Teenage Behavior," Isolation, Withdrawal, Retirement

Ｎone of us is the exact same person at 50 years of age that we are at 20 or 40. Growth, development, and the effects of our life's experiences change each of us over time. Change is a normal and healthy part of our lives as human beings. Behaviors change, attitudes change, and personality can change. The degree of change varies from person to person, but some change is inevitable. People with Down syndrome, too, change throughout their lifetime. Also, just as for people without Down syndrome, there are particular times of life when change is typically most pronounced. This chapter focuses on several stages of life that are likely to result in changes in adults with Down syndrome that may be misinterpreted by others as behavior problems.

ADOLESCENT BEHAVIOR
• •

Adolescence is a challenging time, both for the teen and for the people around her. It is a time to develop one's sense of self and one's independence. The process of finding

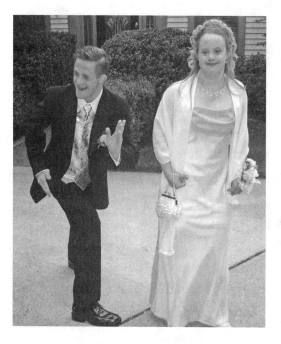

one's self while at the same time "fitting into the crowd" is a difficult balancing act. Mood changes, isolation, experimental behavior, and intermittent assertiveness of personal choice often mark this struggle. For the people around the teen, particularly the parents, understanding and accepting the process are first steps toward surviving this transition. But for parents, acceptance does not always come easily, particularly in the midst of the intense conflicts that often envelop the parent and teen in this period.

For the parents' survival, one of the most useful books on adolescents is by Dr. Anthony Wolf, a father and a seasoned psychologist, who has treated thousands of teenagers and their families in his clinical practice. The title of his book, *Get Out of My Life, But First Could You Drive Me & Cheryl to the Mall...?,* is a testament to his understanding of these issues and his sense of humor. His message to parents is one of hope and surprising simplicity in a period that can be extremely confusing and trying. He says that teens often act the way they do because they are so close to their parents. The drive to establish their identity and independence requires distance from their parents. Of course, teenagers' hormonal surges and body changes, which makes them irritable, moody, and unpredictable, don't help.

Given the difficulty of the teenagers' tasks and the physical changes they endure, we as parents may be getting off easy if all we receive is three or four years of the silent treatment mixed in with intense periodic expressions of anger, hostility, and defiance. They may challenge the rules, but they crave them nonetheless. Wolf assures us that with time, the hormonal surges level off and the drive to establish their own identity and independence may become more reasonable and the teen more responsible.

As a parent, your continued support, and maintenance of rules, helps to guide your teen in the appropriate tasks of this life stage. In the early stage of adolescence (onset of puberty) this will involve teaching about basic but essential grooming and hygiene tasks (deodorants, hair combing, management of menses for females). In the later stage, this will include working on social, academic, and job-related tasks that are necessary for the teen to successfully transition to adult life and responsibilities. Your teen's pride, self-esteem, and identity is built by her increasing ability to "do for self" (what psychologists call competence), at each stage of this process. What helps with this process is the development of cognitive abilities that increase the teen's ability for reasoning and abstract thinking. This helps them to better manage their emotions and to see the need to be responsible for, and not just in charge of, their actions.

SIMILARITIES BETWEEN TEENS WITH AND WITHOUT DOWN SYNDROME

PHYSICAL AND HORMONAL CHANGES

What happens with teenagers with Down syndrome and their families is analogous to teens in the general population (GP). Most teens with DS undergo the same physical and hormonal changes of puberty around the same time (or shortly delayed) as teens and preteens in the GP. As a result, many teens with DS are said by parents to have some of the same bouts of moodiness and irritability as their counterparts in the GP. They, like other teenagers, may also:

- ◆ dress and groom more carefully,
- ◆ take forever in the bathroom, combing their hair, etc.,
- ◆ over-use cologne, deodorants, and hair gels,
- ◆ have problems with pimples and acne,
- ◆ be more interested in members of the opposite sex,
- ◆ and, perhaps, begin to masturbate.

Parents also note gender-specific changes. Boys try to shave (like their fathers, whether or not they have hair) and to wear deodorant for the first time. Girls (like mom) may try on makeup and have to adapt to their menstrual cycle, and for some, the associated discomfort and emotional effects of PMS. In other words, teens with DS appear to respond to puberty and other physical and emotional changes of early teenage development the same way as other teens do.

CONFLICTS WITH PARENTS

Complaints about behavior and emotional issues are often similar to complaints from parents of teens in general. At times, some may display behavior and emotions that are more childlike or regressive in nature, particularly for younger teens in conflicts. For example, they may sometimes use tantrum-like behavior they haven't used since early childhood. Parents also report that whatever issues had occurred prior to the onset of puberty seem to intensify or worsen with these changes, at least temporarily. Like many teenagers, they are generally less patient and tolerant of minor irritations and inconveniences. Of course, they may also resist direction from parents or others in authority.

The effects of these teen era changes may have more of an impact on some people than on others. For some, this process may be somewhat delayed but show up in full force at a later date. Many parents report little or no emotional upheaval from their teens and preteens with DS. However, the same may be said for teens in the GP, who experience these years at varying degrees of intensity and at varying degrees of difficulty for their parents.

DESIRE TO DO THINGS THEMSELVES

One area of similarity is a need for the teen "to do for self." The starting point for the tasks that the teen with DS wants to do for herself may be different because of delays in development. For example, the teen with DS may want to do a grooming or hygiene task without parental assistance, such as showering by herself. Most teens in the GP would have mastered such skills at an earlier age, but may want 'to do for self' in another important area, such as going off by themselves in the community.

Because of the wide range of skills and development in children with DS, some will try to do some tasks for themselves at ages similar to teens in the GP. However, the majority of teens with DS will be at a different level of skill than the teens in the GP. What is similar between the teens with and without DS is that parents often complain that they want to do things for themselves even when they are really not ready or capable of doing the tasks. This often involves testing the limits of freedom, such as how far the teen in the GP is allowed to go from home. Teens often try to go further and further from home, regardless of the possible risks (and the gray hairs they are giving their parents).

Similarly, parents of teens with DS complain that they insist on doing things that they are not quite able to do. This may be aggravated by the fact that many teens with DS are visual learners and they see what other teens in the GP have attained. They may want to be just like everyone else their age, at least in terms of dressing and grooming. This may not always be reasonable or in their best interest. For example, some individuals do not wash private parts carefully enough, or get soap out of their hair, or brush their teeth adequately.

Dealing with these problems may require that parents get very creative. Being too direct or "parental" may cause the teen to shut the parent out. But to allow the teen to do the task inadequately may leave her open to teasing and criticism from peers. There may also be a detrimental effect on their bodies, such as the possibility of gum disease from poor dental hygiene or the development of rashes and painful boils from inadequate bathing. A creative solution for dental care might be to buy electric toothbrushes that are fun and effective. A time-tested strategy may be to find others who are more acceptable to the teen to teach her certain key tasks. These others may include older siblings, cousins, grandparents, etc. The best teachers are often mature individuals whom the teen looks up to. Life skills classes in schools may also be wonderful places to learn.

Regardless of how many classes the teen with Down syndrome is included in, she may still benefit from a separate time with students who have DS or other intellectual disabilities. Although some parents are reluctant to have peers with disabilities congregate together in regular school settings, this is often essential to the teen's own sense of acceptance and self-esteem. (See Chapter 7 for more on this.) Often, the other teens with disabilities are struggling with the same developmental tasks and issues. In these situations, both the teacher and the other peers are instrumental in the learning process. The teen learns from observing others, but there is also no better way to learn than to help to teach others. What may also help in this process is the tendency of teens with DS to follow grooves and routines. Once they learn how to do the tasks correctly, they may continue to follow through with them very reliably. (See Chapter 9.)

DIFFERENCES BETWEEN TEENS WITH DS AND TEENS IN THE GP

ABSTRACT REASONING

As mentioned above, it is normal for teens to challenge the rules, and for their parents to become concerned as the teens' challenges seem to get bolder and riskier the older they get. For example, at an earlier age, teens may want to pick out their own clothes or hair style, but at a later age they may want to stay out later and later with friends. Parents of teens in the GP are relieved to find that as their children mature, they often become more reasonable. This is due to an increase in cognitive skills, resulting in the development of abstract reasoning. With these increased reasoning skills, teens begin to see the reason why parents are setting rules, and not just that the rule is something to challenge. For example, they may see why it is helpful to get in early on a school night in order to be alert the next day, or why it is important to avoid certain people.

In contrast to teens in the GP, teens with DS continue to be fairly concrete in their thinking. This may adversely affect their ability to understand and resolve issues in this life stage. Yet we have found that these teens often have other strengths and attributes that may allow them to compensate for this deficit. For example, many people with DS tend to be very aware and sensitive to others' feelings and emotions. (See Chapter 4.) Contrast this with teens in the GP, who are described by parents as self-absorbed, self-conscious, self-centered, etc. In fairness, this focus on self and others like themselves is to be expected in this stage, given hormonal surges and the need to define one's own identity. This is not to say that teens with DS are not also self-conscious or self-centered—just less so, when compared to other teens.

Why teens with DS have this sensitivity is not clear. It could be a protective mechanism to allow people with DS to survive (by being able to "read" important people in their lives) despite their limitations. We sometimes call this skill "emotional radar." Teachers or caregivers often call this a "wish to please," but most parents are aware that this skill is much more than that. It is an intuitive sense of others that helps them know who to go to and who to avoid. It also allows them to pick up on emotional or physical discomfort in family and friends and to respond to them with help and comfort. More to the point of this discussion, this sensitivity to others, and particularly to parents, no doubt helps moderate many DS teens' anger and rebelliousness. It often allows them to be influenced enough by parents to stay on track with developmentally appropriate tasks, even if they do not have the benefit of abstract thinking.

COMPULSIVE TENDENCIES

A second key difference in teens with DS compared to teens in the GP is that the former often have neat, organized rooms, with clothing and personal items placed "just so." Compare this to parents of teens in the GP who often describe their teens as "slobs," and their bedrooms as "disasters." Even when teens with DS do have chaotic-appearing rooms, there is some order to the chaos—often they have specific piles for specific things. We often estimate that about 90 percent of all teens with DS make their beds and organize their rooms, while about 90 percent of all teens in the GP do not. This is consistent with our observations that obsessive-compulsive behaviors or grooves are more common in teens with DS, just as for adults with DS (see Chapter 9).

The problem with grooves is that they may become more rigid and inflexible, particularly with the type of stress that teens with DS experience during this stage of physical, emotional, and social change. For example, at the start of every school year, and until her anxiety about her new classes and classmates abates, Beth becomes more rigid and compulsive at home. She insists on making her bed "just so" before she eats breakfast, even if she is in danger of missing the bus, refuses to eat her breakfast if her toast is cut "wrong" or her juice is in the "wrong" glass, and repacks her whole backpack if her mother tries to put her lunchbox in to try to hurry her out the door.

On the other hand, even with the stress of adolescence, we have found that grooves may be very productive for teens with DS. They may serve as an effective means for the teen to express her independence and autonomy. As discussed in Chapter 9, grooves and routines are a clear and unambiguous statement of a personal choice or preferences in such key areas as clothing and appearance, social and recreational activities, and music, hobbies, and artistic endeavors. Each person's choices will, in turn, help to shape and define her own unique style and identity, which is of critical importance to the developing teen. Grooves may also be a less antagonistic, clever means for expressing one's independence to parents. This is because grooves do not necessarily require the teen with DS to express anger or a rebellious attitude to maintain.

Regarding this tendency for grooves, we have seen an interesting trend in a group of younger teens with DS. These teens seem to have more experience doing things for themselves and thus have more confidence and assertiveness when dealing with parents and authority figures. As a result, these teens are more like teens in the GP in expressing their feelings and independence. Again, this is generally expressed without the type of impulsiveness and angry outbursts more characteristic of teens in the GP. Interestingly, however, the demands this group makes on parents is often in the form of groove-like preferences and routines, which is not the case for teens in the general population, who tend to be more fickle about their likes and dislikes, adherence to schedules, etc. Parents of teens in the GP are often confused and befuddled by the constant changes, while parents of teens with DS may be mildly irritated by the demands for sticking to set patterns and behaviors. Fortunately, most parents learn to appreciate their child's unique ways and means of "getting there" (even if this means they are slobs or neat-niks, save-a-holics, or whatever).

DELAYS IN TEENAGED BEHAVIORS

A third major difference between teens with and without DS is that the parents of the former may end up dealing with adolescence issues at two separate periods of time compared to only one (albeit possibly long) period for most teens in the GP. There may be certain advantages to having a second period of adolescence, but it may also create a great deal of confusion, if not understood by parents and other caregivers.

Let us explain how this may happen. For teens with DS, the first period of adolescent issues may occur when the teen undergoes the physical and hormonal changes of puberty. This often happens around the same time for both teens with and without DS, in the early teen years. However, most teens with DS do not have the level of skill and maturity needed to do the adolescent tasks that help them make the transition toward adulthood. Consequently, this transition may occur at a much later age, compared to teens in the GP.

We know that the individual's drive for independence is not unique to adolescents. Children strive for independence at all stages of development. For example, a toddler's drive for independence may be as strong as an adolescent's. The difference between the teen and infant is that the infant struggles to become independent *within* the family and the teen struggles to be independent *from* the family. What then defines the stage of adolescence is not the teenager's physical changes, or even her rebellious behavior, so much as her progress toward completing the tasks for this stage of development. Some more mature people with DS may move toward independence while they are still in their teens. This often occurs in just one or several specific areas, such as wanting to get a job or to have more independence in their living situation. However, many people with DS experience the first wave of puberty and the accompanying changes in mood and behavior, but then are not necessarily ready to deal with the tasks of separating from the family until they are older (into their 20s, 30s, or even their 40s). Even then, they may continue to be dependent on parents in certain areas.

This is what is called an "out of sync" pattern of development, because for many people with DS, the maturity of the physical body is not in line (in sync) with the maturity of the mind or of adaptive skills. It's not that the person's physical and mental maturity don't ever get in sync; just that the process may be delayed or modified for years. The fact that this process is out of sync, and may occur when adolescent issues appear to many parents to be long gone, may result in confusion and misinterpretation.

We have seen many people with Down syndrome in their twenties to early thirties and occasionally late teens whose parents were concerned about these changes in behavior. "She doesn't participate in family activities like she used to." "He spends more time in his room." These and other comments by parents reflect a change in their son or daughter.

These changes are a challenge for all families. As described, it is neither unique to having a son or daughter with Down syndrome or to be unexpected for a person with Down syndrome. However, there are a few issues that are more likely to limit a successful transition:

1. Families, support people, etc. may not realize or accept that the person is going through a normal developmental process (because it is delayed) and may misinterpret behavior.

2. Families and others may have difficulty giving the adult with Down syndrome the proper amount of independence.

3. It may be difficult to tell the difference between normal adolescent behavior and behavior that calls for professional intervention.

RECOGNIZING AND ACCEPTING NORMAL DEVELOPMENTAL CHANGES

The older families we see at the Center, whose sons and daughters are now in their 40s and beyond, were often told at birth that their child would not live into adulthood. They were usually told that their child would not walk, speak, or read, and would have other severe disabilities. Even some of our younger families have been given very pessimistic views of their child's eventual development. Not surprisingly, parents who were led to believe that their child would not survive into adulthood, much less develop skills necessary to participate in the world, gave little thought to going through stages of life. The professional prediction was of a static human being, one who would not develop over time.

Many families rejected the concept of a static individual when it came to developing skills. Against medical advice, they took their child home and helped her develop skills that they were told were not achievable. However, seeing the person with Down syndrome as a continuously developing person who experiences the changes associated with going through the stages of life may still be a challenge for them. Even younger families, who were given better and more optimistic information at the birth of their child, often have a difficult time understanding the normalcy of the development of the person with Down syndrome: the pattern is similar, but delayed.

Understanding that the changes are likely to occur is the first hurdle to supporting the person with DS through these changes. When a family asks about the changes that they are seeing, the first question we usually ask is, "Do you remember the teenage years of your other children?" This is usually followed by a look of insight, then a smile and a quizzical frown. Parents understand the challenge of helping a teen develop a sense of self, to "fit in," and to develop independence. It may not always be easy to accept or deal with the process, but parents understand that the process must occur.

We have found that when an adult has limited verbal skills, parents may have even more difficulty understanding that the person's behavior is a part of her drive for independence. Sometimes the person's behavior may be her only reliable means for communicating that this is occurring. For example a mother called us to report that her 33-year-old son, Richard, refused to get out of bed. When we investigated, we found that this man had no contact outside the family and he had little or no independence because his mother did everything for him. His refusal to do anything was his only remaining strategy but it was very effective. By refusing to do anything his behavior sent a message:

◆ to his **mother**,

◆ who called his **sister** (the only relative who had stayed involved),

◆ who looked up our website and called the **Center**,

◆ who investigated the problem and made recommendations for **him** to "have a life."

Although there is obviously much more to this story, the key problem and solution are both here. Richard's mother did agree to let him venture out to a day program and to different programs and activities that did in fact give him a life. She took some convincing because some students had teased Richard when he was in school 15 years ago, and she was afraid for him to be in the community. Still, she heard his message and she was eventually pleased when he was happy with his newfound independence. We have found similar solutions to other situations that were less dramatic but that involved a concern with a "change in behavior." This may be something out of character or even an increase in a preexisting behavior, but the message is clear: "I need more independence!"

When this is the cause and the family sees the solution, they are relieved and pleased by the progress the person has made to communicate and gain some control and independence in her life.

Providing the Right Level of Independence

A challenge for all parents is finding the balance between directing, supporting, and letting go. Parents may be scared to let their child find her way, because when she spreads her wings, she may make mistakes, stumble, and even get hurt. For children *without* Down syndrome, the expectation is that they will eventually be "independent." In contrast, most people with Down syndrome have a greater degree of lifelong dependence, although some are more independent than others. In addition, the independence they achieve will take longer. This makes the already difficult task of "letting go" that much more difficult. For most families, there is never the same sense of "letting go" as there is for children without Down syndrome.

Letting go may also be more difficult for parents of a son or daughter with Down syndrome because the parents may be older than they were when they let go of their other children. Their child with DS is usually the last to leave the nest. Sometimes parents are at a point in life where they don't have the same energy to assist their son or daughter with DS through the process as they did their other children.

The "rules," however, are similar:

1. Understand that the process toward independence will occur.
2. Accept the process.
3. Be supportive. Help her develop as much independence as she is capable of.
4. Allow her to grow toward greater personal decision-making. She can only develop the ability to make decisions by making decisions and experiencing the outcome.
5. Pick your battles. The person has to make decisions as part of the process. Some choices the person makes will absolutely not be acceptable (see #6) and cannot be allowed. However, learning to pick battles takes time and practice. A child needs to make many decisions and experience the outcome over time to learn and grow. A person with Down syndrome will probably need more time for this process. To repeatedly intervene will slow and possibly even stop the process.

6. Keep the person safe. Obviously, allowing a young child to play in the street and get struck by a car is an unreasonable way to teach her that playing in the street is not safe. There are many choices that will similarly not be safe as the person progresses through adolescence and young adulthood. However, many decisions are obviously not "safety-threatening." Offering choices that are all safe can provide guidance. Allowing the person with DS to walk home in the dark by herself may not be safe. However, other choices can be offered, including arranging a carpool with her friends, taking a cab or public transportation, or other choices based on your location.

7. When it comes to decisions that are not dangerous but may subject the person to ridicule, offer encouragement and choices, and discuss your concerns. However, in the end, her choice may be part of the learning process. Peers (and others) can also teach (sometimes in a less kind fashion). Be prepared to support her later without any "I told you so." In addition, she may hear the ridicule and decide she still likes her choice, feel a stronger sense of her independence, and be proud of herself for "not following the crowd."

8. Remember that people with Down syndrome often imitate appropriate behavior much better than they follow verbal guidance. For example, if you want your adolescent to answer questions politely and not ignore you, then you should answer her questions politely, rather than grunting if you are busy or distracted.

9. Recognize that some behavior that starts during adolescence may never be "fixed." For instance, the adult may henceforth always prefer to do things with friends rather than parents. Or she may be more prone to argue for doing things her way. Encouraging independence sometimes includes accepting choices you might not have made. (But then, if she made every choice you would have made, she wouldn't be truly independent.) For example:

Kevin, 23, was isolating himself in his room and interacting less with his parents. His older brother, Steve, who had recently moved out of the family home, made a concerted effort to go out regularly with Kevin to play video games, shoot baskets, or other similar activities. Kevin also became involved in a mentor program and met regularly with the parent of a young child with Down syndrome for a social event. Kevin continued to have less verbal interaction with his parents and to spend more time alone in his room than he had as a child, but he was getting out and enjoying himself. As for many teens, better interaction was seen with people other than his parents.

We would describe Kevin's behavior as "normal." Even when his behavior improved, he still was different than when he was a child. That is not a failure of the intervention. That is the expected outcome. People develop as they go through their life and there are particular times when change tends to be greater and more rapid. The "adolescent period" is clearly one of those times.

PEERS

The desire to be like peers is often part of adolescence. This can be a particular challenge for some adolescents with DS because there may be some things that they cannot do. They see their peers driving, dating without chaperones, going to college, moving away from home, and getting married. The person may feel "left out," sad, or frustrated when she can't do the same things. While this struggle has always been present in families as siblings have matured and done these things, it is now more frequently encountered with regards to peers. As people with DS are included in the local schools and social settings, they have more peers who do not have disabilities and who are participating in these activities. This exposure has many

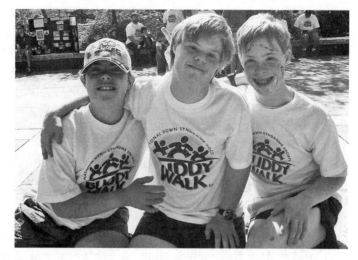

positive aspects, but one possible negative aspect is seeing others participate in activities the adult with DS might not be able to participate in. (See more on this in Chapter 7.)

RECOGNIZING THE NEED FOR PROFESSIONAL HELP

During times of more rapid change, there is greater stress and a greater likelihood of developing a mental illness. Adolescence is clearly one of those times. Depression is the most common mental illness we see, although anxiety may also occur. Sometimes it can be hard to distinguish adolescent behavior from symptoms of depression. For example:

- ◆ While a loss of interest in activities with parents is not unusual, loss of interest in all activities is concerning.
- ◆ Sleep patterns often change in adolescence. Needs for sleep increase and adolescents want to stay up later and sleep later in the morning. However, sleeping all the time or not sleeping at all are concerning.
- ◆ Mood swings are to be expected, but uncontrollable anger and aggression can be signs of a more significant problem. Periodic mood swings may also be a sign of PMS.

Depression is further discussed in Chapter 14 and should be considered if the intensity or duration of the behavior changes or seems unusual or excessive.

WHEN MORE SERIOUS PROBLEMS OCCUR IN ADOLESCENCE

Depression. We have found that there are some teens with DS who respond to the stress of adolescence with depression that includes a more severe form of withdrawal and isolation. When this happens, the anger that is usually expressed between parent and teenager often only occurs when the parent tries to get the teenager to move out of her isolation. This tendency to withdraw and seek isolation may be due to the concept of "learned helplessness" (Seligman, 1975), which also results in a high frequency of withdrawal and depression in adults with DS.

Learned helplessness can occur when the person has limited experience solving her own problems or standing up for herself. As a result, when faced with a major challenge, such as the physical and emotional turmoil of the teen years, she tends to shut down and withdraw into a state of helplessness rather than meet or deal with the challenge. This, in turn, may lead to an internal focus on fantasies, movies, or past events because of the visual memory skills that people with DS have (see Chapter 5). Withdrawing in this way may help to take her away from the conflicts and tensions in their world, but it only delays the resolution of the tasks of this life stage. (See Chapter 14 for more treatment strategies for this.)

Teens in the GP may also withdraw and isolate themselves to a certain extent, but they are also more likely to fight back. The reader may say here that teens in the GP are notorious for shutting out their parents. While this *is* a form of withdrawal, there is, in fact, nothing passive about this behavior, as anyone who has tried to talk to a sullen teenager will attest. On the other hand, teens with DS are more likely to hide and isolate themselves than to express anger directly or indirectly to others through the "silent treatment."

Suicidal Gestures

The "good news" about teens with Down syndrome who are depressed is that they are far less likely to make suicidal gestures compared to depressed teens in the GP. This may be in part because suicidal gestures often involve a high degree of anger/rage at oneself and others, which is less likely to be expressed in teens with DS.

AD/HD. We have seen teens with DS who have more serious behavioral issues. When we look closely, we often find one or more health or neurological problems, which, added to the intense stress experienced in the teen years, make it very difficult for these individuals to control their behavior. Some of these teens have an attention-deficit/hyperactivity disorder, which is characterized by impulsiveness, distractibility, and attention problems. As for children and teens in the general population with AD/HD, the right medication and an academic program adapted to their needs may greatly help to reduce the stress experienced by these individuals. Still, the stresses of the teen years added to the AD/HD issues may present a major challenge for these teens and their families.

Tourette Syndrome. We have also seen that adolescent hormonal changes may trigger the onset of neurological disorders such as Tourette syndrome and bipolar disorder. As discussed in Chapter 21, Tourette syndrome (TS) often involves a constellation of three sets of symptoms: 1) attention deficit and distractibility, 2) motor tics, and less frequently, vocal tics, and 3) obsessive-compulsive behavior. People with TS may be misdiagnosed as having only one of the above disorders or as having another disorder such as oppositional defiant disorder (if the child's tics are viewed as willful rather than biologically based). Misdiagnosis may limit treatment success. This combination of these symptoms and behaviors is debilitating for adults, but for a teen may be especially devastating, particularly when the teen is trying to establish herself in school and amongst peers.

Bipolar Disorder. Bipolar disorder is a mood disorder that includes extreme fluctuations in mood and behavior. This disorder often begins in adolescence and has a devastating effect on the child and her family. Bipolar disorder is more difficult to diagnose in those with DS, especially in adolescence, because the changes in mood may be confused with adolescent behavior. Additionally, teens and adults with DS may be more likely to have a pattern of rapid cycling from up and down states of mood. It is not uncommon for the cycle to occur in as short a period as one day as opposed to weeks or months in the general population. See Chapter 14 for more information.

Autism Spectrum Disorder. Autism spectrum disorder (ASD), which is characterized by difficulties in social and communication skills and behavioral management problems, may become more intense and unmanageable with the onset of puberty. However, many teens with ASD and DS have been diagnosed before adolescence, so although symptoms may be more intense, they are not necessarily new to the families and the professionals working with the teen with ASD and DS. Often, the same strategies for dealing with teens with DS alone are useful for teens with DS and ASD. These teens want independence just like any others, but may need more adaptations to achieve it.

Health or Sensory Problems. Finally, we would be remiss if we did not discuss teens with DS who have health or sensory problems. When we look into why teenagers with DS have behavioral issues, we frequently find health problems, just as we have reported for adults with DS (see Chapter 2 for a detailed discussion of this).

Additionally, sensory integration (SI) issues may also have a profound effect on the teen. SI is the ability of the person to receive and effectively manage and integrate all sensory stimuli, including hearing, vision, touch, proprioception, smell, and taste. Although SI is a relatively new area of study, there is evidence that problems with SI may affect a higher percentage of teens and adults with DS compared to the general population. SI problems may be misdiagnosed as AD/HD and a host of other disorders, and may also add to existing health or mental health problems. For the teen, health and sensory issues may make it even more difficult to manage the stresses of adolescence, and thus may result in the type of behavior issues that are noted in this and other sections of this book. To resolve the behavior problems and give the teen a fighting chance to deal with the intense pressures of the teen years, we need to first diagnose and treat the health or sensory issues.

BEHAVIOR CHANGES IN ADULTHOOD

Although many people with Down syndrome begin acting like adolescents later than usual, the reverse is true when it comes to acting like an older adult. People with Down syndrome seem to age more rapidly. Actually, in childhood and early adulthood, many people with Down syndrome seem younger than their age. However, as they progress through their 30s, they often begin to look and act older than their age. In our experience, we tend to think of people beyond 35 or 40 years old as being 5, 10, 15, and even 20 years older than their chronological age. They begin to have the health problems associated with being older and they tend to "slow down" sooner than others. Therefore, the issues of older adulthood may arise at a younger age.

For older adults *without* Down syndrome, changes or challenges include children leaving home, becoming grandparents, retiring, and dealing with changes in their own or their parents' health. A person with Down syndrome may experience many similar challenges: becoming an aunt or uncle, retiring, and dealing with changes in their own or their parents' health.

As people with DS age, they can continue to learn. Whatever developmental age or level of skills they have attained, they still have the benefit of living and learning. Like other older people, as people with DS age, they are often calmer, more patient and accepting of themselves and others, and able to make more thoughtful and wiser decisions. However, like some older people without DS, people with DS may become reluctant to learn new things or to accept any change. They may also prefer quieter and more sedentary activities. They will often mimic older parents who prefer these activities. If they do not develop Alzheimer disease, people with DS have a memory and cognitive decline similar to that of other older adults in the general population.

Since many adults with DS were born when their parents were older, they are often relatively young when their parents encounter their own aging issues. Interestingly, some of our patients are still processing the issues of adolescence (e.g., siblings leaving home) when they began dealing with issues of older adulthood (e.g., parents declining).

> *Lawrence worked in a rather fast-paced job. As he got older, he found it more difficult to keep up with the pace. Both physically and mentally, the job was a greater challenge. When Lawrence was 48, his father retired and Lawrence saw that as a more attractive alternative to going to work each day. He began to decline to go to work and eventually lost his job. He became very sedentary and now spends most of his time sitting in front of the television controlling the remote.*

Melissa, 44, was brought to the Center by her sisters. They were concerned about depression because she was not interested in doing activities that she had enjoyed for so many years. These activities included going to dances and sports activities such as softball, volleyball, and swimming, through the local park district, as well as track and field events through Special Olympics. She continued to work at her assembly job, but she was not as productive as she had been in the past. Her sisters also found that she did not have as much energy or enthusiasm for longer shopping trips or family gatherings, particularly when a number of younger children were present.

Melissa's sisters were relieved when Center staff found no evidence of depression. Staff explained that people with DS have a premature aging process, which may account for an approximately 20-year difference compared to people in the general population. Like others who were aging, Melissa was moving slower and she was interested in activities that were less taxing and yet still stimulating to her. She liked arts and craft activities and bingo, as well as shorter shopping trips that put less strain on her feet. She also continued to participate in Special Olympics, but switched to bowling, a less taxing activity. In other words, her patterns of behavior would not be unusual for a person who was developmentally at an age closer to retirement.

Why did Melissa's aging seem to be a more positive process than Lawrence's? What families may need to understand is that not only do stamina, interests, and motivation change as people age, but people may also become a little more set in their ways. This is true for people without DS as well, but because so many people with DS have a preexisting tendency for grooves, the tendency may become more pronounced with age. This is not to say that people have to be stuck in groove-like patterns, particularly if these patterns are no longer adaptive for them. We do find, however, that caregivers need to be a little more patient when trying to change grooves. Older adults with DS may simply need more time. Additionally, the longer a pattern continues, the more difficult a change may be. But this is not true for all changes. We have seen many people respond very quickly to changes that they themselves view as positive. For example:

Juan, 39, showed great enthusiasm after he moved out of his aging parents' home and into his new residential facility. His sister, who helped facilitate this move, could not bring herself to tell her parents how happy Juan now was because they had been convinced that he would fall apart with the move. She dealt with this very tactfully by telling her parents that he missed them but that he was making progress (because they had prepared him so well for this move).

On the other hand, we have seen people have enormous difficulty with abrupt changes such as an unplanned move to a group home when a parent suddenly died. This is not true for all people—some do very well with these types of changes. However, a significant number of people do have major adjustment difficulties. We also see that people do adapt, given time and a sensitive caring environment, but this process may take years and much pain.

The message we hope parents will take from this is to prepare for your son and daughter to leave your home well in advance. This will allow the person with DS and you, the parents—who often have more difficulty with this transition than the child—to deal with this productively. More importantly, parents who wait may have no say in where and how their son or daughter will be moved. Our advice and the advice of anyone who has had to deal with a person with DS adapting to an abrupt change is that advanced planning and placement is far preferable to the alternative.

Not Eternal Children

People with Down syndrome are often referred to as "kids" or "children," even when they are fifty years old. The person with Down syndrome is viewed as if she is frozen in childhood. There are many possible reasons for this. Certainly the presence of an intellectual disability leads many people to mistakenly assume that the person with Down syndrome is still a child. While the person may be "child-like" in some respects, there are also generally some very adult qualities, dreams, and hopes.

Another possible reason for seeing people with Down syndrome as perpetual children is related to the kind of world our present-day adults with Down syndrome were born into. Those who were born in the 1960s or earlier had little access to basic health care, much less school, social, and other opportunities, and there was little expectation that they would live beyond childhood. Those who were born a bit later were legally entitled to a public school education (starting in 1975), but still may have faced a great deal of ignorance and resistance to inclusion in everyday life. Families of these older people with Down syndrome sometimes have difficulty seeing the person as an adult because the professionals and community members surrounding them may have had low expectations and because there were more limited opportunities to develop skills.

Today, however, we have a new generation that was born into a world where early intervention and inclusion in school and community are rights. As we watch the new generation of children with Down syndrome grow, I often wonder if we will see a different syndrome with improved health as well as improved cognitive, social, and occupational skills. As we see people with Down syndrome living longer and developing greater skills, it is imperative that we understand and support their development into adolescents and adults and throughout their lives.

RETIREMENT

In the above case of Lawrence, deciding to quit work (retiring) was something he desired that others did not appreciate. He made his wishes known in the only successful way he found.

The age at which people with Down syndrome are ready to retire is as variable as it is for people without DS. Some people with DS are ready to retire in their 40s (considering the premature aging, this

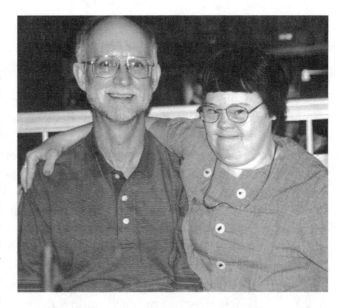

might be comparable to someone else retiring in their 60s). Some people with DS are never ready to retire. There isn't a set age; each person's needs must be individually taken into account.

If the work place has become too great a challenge physically, mentally, or both, it is time to look to do something different. It *isn't* a time to look to do nothing. Although retirement is often seen as doing less, it is actually a natural part of the development process. If families and staff do not see this change as a natural part of development, they can have difficulty accepting it. In addition, state regulations often require some form of day programming for people with Down syndrome who live in a group facility. Therefore, accepting the change is not only an issue of changing the mindset but also of dealing with, and adjusting to, regulations.

If this developmental stage is viewed as "retiring *to* something" instead of "retiring *from* something," there is greater chance of success. A successful retirement program should have the following characteristics: a slower pace, less "work," more recreation, and provisions for changing health needs. It may need to include a place where the person can rest during the day if she needs to.

Retirement programs should not be boring or less than stimulating. We have seen some programs that are shameful—where the adults' only activity is to watch TV or to find their own means for entertaining themselves. Fortunately, as the population of people with DS ages, we have seen a growing number of programs that meet adults' needs while also stimulating and enriching them. The better programs have excellent arts and crafts activities, including some that are taught by professionals (often producing gallery-quality work). These programs also include a regular schedule of outings to restaurants and shopping centers and include healthy doses of cultural, sports, aerobics, and other recreational activities. Many of these programs could complete with any senior program anywhere. People may be retired but they are anything but inactive in these programs and they love it. Many group facilities have developed programs with these characteristics that also meet the regulation that each person living there must attend a day program.

Volunteer work can often meet these requirements as well. We have heard of a number of innovative programs involving volunteer or civic-minded projects for elderly people with DS. For example, one program brings a group of "retirees" comprised primarily of people with DS to a nursing home. The purpose is to help the "less fortunate" in the nursing homes, who are lonely, aged, and sick, by talking and socializing. Staff from these nursing homes report that something magical happens when the group with DS arrives. This should not be surprising, given the sensitivity of people with DS to the needs of others. For the people with DS, there is perhaps nothing so enriching and invigorating as having the opportunity to do for others and especially others who are so appreciative.

Even when excellent seniors programs are available, such as the ones described above, these may not be right for certain people. The key is finding the program that is right for the individual. Does the person want to retire? Is her job too stressful? Would modifying the job meet her needs? Would a different program be better suited? Retirement is not right for everyone and there is no one retirement program that is right for those who are ready to retire.

> *Victor, 52, was getting less and less enjoyment out of work. He found work more and more challenging and frustrating, and his production continued to drop. He still liked to keep busy, however. He enjoyed the slower pace of cleaning the house where he lived. He could rest when he was tired and then start working again. He has quite limited verbal skills so he made his desires known by staying up late at night to clean and then refusing to get out of bed in the morning to go to work. Victor was transferred to the "retirement program" that met in the next building. He was able to spend part of the day cleaning like he wanted, and part of the day socializing with the retirement group. His sleep improved because he was able to do what he wanted to do during the day and didn't feel he needed to be up at night to do it.*

CONCLUSION

People with Down syndrome are not static. This is true at retirement age, during adolescence, and throughout their lives. Their needs, desires, and wants change over time. Many approaches that are successful for people without Down syndrome can be used to provide beneficial and caring support. In addition, however, it is important to remember the differences in people with Down syndrome—such as slower development and early aging—that may require some modification to the support.

Chapter 11

Mental Illness
· · · · · · · · ·
and Its
· · · · · · ·
Precipitants
· · · · · · · · · ·

U p to this point in the book, we have addressed a number of ways that mental health may be promoted and optimized in people with Down syndrome. We have pointed out that good mental health in adults with Down syndrome does not necessarily look the same as good mental health in others, due to common behaviors such as self-talk or the "groove" and differences in language and memory abilities. These differences are sometimes mistaken for signs of mental illnesses, but are generally nothing to worry about if parents and professionals react to them appropriately.

On the other hand, sometimes adolescents and adults with Down syndrome *are* affected by mental illness. A mental disorder (mental illness) is defined in the *Diagnostic and Statistical Manual of Mental Disorders, Fourth Edition, Text Revision* as:

- ◆ A clinically significant behavioral or psychological syndrome or pattern that occurs in an individual.
- ◆ It is associated with present distress or disability or with a significantly increased risk of suffering death, pain, disability, or an important loss of freedom.

- ◆ The syndrome or pattern must not be merely an expectable and culturally sanctioned response to a particular event (such as the death of a loved one).
- ◆ Whatever its original cause, it must be considered a manifestation of a behavioral, psychological, or biological dysfunction in the individual.
- ◆ Neither deviant behavior or conflicts that are primarily between the individual and society are mental disorders unless the deviance or conflict is a symptom of the dysfunction in the individual (DSM-IV-TR, 2000).

Types of mental illnesses include:
- ◆ **Mood disorders** (disorders in which disturbance in mood is the predominate feature) such as depression, bipolar disorder, dysthymic disorder, and mood disorders due to a general medical condition;
- ◆ **Conduct disorder** and **oppositional defiant disorder**;
- ◆ **Schizophrenia** and **other psychotic disorders** (disorders in which the symptoms of delusions or hallucinations are the primary features);
- ◆ **Anxiety disorders** and **obsessive-compulsive disorder**;
- ◆ **Impulse control disorder** (failure to resist an impulse, drive, or temptation to perform an act that is harmful to the person or others and is not caused by another mental illness).

Mental illnesses are fairly common in adults in general, occurring in an estimated 26 percent of adults in the general population in the United States (Kessler et al., 2005). About 9.5 percent of the adult U.S. population have a depressive disorder in a given year. Major depression is the leading cause of disability in the United States. Adults with Down syndrome seem to be a little more likely to contend with a mental illness during their lives. One researcher reports a lifetime prevalence of 27.1 percent of people with Down syndrome developing mental illness (Chen). The data from our Center suggest a prevalence closer to 35 percent (but many of our patients are referred specifically because they are having problems and, therefore, our rate would be expected to be higher). About two-thirds of the people we see don't have any mental illness. They are doing well and we have learned a great deal from them on maintaining mental health, as has been discussed in previous chapters.

PRECIPITANTS TO MENTAL ILLNESS

◆ ◆ ◆ ◆ ◆ ◆ ◆ ◆ ◆ ◆ ◆ ◆ ◆ ◆ ◆ ◆ ◆

In general, there are two ways that mental illness may be precipitated in anyone: either through physical causes, such as biochemical or structural differences in the brain or an illness, or through what laymen usually refer to as "stress" ("stressors"), or a combination of these factors.

In Chapter 13, we explain some of the structural and chemical differences in the brains of people with Down syndrome that can make them more susceptible to some mental illnesses. For example, differences in the transport of serotonin may make people with Down syndrome more likely to have symptoms of depression. In Chapter 2, we discuss many of the physical problems that can lead to mental health issues in adults with Down syndrome. In this chapter, we will focus on the stresses that can sometimes lead to mental illness in people with Down syndrome.

STRESS

It is interesting to note that hypertension (high blood pressure) is uncommon in people with Down syndrome. When we share this finding with others, frequently their response is "that's probably because people with Down syndrome have no stress in their lives." This is a myth. Not only do people with Down syndrome have stress in their lives, they perceive it and it can affect them.

There are clearly some challenges in life that some people with Down syndrome don't have to deal with. For example, it is rare for an adult with Down syndrome to worry about how he is going to afford housing. However, this is not to say that their lives are without stressors. Sometimes adults with Down syndrome are expected to deal with challenges that other adults are not. For example, many of our patients live in residences in which there may be several other people who have undesirable habits, are awake at night, or whom they just don't like. However, they may have very little room to negotiate a change or to live with whom they would like. Furthermore, the intellectual disability secondary to Down syndrome often limits the person's ability to cope with stress. Therefore, at times an adult with Down syndrome may experience just as much, if not more, stress as anyone else, but may have less ability to cope with the stress.

The presence of stress in someone's life usually does not trigger a mental illness. Appropriate support, removing oneself from the situation, participating in activities that reduce stress, and other strategies help prevent the development of mental illness. However, it is often necessary to recognize the stress in order to actively develop strategies to deal with it. Adults with Down syndrome may not recognize their own stress or may not be able to verbalize their concerns. Care must be taken not to downplay stress in a person's life because he doesn't verbalize a concern. It is important to recognize that the person with DS may be experiencing stress and may need assistance to develop healthy strategies.

Common stresses that can precipitate mental illness in adults with DS include:
- learned helplessness,
- lack of opportunity,
- lack of respect,
- expected, but stressful events,
- unexpected, stressful events,
- grief.

Common Sources of Stress

. . . .

Learned Helplessness

One particular precipitant to mental illness (especially depression) is a condition called learned helplessness. This occurs when a person has experienced failure, leading to a sense of futility, hopelessness, and a tendency to give up in future situations. For example, if a baby or child repeatedly cries but no one responds, he eventually learns it is hopeless and stops crying. Essentially, he gives up. He has learned to be helpless and may not even cry in new situations where others may be more likely to respond. We have seen a number of adults with Down syndrome who were frustrated or unhappy with their situation. After repeated, unsuccessful attempts to communicate their concerns or have their concerns taken seriously, they developed a sense of despair and gave up. Often, they not only gave up trying to make that particular change, but also became apathetic in general, as well as depressed.

Sometimes a person's limited language abilities keep him from expressing his concerns understandably. Other times, the people who hear the concern may not take him seriously or may see his concerns as unimportant. Limited resources may also be a challenge. For example, if the person does not like his group home, but there are no other choices, no change is likely to occur.

> Zachary, 22, became depressed. His parents had worked very hard to get him into a workshop, but Zachary did not like the job and felt trapped. He had a limited ability to communicate his desire to leave the workshop. With time, the problem became clear and his parents worked to find him a new job. The new job was very similar to the previous one, but Zachary was much happier. Much of his happiness seemed to be related to his sense that he could have an impact on his environment.

For an environment to be supportive, it must be responsive. Listening is the first step in providing support or care. Without understanding the problem, one cannot offer a truly beneficial solution. Clearly, it can be a major challenge to understand the needs of a person with Down syndrome who has minimal communication skills. While this book outlines a number of issues that are common to people with Down syndrome, it also points out that each person with Down syndrome is an individual and has unique needs, desires, and hopes. When someone expresses these needs but is not listened to, it can be very frustrating and eventually cause despair.

Think of this analogy if you want to understand how frustrating it must be to have people not listen. Imagine entering the department store with a nice shirt that you recently purchased. After waiting in a lengthy line at Customer Service, you reach the front and place the shirt on the counter. Before you have a chance to say anything, the clerk smiles, takes the shirt, and hands you your money back for the returned item.

You are pleased with the clerk's politeness, cheerfulness, and eagerness to help. On the other hand, as you see your shirt being carried away to be returned to the shelf, you become frustrated. The purpose of your visit to the store (that you didn't get to voice to the clerk) was to get the security tag removed from the shirt because it had not been removed when you purchased it. You really liked the shirt and now it is being taken away. The service was great; it just wasn't what you needed.

Anyone who has his attempts to change or affect his environment ignored or misinterpreted can become frustrated. If this happens recurrently, it can be a significant precipitant to mental illness.

LACK OF OPPORTUNITY

Lack of opportunity can be very stressful, frustrating, and challenging to self-esteem (see Chapter 7). Opportunity is not just something to do or something that fills our time. It is an interesting challenge that allows us to feel creative and excited. For some adults with Down syndrome, the tasks or jobs available do not begin to fill these criteria. For some, there may be no tasks or jobs available at all, due to lack of funding and other reasons.

The individual defines the fulfillment that the task or job provides. Therefore, what may seem boring or unfulfilling to you may be quite fulfilling for someone with Down syndrome. The opposite is also true. Unfortunately, frequently adults with DS have little input into the work they do and this can lead to frustration.

Living situations can also be a source of frustration or stress. Many people with Down syndrome have limited living situation opportunities. Funding issues, the need to rapidly find a home after the death of parents, and other issues all contribute to lack of available and appropriate living situations. Certainly, it is ideal if families can investigate opportunities well in advance, but this does not always occur. In addition, there are often fluctuating funding issues. A well-made plan can become problematic at the time of need because of a change in funding by the state or other provider.

Many adults with DS continue to live in their family home with their parents and/or siblings and it works very well. Many move to group living arrangements and that works very well for them. However, sometimes when someone wants to move out of his family home, no opportunities are available. Others have moved into group facilities and the fit is wrong. Once again, individual assessment and planning is important to optimize the situation and minimize stress.

Even when living in a fine agency-supported home, there can be stressors. While we enjoyed living in a dorm in college, there are issues that would make living there forever a challenge. Noise issues, tolerating others' habits, and compromising to meet the needs of all individuals can all present problems. Although these are issues in any family, sometimes a group facility has a large number of individuals who make it more challenging. In addition, difficulties with language and the ability to express concerns (see Chapter 6) can limit the ability to deal with these problems.

The challenge for the family or staff supporting people with Down syndrome is to make the living situation the "home" of the person with Down syndrome. This is

Inclusion and Choice

Full inclusion is the drive in schools for people with intellectual disabilities to participate as much as possible in regular schools—attending classes with typically developing students and having as much access as possible to the regular curriculum. Inclusion is increasingly being recognized as a goal for adults with intellectual disabilities as well. To be included in our society, one should be able to participate. One of the highest hallmarks of participation in our society is having choice. Unfortunately, many adults with DS are not included because they do not have choices. Often, financial/funding issues or society (or professionals) limit them because only one way for individuals with Down syndrome to do something is recognized.

important for family members to remember. When a person with Down syndrome goes to live with a brother or sister, the family also faces the challenge of making it the home of the person with Down syndrome. Staff members at group homes have the same challenge.

For some adults with DS, lack of opportunity may also be a problem in the areas of education, recreation, and travel. As in the other areas, the first step is to recognize that these may be areas of stress for the person with DS. Once the problem is recognized, the adult needs encouragement to continue to find and develop opportunities to optimize participation in these areas.

LACK OF RESPECT

Unfortunately, another stressor for people with Down syndrome is dealing with people who do not respect them. It is stressful to deal with people (both children and adults) who make derogatory comments or call them hurtful names. Unkind or unscrupulous individuals can be very hurtful. Even kind or well-meaning people can cause discomfort by not recognizing or appreciating the skills of a person with Down syndrome.

> Bill, age 27, loves his job at the grocery store. However, the customers sometimes upset him. It is easy to see how the rude customers who call him "retard" are a real stress in his life. The other customers who are a challenge for Bill are the ones who assist him with the bagging. Bill takes real pride in his work and interprets this assistance as indicating they do not feel he is capable. Despite all the benefits Bill gets from his job, not the least of which is improved self-esteem, his daily interactions with customers could be precipitants to mental illness. Bill has opportunities to discuss his day with the staff of his group home each evening after dinner. He receives support and then participates in activities that he finds relaxing. He continues to do very well despite the challenges at work.

Here are some ways you can assist an adolescent or adult with Down syndrome deal with perceived or real disrespect:

- ◆ Have him ask himself why the person might be acting that way. Help him determine whether the person means to be disrespectful or whether he is merely perceiving it as disrespect.
- ◆ Help him understand that the person who is purposefully being disrespectful is the one with the problem. Encourage him to ignore it as best as possible or to address (or have someone else address) the person who is being disrespectful if it is a situation that can be changed.
- ◆ Encourage him to talk about episodes in which he feels he has been treated disrespectfully. Acknowledge and affirm his feelings and support him in dealing with them. Encourage and support him in the development of self-esteem in other ways (see Chapter 7).
- ◆ Help him develop strategies to deal with how he feels. These may include relaxation techniques, physical exercise, and other strategies.

EXPECTED BUT STRESSFUL EVENTS

There is little doubt that the environment and the passage of time will present situations that can be stressful. Some of the events and the timing are certain or to be expected, such as graduating from school and entering the work environment. Other events are less predictable. An illness, the death of a family member, divorce, and other life events are all relatively unplanned. Preparation is helpful for the person with Down syndrome to deal with both expected and unexpected events.

Remember, change can be difficult for many people with Down syndrome. A particularly difficult event is when a sibling moves out of the house, leaves for college, and/or gets married. These changes tend to affect the person with Down syndrome in two ways. First, he experiences the sibling's move out of the family home as a loss and goes through a grieving process. Second, he often senses that these are normal events that he will never participate in. For instance, Joan, after becoming upset at her sister's wedding, said, "I'll never get married and have children." As a person with Down syndrome enters adolescence and adulthood, the differences between his life and the lives of siblings or nondisabled peers can become more evident.

The grief of the loss experienced when a sibling moves should not be minimized. It certainly is not minimized in the minds and hearts of many people with Down syndrome. As outlined below in the section on Grief, there are a number of ways to assist people with Down syndrome in this process. Obviously, a significant difference between a family member moving and a family member dying is that when the family member has moved out of the home, physical contact with the person is still possible. Involvement of the family member in the life of the person with Down syndrome helps with the loss. Consistency and regularity are essential. There is no question that people with Down syndrome are generally hurt by unfulfilled promises (for example, when a family member misses a scheduled event.) In addition, the tendency toward order and repetition (see Chapter 9) make irregular visits particularly difficult.

Improving the availability of opportunities and inclusion in society are clearly part of the solution to concerns related to having fewer opportunities. However, many people with Down syndrome have challenges that prevent their life activities from being just like those of siblings or peers. Accentuating the positive aspects of the person's life, seeking opportunities that mirror the opportunities of siblings or peers, and strengthening self-esteem are all beneficial approaches.

ACCENTUATE THE POSITIVE

Everybody has some limitations. Certainly, a lack of height, an inability to jump, and poor ability to shoot a basketball eliminated that career choice early in the second author's life. However, with the encouragement of family and others, strengths were discovered and accentuated and meaningful activities were found. Likewise, many of our patients with DS are found to have untapped skills. Artistic talent, musical flair, incredible memory, a real sense of order, and others are all gifts that can be real assets. These strengths that can be part of a very fulfilling life are further discussed in Chapters 4, 5, and 7. Assessing, guiding, teaching, and, particularly, modeling the use of talents can lead to great satisfaction.

SEEK SIMILAR OPPORTUNITIES

Seeking opportunities that mirror the opportunities of others can be very beneficial. We know several adults with Down syndrome who have expressed interest in being able to drive a car, get married, and/or move out of the family home and then have accomplished those goals. As people with Down syndrome become further included in society, opportunities to achieve these sorts of goals are increasing. However, not all people with Down syndrome can realistically be able to participate in all opportunities. Again, assessing interests and capabilities, guiding the person to alternative opportunities, and then teaching and modeling them can lead to life satisfaction and self-esteem and acceptance of the changes occurring in life.

> *Darryl, an 18-year-old, man with Down syndrome, was frustrated about not being able to drive. He had participated in driver's education, but did not have the manual skills or judgment to drive. As his family worked through this with him, they discovered that the lack of independent travel was a significant part of his frustration, so they worked on teaching him how to use public transportation. Darryl has found it particularly satisfying that his family no longer drives everywhere but sometimes uses public transportation too. When his older brother comes home from college and they go to a movie, museum, or other outing, they usually take public transportation. Darryl takes the lead role in use of the public transportation because his older brother is not as familiar with the system.*

While lack of skills or opportunity are challenges to overcome, promoting healthy self-esteem is still ultimately the goal as changes in life occur. Further information on promoting self-esteem is discussed in Chapter 7.

PREPARING FOR EVENTS

As with any events that are planned, calendars and schedules are very helpful in allowing the person with Down syndrome to prepare. As indicated in Chapter 5, visual memory is often stronger and visual cues are often more beneficial than verbal. Therefore, using a calendar or schedule with pictures is very useful. We have often found that a photograph of the upcoming event works best, especially if it shows the person himself participating in the activity.

> *George, age 28, had severe atlanto-axial instability. He required traction for several weeks before the surgery to optimize the alignment of his neck. This was really a challenge for him to bear. A picture that indicated the proposed date of his upcoming surgery was placed on his calendar. For George, a symbol that signified surgery worked for him. This helped him deal with the time in traction.*

In addition, advance warning is often necessary. On a day-to-day basis, giving a warning before transitions is a good idea. For example, it can be helpful to tell the person five or ten minutes in advance that it is almost time to stop work and get ready to go home. Giving the warning too far ahead is often not helpful because the person forgets or becomes re-involved with the job. Too little or no warning does not allow him to prepare for the transition.

Warnings for larger transitions, such as a move or changes in family, are also appropriate. A picture that signifies the event can be placed on the day on the calendar. Perhaps a picture of the adult with DS standing in front of his new home would work well. Pointing to the date and counting off the days as they go by may also be helpful. Again, giving a warning too soon can be problematic (although how soon is "too soon" varies from person to person).

Often, parents or others delay telling the person with Down syndrome in hopes of preventing him from perseverating about the upcoming change. However, he often learns about the change by overhearing conversations anyway. In addition, many people with Down syndrome have a much greater "sense" of upcoming events or change than is assumed. They have a radar detection skill that helps them perceive changes in others' demeanors or in events or activities. In those situations, it is better to have an open discussion and to assist the person with the transition than to delay telling him. Otherwise, he may jump to the wrong conclusion about what is going to happen or why, which may cause more worry. He may also come to the correct conclusion, but, because he is not supposed to know, he may not get an opportunity to address his feelings about the situation.

Many times we have heard that a patient's behavioral change or alteration in mental health began some time before an upcoming event. "He hadn't even been told about the change yet when his depression started." He was apparently already aware, however, and was struggling with the change. Always consider the incredible ability of many people with Down syndrome to "pick up" on events they have not been told about.

UNEXPECTED, STRESSFUL EVENTS

If an event is unplanned or unexpected, clearly many of the recommendations outlined in the section on planned or expected events are not applicable. However, there are still a number of similarities.

Many unexpected events, such as a death, illness, or divorce involve a sense of loss. The death of a family member, friend, or care provider can be particularly challenging; the grieving process is therefore discussed in some depth in the next section. Many of the strategies used to support a person with Down syndrome through the grieving process can be used for other unexpected events.

A key principle is to assess "where the person is" and help him from there. Ask what he knows or understands about the loss first. This can eliminate a great deal of confusion as to how to help. If the person is nonverbal, strategies discussed in Chapter 6 may be helpful.

Loss is a form of transition, and transition can be difficult for many people with Down syndrome. If possible, warn the person of the transition that is coming and then let him proceed at his own pace. Careful observation of his response—whether spoken or conveyed through his body language—helps avoid overwhelming him with information. Share what he is ready for and able to grasp and come back as the need and readiness present themselves.

When the loss does not involve death, there are often continued opportunities for the person with Down syndrome to interact with the individual(s) undergoing changes. It is once again essential to assess the person's ability to deal with the changes. A question often arises as to whether a person with Down syndrome should visit a sick family member. We generally encourage regular visits. Rarely, the changes in the ill person can become too disturbing for the person with Down syndrome. In these situations, the person with Down syndrome must reduce or eliminate visits.

It can be helpful to provide pictures of the person with Down syndrome together with the person (or people) that he appears to be losing due to illness or other events. The strong memory that so many people with Down syndrome possess can be a blessing here. The pictures help them remember happier times, which can be a real comfort.

A calendar or schedule, especially one with pictures, can help the adult with DS deal with the aspects of the loss that can be anticipated. For example, if treatment start and stop days or a surgery date can be placed on the calendar, it can give a timeframe or some sense of order.

Similarly, if the person with Down syndrome becomes ill or needs surgery, as discussed previously, a calendar can be used. Adding structure or increasing the predictability as much as possible helps the person with Down syndrome deal with the

Dealing with Divorce

Divorce has aspects of both unexpected and expected events. Usually it is not something that is suddenly sprung on the person with Down syndrome. Often, even if he hasn't been told of problems, he is aware of them. Therefore, in preparation for divorce, here are some helpful tips:

◆ Reassure him that it is not his fault.
◆ Reassure him that his parents still love him.
◆ Reassure him that he will continue to have a home, will be taken care of, and will see both of his parents.
◆ Don't put him in the middle of the two parents. Don't put him in a situation where he is "turned against" one parent or the other.
◆ Maintain his schedule as much as possible.
◆ Give him permission to discuss his concerns and provide him opportunities to do so.
◆ Encourage activities that help to reduce stress.

illness. It is important to explain the treatment or procedures at a level that is understandable. For example, for our patients who are anxious about coming to our office, we have a book with pictures and words that "walk a person through an office visit." The book includes pictures of history taking, examination, blood drawing, and other aspects of the appointment. Copies of the book are available to our patients to take home and use before the appointment.

There are many changes or losses in life that can challenge adults with Down syndrome. Helping them put these losses in a structure and optimizing predictability is usually helpful. Using strengths in memory and visual learning skills to help a person with Down syndrome deal with loss can improve the benefit of the intervention.

It is important to realize that even good change is still change. Good news such as a job promotion, being asked to go on a trip with a friend, or the birth of a new niece or nephew can all be very positive events in the life of a person with Down syndrome. However, they can also cause stress. Using the strategies outlined above can help prevent these positive events from becoming negative events.

GRIEF

Grieving is a very individual process. People grieve in a variety of ways. However, there are some common features that we have seen in people with Down syndrome. First, people with Down syndrome often have a delayed grief response. Second, they need to grieve in their own way and time. And third, their strong memories often complicate the grieving process. Difficult or prolonged grieving can sometimes lead to mental illnesses such as depression.

Delayed Grief Process

The grieving process may be delayed in people with Down syndrome. It is not uncommon for us to see a person with Down syndrome do well for six months or more after the death of a loved one and then to start expressing his grief. Sometimes someone will do fine for a long time and then another loss will occur that triggers the grief response. For example, a very significant person (such as a parent) will die and our patient seems to do fine. Then, months or sometimes years later, what appears to be a less significant death occurs (for example, a person far removed from our patient or the turtle at the group home dies), and then our patient expresses grief about the previous, more significant death. We have seen several such instances in which an adult with Down syndrome suddenly started talking about the loss of the significant person in his life after several years.

In her pamphlet, "Mental Retardation and Grief Following a Death Loss," Charlene Luchterhand, MSSW, offers some possible explanations for the delayed grief (Luchterhand, 1998). The person may not have been given the opportunity for grieving, may take longer to sort through his feelings and emotions, and may not have had the skills to understand the process and how to go through it.

In addition, we have often wondered about the ability of many of our patients to comprehend the concept of time. Sometimes, in describing the death of a family member, an adult with DS will talk as if it happened in the last few weeks when it actually happened many years before. We have seen this difficulty with time around other issues as well. Therefore, what may appear to others as an unusual time to be grieving may be connected to differences in how time is perceived. (See Chapter 4.)

> Joel, 26, was quite healthy when he came to see us. His parents had recently updated their will and decided to purchase their cemetery plots. They were relatively young and healthy and there was no immediate anticipated use of the plots. While they were buying their plots, they also purchased a plot for Joel. He had become very upset and eventually required antidepressant medication because he was so frightened by the message he perceived in this purchase of a plot for him. He had great difficulty grasping that the purchase was for a later, undetermined time. He was full of fear that he was going to die in the near future despite being healthy. Planning for the future was a concept beyond his skill level.
>
> If Joel had been given a clearer explanation before the plots were purchased, he may not have had this reaction. On the other hand, if his parents could have predicted how he would respond to the news, given his response to other, similar events, a better approach may have been not telling Joel at all.

Memories

People with Down syndrome often have incredible memory capability. This ability can serve them well but can also cause problems because of the remembrance of painful times. For many people without Down syndrome, the grief process involves the easing or forgetting of the pain while remembering the person. However, the intense memory of many people with Down syndrome can make this process difficult. Using strategies that help the person with DS remember happy times with the deceased can be helpful. This is discussed in more detail in Chapter 5.

THE RIGHT TIME TO GRIEVE

In helping a person with Down syndrome through the grieving process, it is generally best to provide assistance at the time when he is ready for the help. We have often found that having a person attend a "Grief Group" at a designated time can be troubling for many of our patients. At 4:00 on Tuesday afternoons, he may not be ready to discuss the death of his mother. In fact, attending the group at that time may actually bring back painful memories and cause him to perseverate on the pain. Scheduled grief groups may work for some, but for many, they just bring back the pain that they had been able to set aside for a time.

Usually, it is more helpful, although more challenging, to allow a person to work through his grief when he is ready and interested. When everyone is dressed and heading out the door for an event and he brings up the recent death of his mother, it may not seem like the most convenient time; however, it is likely to be the most successful time. We recommend letting the person with Down syndrome guide the discussion: in his time, in his way, in his place.

When the person is interested in talking about the deceased, it is important to allow that opportunity. Particularly if the person's network of family and friends is small, talking about the deceased loved one may help him feel connected to the loved one through memories.

Literal Thinking and Grief

As discussed in Chapter 4, most people with Down syndrome seem to be rather concrete and literal in their thinking. This concrete thinking can help them to get through their day, to achieve in their jobs, and to make sense of their world. However, some degree of abstract thinking is also helpful in many situations, and not having that ability can be problematic, especially if others do not recognize those inabilities.

Scott was 34 when his mother died. He was placed in a grief group at his group home. The group was called the "Mourning Group." The group met every other Wednesday afternoon. We were never able to figure out if it would have been helpful to Scott. He got so locked into the fact that the group met in the afternoon despite being called the "morning" group that he would not participate.

HELPING THE GRIEVING PERSON

Ms. Luchterhand offers the following guidelines for helping an adult with an intellectual disability grieve:

- Be with the person. Spend time with him.
- Talk about the death and the person who died.
- Share feelings.
- Encourage the person to attend the visitation/wake and the funeral or memorial service.
- Try to prevent other losses.
- Allow the person to make choices (about how he needs to grieve).

She also offers the following advice when teaching about death:

- Use simple words and avoid words that have more than one meaning (e.g., "fell asleep").
- Teach by using examples in everyday life (such as the death of an animal or a famous person).
- Use many examples over time.
- Allow the person to see how you deal with losses in your life.
- Allow him to show emotion.
- Encourage questions.
- Talk about stages of life: birth, childhood, teen years, adulthood, aging, death, etc.
- Identify someone who can lead a class or group to talk about death and grief and then ask the person if he wants to attend, assuming it's the right time for him.
- Describe what is good about death (no longer suffering; if after-life is part of his religious beliefs). Don't, however, introduce religious concepts that he's not familiar with.
- Help the person feel safe now. Reassure him that he and other family members are healthy (in a truthful way).

Based on our experience with grief groups, we do advise determining whether participating in a group would most likely be helpful or problematic for the adult with Down syndrome. Does the person tend to perseverate on other issues? If someone else mentions the death of his loved one, does it seem to help him or cause him more problems? Has he previously done well in structured groups? Trying to answer these questions may give some insight into whether a grief group would be beneficial. Sometimes, however, if you are uncertain, doing a trial in a grief group for people with DS or other intellectual disabilities may answer the question one way or the other.

Another strategy we have found very helpful is making a book with pictures of the deceased. It is particularly helpful to have pictures of the person doing enjoyable activities that are good memories for the person with Down syndrome. It is also generally helpful to use a picture that shows the deceased and the person with Down syndrome together. The goal is to help the person ease and "forget" his pain while remembering the person and focusing on the happy memories. While being very careful not to trivialize the grief or to "sweep the pain under the rug," it can be very positive to redirect the grief toward happy memories.

Avoiding other losses is only partly under our control. Obviously, we do not have complete control over many losses in our lives. However, we do recommend avoiding or delaying changes or losses, if possible, such as moving, or job changes, during the time of the most intense grieving.

Even the fear of another loss can be very disturbing. This is particularly true of the fear that others close to him will die. We have often heard this concern in our patients who feared losing another parent, a sibling, or other person who is close. Reassuring the person with Down syndrome and remaining in close contact can be helpful in diminishing these concerns.

Sometimes grief goes on for a prolonged time, severely interrupts a person's life, and can lead to depression. It is imperative to try to help the person work through his grief as outlined here, but if the grief becomes prolonged and appears to be more than just a grief reaction, further assessment and treatment may be necessary. Assessment for mental illness is discussed in the next chapter.

Remember, grieving is a unique process for each person. What is beneficial for one person may not be for others. The aspects of grieving that are common in the people we have seen are certainly not universal. Often someone who knew the person with Down syndrome before the loss can best determine how to help him grieve. In addition, careful observation with an open, compassionate heart and a willingness to respond when he asks for help is key to assisting the person with Down syndrome.

While every person may grieve differently, it can be useful to learn how other people have helped a person with Down syndrome deal with grief. In response to an article on grief in our newsletter a few years ago, Sheila Hebein, the Executive Director of the National Association for Down Syndrome, sent us the following letter:

> My son, Chris, has had many losses to deal with in his life. His first one came when my father died, but Chris was only 5 at the time. Then he lost his paternal grandmother (Nona) when he was 11. He had been extremely close to her, but we were open with him and answered his questions as honestly as we could. He was at the wake with the rest of the family. He also participated in the liturgy by taking up the gifts with two of his cousins. Since he has been an adult, his paternal grandfather died and again, he was very close to him because grandpa lived with us on and off for several years. Chris was 19 at the time and we involved him in every way we could. He was with the whole family throughout the wake—I believe he was the only grandchild who didn't leave to get something to eat. He would go back to the casket and touch his grandpa's hand and kneel and pray. He was a pallbearer along with his cousins and we talked frequently about grandpa at home.

Four years ago, my Mom died in England and Chris wasn't able to attend the funeral, but we talked about "Nana" a lot. Then my sister's husband died and that also was very difficult. We went to the funeral in New Hampshire and Chris was with his cousins and participated in all aspects of the funeral. We have spent many family vacations in New Hampshire and I usually make videotapes because all our family members live out of state or out of the country and the tapes have helped Chris "stay in touch" with everyone. He played the tapes of his Nana, his Uncle, and his Grandpa often after they died and I think that helped him.

However, the past year brought several more significant losses. One of Chris's former teachers died—she belonged to our church where Chris is an altar server. Arlene struggled with cancer and when we last visited her before she died she told him that she was counting on him to serve at her special (funeral) Mass and he promised that he would. It was such a sad day. Chris managed to get through it, although he did shed tears during and after the funeral.

Another big loss for him (and for us) was when my husband's brother died. Uncle Jim was a priest in Upper Michigan and he was on a ventilator in intensive care during the New Year's holiday. We spent 4 days with him at that time and Chris would pray with him, moisten his mouth, and just sit quietly with him. At one point he was sitting with his Dad in the waiting room and he started to cry. He said, "I'm afraid my Uncle Jim is going to die." At that time we didn't think Jim was going to die, but 3 weeks later he did. Again, Chris was involved in all aspects of the funeral. Because Jim was a priest, the Bishop celebrated the Mass and there were over 50 priests, all in their white robes. It was truly a celebration of Jim's life. Chris played the piano during the Mass and during the visitation time in church. He was also a pallbearer with his cousins.

Chris was very close to his cousin Julie who lives in England and 3 years ago he was an usher in her wedding. In April, Julie had her first baby who died when she was just 2 weeks old. That was very hard for Chris, because he had been looking forward to seeing the baby when we went to England in June. I was touched by his openness with Julie and her husband, Ciaran. He put his arms around her and said, "Julie, I'm so sorry about your baby, Sinead" and at another time I heard him talking to Ciaran and telling him how sad he was that he lost his daughter. Some people would tell him to not talk about this terrible loss because it would upset Julie and Ciaran, but I think it's healthy and helpful to express your feelings and I know his sensitivity and love moved them. I also know that they are thinking about Sinead all the time anyway and Chris was able to shed some tears with them.

In most instances we tried to prepare Chris for the death of our loved ones. Whenever possible, we took him to visit them in the hospital or at *home and we told him how very sick they were. I think that helped prepare Chris to deal with the loss.*

Chris is a very spiritual person and we have shared our faith with him. Therefore, I know he truly believes that when a loved one dies, they go to heaven. Every day he prays for the people he loved and has lost. When we visit the graves of our loved ones, he prays with his arms outstretched and asks the Lord to take care of his Nana and Granddad and baby Sinead or his Nona and Grandpa and Uncle Jim. I think that by openly talking about them and praying for them, it helps him and us.

Chris has a pretty good sense of time, but I know that not all of our adults do. I'm not so sure that time matters so much when you are thinking of someone you loved and have lost. If the person is thinking about them then I think it's probably OK to talk about them. If someone seems to be "stuck" and only thinking about a person who died several years ago, it might be helpful to acknowledge that you miss the person too. You could perhaps say a prayer together and then try to focus on something else, but I do think it is important to validate the person's feelings and not dismiss them. My nephew was killed several years ago in a car accident when he was 25 years old. My sister can still barely talk about Neil without crying, and I wouldn't dream of telling her that she should move on. We are all different and deal with loss in our own way whether we have Down syndrome or not.

There are many stresses in life that can precipitate mental illness. Some of them are relatively small issues that are part of daily life, some are larger but expected, and some are larger but unexpected. Many strategies can be used to help a person with Down syndrome manage his stress. The first step is to acknowledge the possibility (and probability) that a person with Down syndrome will have stresses in his life. The second step is to listen to his concerns and help him devise ways to manage the stress. Additional methods outlined can be used based on the individual's needs and personality.

Chapter **12**

Assessment

· · · · · · · · · · ·

of

· · · · · · · ·

Mental Illness

· · · · · · · · · · · · · · ·

In Chapter 1 we discussed in a general way how we assess the mental
health of an adolescent or adult with Down syndrome, whether or
not a mental illness is suspected. When it seems likely that a mental illness *is* present, we
proceed further with the interview. More detail is sought with regards to the chronological order of events, possible precipitants, family history, previous treatments, the effect
the change has had on the person and the family, and other questions about the illness.

Assessing a person with Down syndrome who has a mental illness or a behavioral
change can be quite challenging. A number of barriers can limit the ability to obtain
an adequate history. The impairment of language skills, conceptual thinking, and
overall cognitive functioning are all hurdles to be overcome. This is because a large
component of the diagnostic criteria for mental illnesses devised by the American Psychiatric Association relies on the self-report of subjective feelings. (These criteria are
described in the *Diagnostic and Statistical Manual of Mental Disorders,* fourth edition,
text revision, or DSM-IV-TR.) For example, people in the general population with depression often report sadness, a lack of energy, a loss of interest in things enjoyed previously, and feelings of guilt and worthlessness. People with anxiety will often report
feeling anxious and fearful in certain situations.

For people without intellectual disabilities, standardized questionnaires are available to help diagnose mental illness. These questionnaires essentially help the practitioner assess the individual on the basis of the DSM-IV-TR criteria. Generally, people with Down syndrome have difficulty answering the written questionnaires.

Because it is often difficult to obtain a clear history of emotional or behavioral changes in people with Down syndrome using conventional methods, we try to gather the information through a multi-pronged approach:

1. We obtain as much history as possible from the adult herself.
2. We ask parents and other caregivers for information about the history of the emotional or behavioral change.
3. We observe the person's behavior.

OBTAINING A HISTORY FROM THE ADULT WITH DOWN SYNDROME

As mentioned above, most people with Down syndrome have trouble sharing, or answering questions about, subjective feelings. Even some people with Down syndrome who have good verbal skills have difficulty sharing feelings. As discussed in Chapter 6, this can be an even greater problem if the adult with Down syndrome is speaking to an unfamiliar person. Nevertheless, we recommend getting as much history from the adult as possible. Although he may not report subjective feelings, he often provides very useful information. For example:

> We were assessing Randy for aggressive behavior. No one had previously asked Randy why he thought his behavior had changed, but he reported to us that Alvin's behavior was the cause. Alvin was entering Randy's room in their group home each evening after the staff went down to the office. Alvin was irritating Randy and taking his belongings. Randy did not take any action when this occurred, but would ruminate overnight or perhaps for several days. Then he would retaliate in an aggressive, physical manner in front of the staff. (Because he has limited verbal skills, he did not know how to report Alvin's activities to the staff, and the staff had not asked him.) Without the history provided by Randy, the staff had labeled his behavior as an "unprovoked outburst." The history obtained from Randy was invaluable in addressing his behavioral challenges.

When obtaining a history from a person with Down syndrome regarding a change in behavior or possible mental illness, we recommend the following:

◆ Bring her out of the situation, if possible. For example, if there is an inappropriate interaction between two people, separate them to help diffuse the situation and allow for privacy to ask her questions.

Unprovoked Outbursts

The term "unprovoked outburst" often causes us to have a "provoked outburst." All too often, the term is used to eliminate the responsibility to thoroughly assess the environment and aspects of the individual's life that may contribute to her behavior. True, sometimes a person with Down syndrome will behave in an inappropriate manner with no apparent cause. However, as we have previously described, people with Down syndrome may see the world differently than others. For example, the strong memory of many people with Down syndrome, a tendency to ruminate about events, and the different understanding of time, all may contribute to a response that seems unrelated to a given event. Therefore, the label "unprovoked" may be much more the observer's lack of understanding than it is the person with Down syndrome's random loss of control. The implication of the term "unprovoked outburst" is that the person with Down syndrome has to be "fixed" and the environment has no role in either the cause or treatment of the problem.

◆ Reassure her. "Tina, you know I love you but this behavior is not like you, and, I think you know, not appropriate." "Julie, you seem so unhappy lately. I am concerned about you and want to help."
◆ Start with an open-ended question. "Can you tell me what happened?" "Can you tell me what is bothering you?"
◆ If she is not able to answer open-ended questions, try to probe with more direct questions without giving her an answer (which may or may not be the real problem). Be careful not to inappropriately lead her. For example, if you have observed that Rosie has difficulty in the class that follows physical education class, it would be appropriate to ask, "Rosie, has something been happening in physical education class?" A question that would probably be too leading is, "I bet George is bothering you in physical education class. Right?" As previously discussed, many people with Down syndrome do seek to please others, and will often answer questions in the way they think you want them answered. Leading questions will, therefore, often be answered in the way they are being led.

If the patient cannot provide a history verbally, attempts should be made to get the history in other ways. As described in Chapter 9, Gary had spontaneously drawn pictures with a strong sexual content. The drawings led to a determination that he had been sexually abused. We were able to intervene based on this information. Many of our patients write extensively. The context of the writings may also provide valuable pieces of history. It may also be beneficial for some individuals to ask them to draw or write about what is bothering them.

Obtaining a History from Parents/Caregivers

Although the history of subjective feelings obtained from an adult with Down syndrome is usually limited, close family members are quite often able to observe key symptomatic changes in behavior. For example, we find that most people with Down syndrome do not report sadness, but their families find a definite change in personality which we call a "loss of spark, life, and vitality." Most people with DS also do not verbally report a loss of energy or a lack of interest in doing previously enjoyed activities, but close family members usually observe this behavior change. Additionally, we have rarely heard a person with DS say that they feel worthless and thus we have not used this in our criteria of depression. Likewise, most of our patients do not verbalize feelings of anxiety, but body tension and other indications of anxiety are still usually quite obvious to family observers. (For more on the criteria for depression and anxiety, please see Chapters 14 and 15.)

Another way that families can learn important information is by listening to self-talk. We have seen a number of adults with Down syndrome who were not able to provide clear answers to questions regarding the issues that were bothering them. However, their families often observed them talking about the issues through self-talk (see Chapter 8). Interestingly, many families have also found that the person with Down syndrome speaks more clearly when self-talking than when speaking to someone else.

An additional piece of history that family members can provide is the family medical history. Many mental illness conditions run in the family. The family history may therefore give further insight into causes for the change in the mental health of a person with Down syndrome. In addition, sometimes the response of a family member to a particular medication may guide the decision as to what medication should be used.

Another important piece of information parents and caregivers can provide is how the person with DS has responded to previous medications. When we learn that a particular medication did not work, we ask ourselves, "Is the diagnosis correct? Is the medication correct? Are there other factors we have not considered?" For example, imagine that someone has a problem with depression but we do not obtain the history of mania that she also has. In this situation, prescribing an antidepressant for depression may induce mania. If that occurs, it can be a valuable piece of history. In addition, because obtaining the history is challenging, ongoing reassessment and history-taking is essential (particularly if the treatment is not successful) to determine if there are pieces of the history that were either previously overlooked or were not recognized as significant.

Difficulties in Interpreting Second-Hand Information

Despite our efforts to obtain as much history as possible from our patients, much of the information must still come from family or care providers. Unfortunately, this adds a level of interpretation. The observer brings her own biases, interpretations, and the possibility for error in reporting. In addition, another individual may assign a different level of importance to a behavior than the person with Down syndrome would. This may lead to under- or over-reporting of behavioral changes. This can be particularly problematic when the observer is unfamiliar with people with intellectual disabilities. The observer may interpret the common, typical behaviors described in Section 2 as abnormal. This may cloud the whole perception of the events or presentation. Furthermore, frequently we will get completely different histories from families, residential staff, day program staff, and other service providers. These challenges make it necessary to obtain as much history as possible from multiple sources and try to sort out the discrepancies.

DO'S AND DON'TS IN REPORTING THE HISTORY OF A BEHAVIOR

When observing the behavior of a person with Down syndrome, we recommend these tips:

- *Write your observations down.* It can be difficult to remember the specifics and often a connection to a cause will only be seen after reviewing the notes.
- *Record chronological events.* When did the symptoms first start? What changes were seen over time? If it is episodic behavior, what is the order of events during any given episode?
- *What else was occurring at the time the behavior occurred?* What else was occurring in the family, at work, at school, with friends? For episodic events, it is important to look at the surrounding events, people, etc. As previously discussed, because many people with DS have such strong memories, it is important to observe for clues that may seem unimportant at first glance but may indicate a cause. For example, could there be a smell, an object, or some other trigger that reminds the person of a negative event in the past?
- *Be as objective as possible.* Avoid subjective observations such as, "He acts like he hates me." When observing, just as when interviewing, one must take care not to lead the observation in an inappropriate direction before there is an understanding of the problem.

MAKING OBSERVATIONS

In addition to obtaining as much history as possible from the patient, as well as from family and care providers, we often find it necessary to do some observation of our own. Sometimes we obtain the best information by watching or being with the person in her home or work setting. As noted in earlier chapters, language difficulties, memory, the concept of time, and other issues for people with Down syndrome may make the history unclear. Putting the verbal history in context by visiting the person in her usual environment can be invaluable.

Jason, age 34, was brought to see us for outbursts of aggression. A visit to his home at 7:30 a.m. quickly revealed the cause of the problem. Jason's bus arrived that day on time at 7:50 and he became agitated when we continued to talk and tried to briefly delay him from getting on the bus. There was a clear compulsive component to his behavior. After discussing my observation and questioning the staff again, the staff did report (which they had previously denied) that Jason had many compulsive behaviors that interfered with certain activities. For example, he needed to finish one task, such as putting away items in his room, before moving on to another task or activity. If a staff person intervened to try to divert him to another task before he was finished, he could become aggressive. With this clearer understanding of Jason's problem, we suggested staff organize his activities to minimize times that he was kept from completing tasks, and Jason improved nicely.

We generally prearrange a visit. We recommend arranging this with the family or staff and ensuring that the person with Down syndrome be informed. Occasionally, if we have arranged to see one person at a group facility (residential or work program), we might either be asked to observe someone else or we might inadvertently see someone else. In any case, we recommend asking if the behavior observed is typical. Observation itself might alter behavior and it is important to know if the behavior is not what is typically seen.

CONCLUSION

The assessment of mental illness in an adolescent or adult with Down syndrome can be difficult. It can be challenging and time-consuming to try to obtain a clear history from the individual, to get a history from a variety of people, or to directly observe the person, if necessary. However, careful, ongoing assessment using the multi-pronged approach is essential for understanding the nature of the person's problem and for developing the therapeutic plan that will be outlined in the next chapter.

Chapter 13

Treatment Approaches for Mental Illness

Once a mental illness is diagnosed, the next step is to develop a treatment intervention. Chapters 14 to 23 discuss the specific treatments that are often effective for adolescents and adults with Down syndrome who have been diagnosed with particular mental illnesses or disorders. However, because many of these treatments involve either counseling or the prescription of certain classes of medications, we will provide an overview of general issues related to these treatment approaches here, in order to avoid repetition from chapter to chapter.

PART I: WHEN COUNSELING IS NECESSARY

Counseling may be extremely helpful to some adolescents and adults with Down syndrome. Under the right circumstance, counseling from a trained, sensitive, and knowledgeable therapist may:

- give people support and encouragement,

◆ enhance pride and self-esteem,
◆ help people to identify and resolve life problems,
◆ be a useful part of the treatment for more serious problems such as depression, anxiety, obsessive-compulsive disorder, etc.

This sounds wonderful, and it can be, but a number of conditions need to be met for people with Down syndrome to benefit from counseling.

For an adult with Down syndrome and his family or other caregivers to make an informed judgment about the need and efficacy of counseling, they need to know more about what counseling entails. If they decide to try counseling, they need to ensure that:

1. Counselors have adequate education, training, experience, and sensitivity.
2. There is a good fit between the personality of the counselor and the person counseled.
3. Counseling is a safe and secure process.
4. The counseling process has meaningful goals, and a means to obtain these goals and assess an outcome.

COUNSELORS

◆ ◆ ◆ ◆ ◆ ◆ ◆ ◆ ◆ ◆ ◆ ◆ ◆ ◆ ◆ ◆ ◆ ◆

Counselor is a generic term we are using to refer to any professional who is trained to identify and help resolve any emotional and behavioral problems that people have in their lives. A number of different professionals are trained to do counseling, including:

◆ Social workers (M.S.W., D.S.W., or Ph.D.),
◆ Psychologists (Ph.D. or PSY.D.),
◆ Counselors, (M.A., M.S., or Ed.D.),
◆ Psychiatrists,
◆ Pastoral counselors (M.Div., D.Div., or Ph.D.) and
◆ Marriage and family therapists (M.F.T.).

In most cases, it does not matter what type of professional you seek to do counseling. Their ability to establish rapport as well as their training and experience are what matters most. The ability to use a specific approach to counseling also depends more on the counselor's training than on their profession. For example, behavioral counseling began over 40 years ago in the field of psychology, but this approach is now used by all the different counseling professions. As a second example, marriage and family counseling began approximately 30 years ago by counselors from all different professions and it continues to be practiced by all of these fields as a specialized area of training and practice (see below for more on this approach and an example). There is also a relatively new field of counseling which specializes in this approach, and this is represented by marriage and family therapists or MFT's. Both MFT's and other counseling professionals who are adequately trained in this approach are able to do this type of counseling. Like behavioral and marital/family counseling, most other counseling approaches and techniques may be used by all the different counseling professionals if they are trained in these approaches.

There are, however, several professions which do specific tasks that are unique to these professions.

◆ **Psychologists** are trained to do counseling but they also have unique expertise in psychometrics. This is the use of standard tests and instruments to measure different areas of mental and behavioral functioning. There are many different types of standard tests (Neuro-psychological batteries, personality tests, adaptive skills and maladaptive functioning measure, AD/HD tests, etc.). However, the tests that are often referred to as "Psychologicals" are the standard IQ tests that measure a person's level of intellectual functioning. These types of IQ tests are often required by state governments for people with Down syndrome and other disabilities to establish the degree of the person's mental retardation.

◆ **Psychiatrists** also have somewhat of a unique role in the mental health field. Psychiatrists are physicians (M.D.) or Doctors of Osteopathy (D.O.) who are trained to treat people with mental health problems. They often have training in counseling but many specialize in the management of psychotropic medications. This is the class of medications for the treatment of mental health problems, such as antidepressants, anti-anxiety, or antipsychotic medications. To complicate matters, physicians who are not psychiatrists are also able to prescribe psychotropic medications[1], and many do so in their practice. This is particularly the case for the conditions with more commonly known symptoms, such as depression and anxiety. Physicians may also refer a patient for a consultation with a psychiatrist, just as they would to any other medical specialist. Additionally, many people may initially consult with a psychiatrist to help diagnose and recommend a medication for a mental health problem. Afterwards they may have their own primary doctor refill their prescription and follow them medically for the condition.

Does the presence of a more serious mental health problem require the treatment of a psychiatrist or physician?

The answer is both Yes and No. Counselors who diagnose mental health conditions in their practice and who are not able to prescribe medications will quite often

---

[1] Depending on the state, nurse practitioners (CPN) or Physician Assistants (PA) are also able to prescribe medications.

refer to a physician for a consult on a psychotropic medication. In these cases the counselor often continues to see the person in counseling while the physician manages the medication. Likewise, many physicians who prescribe medications for mental health problems will refer to a counselor for ongoing counseling. In either case the patient benefits from the combination of both medication and ongoing counseling. Research has consistently shown that either medication or counseling may be beneficial, but the combination is far more effective in resolving these types of problems and symptoms (Frank et al., 1990).

Payment for Counseling Services

We would be remiss if we discussed counseling without talking about how people pay for this service. The truth is that counseling and mental health services are woefully under-funded by insurance and government sources in the United States. Third party private or government insurers may not pay for this service, and when they do, they often pay no more than a third or a half of what the service costs. Certainly, payments are well below what is paid for a comparable expense involving a medical problem.

Still, there has been great progress in this area over the last 30 years or so. Awareness of, and payment for, these types of problems has grown exponentially. These changes have been spearheaded by the families of people with mental health problems. Additionally, most of the counseling professions have advocated for third party payment for their services. Most insurance companies that do cover mental health services cover counseling provided by social workers, psychologists, and psychiatrists; some also cover services by other professionals. However, each insurance policy is different. You need to call your own provider to determine what type of coverage you have. If services are limited, it may be possible to change to a different coverage when there is open enrollment or to work with your employers to advocate for expanded coverage of mental health services.

EDUCATION AND TRAINING

Individuals with DS need fully qualified counselors. Just because their thoughts and feelings might seem less complicated than those of others their age does not mean that someone who is not a counseling professional would be a "good enough" counselor for them.

Like other adolescents or adults, people with Down syndrome should receive counseling from individuals who have, at a minimum, a master's degree from an accredited program in their chosen profession (four years of college and at least two additional years of a specialized master's program in a counseling field). They must also have a license in their chosen profession from the state in which they practice.

In most cases, state licensure is dependent on passing an accrediting exam and a required number of hours, supervised by a senior clinician, after the completion of a formal educational program. Training and subsequent work experiences should be documented in a resume and the counselor should be able to furnish this and a copy of their diploma to anyone seeking counseling.

In the disability field there are a number of different types of case managers, including Qualified Mental Retardation Professionals (QMRP's). There are also managers and direct caregivers in residential living situations and at work sites. These individuals have critically important roles and they are often very caring and sensitive people, but they have not had training or education to do counseling and therefore should not be considered appropriate for this role.

PERSONAL ISSUES

Counselors should be sensitive, insightful, and caring human beings. Additionally, the counselor's life experience may be an important factor in the success of counseling. Counselors who have "been there" (having experienced different aspects of life: marriage, raising children, grief, etc.) are often more aware and less judgmental than those who are younger or less experienced. In fact, researchers have found that successful therapists tend to be more experienced and try a variety of approaches to suit the person and his problem. Younger therapists may need to be more rigid in their approach simply because they do not have the life or treatment experience to try different things that work. Fortunately, young counselors are often supervised by more experienced therapists. This type of arrangement may offer the "best of both worlds"—the energy and enthusiasm of a youthful therapist coupled with the wisdom of a seasoned supervisor.

Another question is whether the counselor should have previous experience working with people with DS. In our experience, a counselor who has this experience may help the adult with DS have a more positive counseling experience. This will happen if the person with DS feels the counselor truly understands and appreciates him, both for his strengths and weaknesses. The counselor who "knows," asks the right questions and responds to the right issues; this says "I understand" to the person being counseled.

On the other hand, it may be very difficult to locate a trained counselor who has experience with adults with Down syndrome. In this case, finding someone who is willing to learn might be the best option. In fact, when we first started this Center, we had very little experience or understanding of the people we are now serving. We did, however, have a great deal of respect for the knowledge of family caregivers. We listen and respect the opinions and ideas of caregivers who have spent so much time, energy, and effort trying to understand and advocate for the person in their care. If a counselor is able to bring his or her own expertise and still be open to learning from the family, then this collaboration has an excellent chance of working. In contrast, if the counselor seems to look down on the person with DS or lack understanding or respect for him or the caregivers, then he should be avoided.

Conflicts of Interest

A cardinal rule in the counseling field is that a counselor cannot have a "dual role" with the person counseled. This means the counselor can only play the role of counselor for the person being counseled. He or she cannot be a friend, parent, caregiver, manager, supervisor, salesperson, and certainly not a lover or sexual partner. Residential or work site staff or managers, even those who have training and experience as counselors, cannot be counselors to the people they work with or supervise. This simply does not work.

It may get a little confusing when staff who are assigned to work as case managers or direct caregivers are called "advocates" or even "counselors." While they may appropriately advocate for the person's needs and services and assist the person in their care, they cannot serve as his counselor. This must be left to counseling professionals in order to maintain the integrity and security of this process. (See the sections on Safety and Confidentiality below.)

Safety Issues

Counselors may be caring human beings but they must also carefully maintain a professional role and boundary to ensure the safety and security of the counseling experience. Public awareness of safety concerns has been growing in light of allegations of abuse leveled at religious persons and others who care for children. Families are also justifiably concerned with the safety of family members with DS who are dependent on the care of others.

There may be some relief to know that safety and issues of confidentiality have been the focus of the counseling field for as long as there have been counseling professionals. Just as medical professionals are careful to have nursing staff present during a medical procedure, counselors should be careful when they do individual counseling. For example, one way to help ensure safety during individual counseling sessions is to leave the door open several inches. The person in counseling is not heard outside the door (to protect his confidentiality, see below) but other counselors or family members are able to see in.

Sometimes it is wise to have a second staff person present during counseling sessions. For example:

> Teresa, a 28-year-old woman with DS, came to counseling with issues around sexuality and dating. She had many questions about sex and her relationship with her boyfriend. Her questions showed a great deal of misinformation and confusion about what "sex" entailed. As an example, she asked whether she was pregnant when she had her period. Also, could she get pregnant by kissing her boyfriend?
>
> Although Teresa was very verbal and capable in managing daily living skills and a job in the community, she was immature in certain areas and did not have a good sense about what was private. She would ask anyone

she encountered questions about sex. This included customers at work and strangers at social events. When her mother learned this, she was appalled and tried to answer her daughter's questions. Unfortunately, she was not terribly comfortable with discussing these issues and her daughter did not seem to understand her explanations. Shortly after this, her mother brought Teresa to get help at the ADSC.

While at the Center, Teresa had a complete physical exam with Janet Bilodeau, LNP (the Center's experienced Nurse Practitioner) and she and her mother had a meeting with Dr. McGuire (counseling staff) to discuss the inappropriate behavior. Although Teresa requested individual counseling sessions, she agreed to have a female staff member present with Dr. McGuire. This staff person was Jenny Howard, who has been the Center's outreach staff for many years. Jenny was helpful with regard to safety issues (for the benefit of both Dr. McGuire and for Teresa) but she was also helpful in bringing a female perspective to the discussion.

In order to manage her problem social behavior, Teresa agreed to write down any questions she had about sex and dating and to discuss them only when she met with ADSC staff (or her mother). A sex education meeting with Jenny and Janet was also set up for her. Interestingly, in the course of the counseling and the sex education, Center staff learned that Teresa did not actually want to have sex, but just to be affectionate with her boyfriend. Over time, these and other issues were sorted out to the family's and Teresa's satisfaction.

As this example illustrates, careful attention to safety issues protects the integrity of the counseling process while still allowing the discussion and successful resolution of even the most sensitive personal problems and issues.

CONFIDENTIALITY

Confidentiality is also a key issue in counseling. How can someone feel free to talk about sensitive personal issues ("to spill their guts"), if this information is not kept private and confidential? The counseling profession is clear about this issue for adults in the general population. Counselors are allowed to discuss facts of the counseling with a supervisor (who must also maintain strict confidentiality). Otherwise, the only time confidentiality is breached is when the person being counseled makes a credible threat to hurt himself or someone else, or when the person allows limited information to be given, such as to his insurance company for payment purposes.

Confidentiality is more complicated for adolescents in the general population. In a strict legal sense, guardians are allowed access to records up until the adolescent is the age of majority, which is 18 in most states. However, in order to establish trust, parents invariably allow teens 14 and older (and even 12- or 13-year-olds, if very mature) to have confidentiality, barring some serious safety issues (threat to self or others).

The issue becomes far more complicated for adults with DS. Chronologically, they are adults, but developmentally they are often more like children or young teenagers. The legal issues are also confusing for many families of people with DS. In fact, adults with DS who have legal guardians (established through the appropriate court) are subject to the same rules as children in the general population. Guardians have access to their records. On the other hand, adults with DS (over the age of majority) who have no legal guardians are considered their own guardians, and thus, have all the legal rights of other adults. We have found that this sometimes presents problems, such as when people who are their own guardians do not agree to needed medical treatments. However, we have not experienced this as a major problem when counseling people. In most cases, once their rights are carefully explained, adults with DS agree to share relevant information with caregivers. This is fortunate, because it is rare for us to do individual counseling without the ongoing involvement of caregivers.

We like to involve caregivers because expressive language limitations make it difficult for many people with DS to communicate relevant issues and concerns to the counselor. Individual counseling is not useful if it is conducted in a proverbial vacuum. Therefore, gathering information from caregivers in different environments may help to keep the counseling focused on the adult's real needs and issues. The more information available to the therapist, the more understanding and helpful the therapist may be.

Because of a need for more open communication between the counselor and caregivers, the issue of confidentiality must be explained very clearly to the person with DS and his caregivers before the start of counseling. Whenever possible, the counselor must respect the needs and wishes of the person with DS. For example, some individuals are dealing with adolescent-like issues of independence with parents (often delayed into their 20s or 30s for people with intellectual disabilities). In these situations, we may try to negotiate more privacy for the person with DS from caregivers (just as counselors of adolescents in the general population do), even if the caregivers are the guardians. Additionally, if parents are given information or progress reports on the counseling, we try to get permission to do this from the person with DS. Although this is not legally necessary if someone has a guardian, it is necessary to maintain trust in the therapeutic relationship.

We are also careful to ask the person in counseling first before discussing any information with his parents or other caregivers. It may be helpful for the person with DS to be present when this information is discussed with the caregiver, either in person or by phone. Again, this helps to maintain trust and confidence in the integrity of the counseling process. We have not had any problems creating a collaborative relationship between all parties when we have dealt with these issues openly and sensitively from the start.

THE WRONG COUNSELOR FOR ME?

Some counselors have gone through clinical training and internships, have extensive life experiences and even experience with people with DS, but still may not be the right counselor for a particular person with DS. Perhaps they are not very insightful in general, or in a specific problem area, despite their training or experience. Or they may lack the ability to understand and convey a sense of warmth and caring to the person they are counseling.

Even when counselors are trained, understanding, and sensitive, they may still not be the right person for the job. The truth is, we all have our unique styles and personalities, and personalities may clash between counselor and the person counseled, just as between people in any sphere of life. Counseling is as much art as science, and much of the art involves the personal style of the counselor.

Counselors are very aware that personality is a critical component in counseling and they will often recommend that the patient interview them before starting therapy. Many also recommend a trial period before a commitment is made for counseling. For families seeking a counselor for a family member with DS, it is highly recommended that they sit in on at least one session in order to see if the counselor is the right person for the job. Issues of personality and style can only be determined through face-to-face contact. When they observe the counseling process, families need to trust their intuition and their sense of whether or not the counseling feels right for themselves, but especially for the family member with Down syndrome.

Additionally, most people with DS will have a definite feeling about a counselor they are seeing. The question is not *whether* the person has these feelings, but how to gather this information from him. As discussed in Chapter 6, people with Down syndrome often try to avoid being negative or critical, but someone who knows them well can usually determine their true feelings from the degree of their response (enthusiastic to less than enthusiastic). If the adult with DS gives a half-hearted endorsement or response to the counseling, then this should be looked at very closely. Perhaps the person needs some time to get used to the process of counseling because it is new. However, if his response continues to be half-hearted or lukewarm after a number of sessions, this may mean that the counselor is not a good fit for the person's needs and personality. Any good counselor will have not have a problem referring to another counselor who is a better fit due to personality issues.

TYPES OF COUNSELING HELPFUL FOR ADULTS WITH DOWN SYNDROME

◆ ◆ ◆ ◆ ◆ ◆ ◆ ◆ ◆ ◆ ◆ ◆ ◆ ◆ ◆ ◆ ◆ ◆

SUPPORTIVE COUNSELING

As part of any multidisciplinary evaluation at the Center, a psychosocial assessment is completed by counseling staff (Dr. McGuire) to gather key information on the person's social and adaptive skills, as well as his network of family and peer support.

During this assessment, the person's caregivers often ask him if he would like to talk alone with Dr. McGuire. They explain that this may be a way for the person to express his feelings, "to get things off his chest," etc.

Although many people with DS do not feel a need to talk alone, some do. Interestingly, quite a few of the individuals who want to talk have no current or urgent problems or issues. Instead, they often want to discuss some meaningful experience or event from the past. Common themes include being hurt or treated unfairly by another, being jilted by a love interest, or losing someone close. The issue may also appear fairly insignificant to others, such as an accidental breaking of a dish. Many times these counseling themes involve a repetition of the same story over and over.

Regardless of how seemingly insignificant or repetitious the issues, we take the counseling process very seriously at the Center. We listen very patiently and respectfully, ask for clarification when needed, reflect on the feelings expressed, and give advice when appropriate. In our experience, and from what families have told us, being able to express themselves to someone who really listens to them is extremely important to adults with DS and enhances their self-esteem. For these individuals, the verbal message is less important than the communication of some feeling which is heard and responded to with respect and understanding.

This type of counseling is called supportive counseling, and despite the apparent absence of an urgent problem or issue, the process can be very beneficial to the person counseled. This approach is used only if the person is offered and accepts the invitation to talk to an experienced counselor. In our experience, those who accept this invitation often feel they are able to say what they need to in one or two meetings, although some people continue for a more extended time. After the counseling is completed, we try to "check in" with the person with DS with brief individual meetings when he returns for routine medical follow-ups. This often helps to keep a therapeutic connection between the counselor and the person with DS long past the initial counseling sessions. Additionally, and perhaps most importantly, this gives many people enough of a positive experience with counseling process that they ask to come back to talk when there are new issues and concerns that are bothering them.

Good counseling always involves elements of supportive counseling, in terms of sensitivity to the person's thoughts and feelings, regardless of the verbal message. The counselor communicates a message of human kindness, understanding, and respect. This message may be communicated to someone who is nonverbal or who has limited verbal skills just as well as to someone who has good verbal skills. The process of respectful listening and responding is extremely beneficial to all, regardless of their expressive language skills. We know this is the case because people have communicated in clear nonverbal messages their wish to continue the counseling. For example, some people use the sign for talk, while others improvise this by moving their hand outward from their mouths. Still others put their hand over their chest, indicating a need to express feelings (from the heart).

INSIGHT-ORIENTED VERSUS BEHAVIOR CHANGING APPROACHES TO COUNSELING

All good counseling includes some type of learning or insight about oneself or one's behavior. Even in supportive counseling, the person may learn that he is valued and that he has more skills and resources than he had assumed. Often, supportive counseling is sufficient. Other times, more extensive measures may be needed. In these cases, the goal of counseling is often the identification and change of maladaptive ways of thinking and behaving which are creating problems for the person.

INSIGHT-ORIENTED APPROACHES

Some counseling approaches emphasize the need to change how people think. These are often called insight-oriented approaches. Proponents of this approach assume that if people understand the cause of a problem, they will be motivated to behave more adaptively. For example, for Teresa, one key insight was that it was inappropriate to address questions on sexual issues to anyone other than the counseling and medical staff at the Center.

Other approaches emphasize changing behavior as a way to gain insight. For example, many approaches use carefully designed tasks to stop maladaptive patterns of behavior. The assumption in these approaches is that it is easier to gain insight once someone does a task and sees the positive result. In reality, insight and behavior change approaches work hand in hand and it is not uncommon to see components of both in any counseling situation. To return to the example of Teresa, we can see that she gained insight into her problem behavior (discussing personal sexual issues inappropriately) both before and after she did the assigned task (which was to discuss these issues only with staff at the Center).

BEHAVIOR-CHANGING APPROACHES

There are also a host of approaches which emphasize behavior change and not insight. These so-called behavioral approaches include the behavior modification and applied behavior analysis approaches. Behavioral counselors identify behaviors in people's lives which create problems and then reinforce more desirable alternative behavior. Behaviorists often break the problem down into more manageable steps of change. Behaviorists are also known for systematically tracking the frequency of the targeted behavior to evaluate any changes.

Behaviorists have not been known for their supportive counseling techniques, but they need to be sensitive to the thoughts and feelings of the adult with Down syndrome and his family in order to develop a working relationship with them. For example, when designing a behavior plan, successful counselors listen carefully and respectfully to caregivers in order to identify problem behaviors and issues. Since caregivers are often the ones who reinforce the adult's behavior, the counselor needs their full cooperation and acceptance of the plan. He or she needs to give some insight and rationale for the use of the approach and the expected change in behavior.

Equally important, the successful behaviorist will work very hard to obtain the understanding, acceptance, and cooperation of the person with DS. At the very least, the behaviorist must carefully consult the adult regarding what reinforcers are most desirable. Helping the person develop an investment in the process is not only respectful, but also greatly increases the chance of success. This is because the person feels he has a hand in managing his own behavior. Along these same lines, adults with DS may be able to use charts to monitor their own behavior rather than just rely on caregivers to do the charting. These and other strategies make the behavioral approach more palatable for caregivers and the person with DS. There are a number of good examples of this approach throughout the book. See for example the story about Janine on page 300.

COMBINED APPROACHES TO COUNSELING

Several counseling approaches combine insight-oriented with behavior-changing strategies. Here we describe the two that we have found to be especially effective in working with people with DS: the social learning and the cognitive behavioral approaches.

SOCIAL LEARNING APPROACH

The social learning approach is one of the most popular approaches in the counseling field. This approach has been shown to be effective with a wide variety of problems, including depression and anxiety. Through this approach, people change problem behavior by first watching others do a task, and then learning to do it themselves, through a technique called modeling.

We have found this to be a particularly effective strategy for people with Down syndrome because they tend to think in visual images and to have excellent visual memories. As discussed in Chapter 5, this is why people with DS tend to remember past events in great detail. The ability to learn through visual observation and recall is also very impressive.

In Chapter 16, we give an example of an adult with DS using the social learning approach to model a desired behavior change first demonstrated by his sister. The adult, Charles, had developed a habit of buying the same toiletry items over and over, even though he already had more than enough of them at home (such as ten bottles of shampoo). After his parents died and he moved in with his sister, she consulted with us to learn how to break him of this habit. The first step was to have Charles look in his bathroom cabinet to see what items he truly needed. His sister then helped him find a picture or make a drawing of the item he needed. Afterwards, he took this picture to the store to help him locate and buy the item.

The new routine gave Charles a sense of independence and purpose for the shopping trips. His sister was also very pleased because it helped him develop independence while keeping him from buying and hoarding items unnecessarily. His sister followed up the shopping trips by watching him put the acquired items away in his cabinet. She would then heap praise on him for a job well done. After doing this routine together for several shopping trips, Charles began to do the task by himself.

Perhaps the most interesting and innovative use of the social learning approach is to use a photograph or a video playback of the person himself. This approach is called self-modeling. As discussed in Chapter 4, people with DS are drawn to photographs and videos of family and friends, but are especially interested in images of themselves.

For example, we find that our patients with DS are far more likely to follow an aerobics exercise routine if they watch a tape of themselves doing the routine. Another example of the social learning approach is the story of Brian, who refused to see his brother after his brother could not come to a holiday gathering (Chapter 5). In order to get the two brothers together, his sister followed our advice to show Brian pictures of positive past family events which included both brothers. Not surprisingly, the pictures that had the most influence on Brian included pictures of himself with his brother.

The person's image of himself also has great potential as a motivator for appropriate behavior. The beauty of a videotape or DVD is that it may be edited to show desired behavior that the person is not engaging in at present. For example:

> Rosemary, 34, had been independent in completing basic self-care tasks, but she began to refuse to leave her house to go to work in the morning. After a thorough evaluation, we determined that this was due to a number of factors including a hypothyroid disorder, fatigue, and a conflict with a young staff person where she worked. The hypothyroid problem was treated and her fatigue was resolved by moving Rosemary in with a new roommate who did not keep her up late at night. The conflict with the staff person was resolved by having a different staff person deal with Rosemary in the morning.
>
> After these changes were made, Rosemary's morning routine went more smoothly, but she still required constant prompting to complete her routine in a timely manner. We believe this was because the problem had gone on long enough to become a habitual pattern for her. We suggested that staff videotape her morning routine, which included the constant prompting from staff. Following our directions, the staff then edited the tape with two VHS machines (Dowrick, 1991). The edited tape left out all staff prompting and approximated a normal speed for completing her morning routine. We then asked the staff to show Rosemary the edited tape in the morning after she woke up.
>
> The first morning Rosemary was shown the tape, staff were very surprised by the result. Not only was she mesmerized by the tape, but she then went on to follow her routine at a much faster pace and without needing much prompting. For the next few days, she continued to watch the tape every morning and then to move at a faster pace, until, by the end of the week, she was moving at the same speed she had moved prior to the onset of her problem behavior. Interestingly, the only change that she exhibited from her former routine was to look at the tape every morning. She continued to do this long after the problem was resolved.

COGNITIVE BEHAVIORAL APPROACH

The cognitive behavioral approach is also very effective with people in the general population and people with DS. This approach emphasizes changing thoughts which influence someone's mood and behavior. This approach has been especially effective for treating depression. Research has shown that people who are depressed have negative thoughts about themselves ("I am worthless"), about their ability to affect the world ("I cannot do anything"), and about the world (a cold and insensitive place). It is easy to see how this then affects their self-esteem and makes them highly susceptible to depression. In the cognitive behavioral model, the counselor helps people to identify negative thoughts and change them into positive thoughts and behavior.

Sometimes a person's negative thoughts have some basis in fact, such as when he cannot do a task due to limited skills. For a person with a strong bent toward negative thoughts, "failing" in a task often supports his own beliefs that he is bad or deficient in some way, which may then lead to depression. In some cases, the failure may simply be due to lack of instruction with the task. Once the person learns to do the task, he is successful. In other cases, the task may be beyond the person's capability. In these situations, the person is encouraged to do a task that is more appropriate for his skills. In either case, once he is taught to do a task successfully, or encouraged to do a appropriate task successfully, he is then encouraged to listen and accept positive feedback from others. In addition, he is encouraged to practice making positive comments about his success to counteract any continuing negative thoughts and behaviors.

When using this approach with someone in the general population, a therapist will carefully examine the person's thought patterns to look for negative and self-defeating thoughts that result in a problematic response to a challenge. For example, the therapist will ask the person what he would say to himself when he tries to deal with a problem (e.g., "I cannot overcome this challenge"). The counselor will then help the person to substitute a more positive statement into his thought patterns ("I have the strength and skill to meet this challenge"), which is more likely to result in a positive solution. This approach can also be used for very verbal people with Down syndrome.

We have found that for people with DS who are less verbal, self-talk (see Chapter 8) is an excellent vehicle for examining negative thoughts. Caregivers often know or are able to learn the content of the person's self-talk. When negative self-talk messages are identified, the counselor at ADSC helps people to substitute phrases that are more positive, just as counselors do with people in the general population. A good example of this is seen in the case of Ben, discussed in detail, below. When people have more positive thoughts, they behave more positively. They then receive more praise and feel increasing pride and self-esteem, leading to more positive thoughts and behaviors (on and on in a more positive spiral).

To provide a more realistic look at the types of problems we see at the Center and how we might use a combination of different counseling approaches to resolve a problem, let's look at the example of Ben:

> *Ben, 18, lived with his parents and older brother and attended a transition program which emphasized community work skills. He was able to communicate effectively with familiar others, but sometimes had problems verbalizing his feelings. According to his family, everything*

was fine until he began his second year of the transition program. At that time he showed symptoms of depression, anxiety, and of an obsessive-compulsive disorder. In place of his usual good nature, he was moody, tense, and irritable. He became withdrawn and started refusing to go to social and recreation activities he had previously enjoyed. He also stopped doing the free time activities he "loved" such as listening to music, watching favorite movies, or playing video games. His family also noted that his appetite had decreased and he had a great deal of difficulty falling or remaining asleep at night. He was listless and appeared to have little energy during the daytime.

Ben's family also became concerned with his increasingly odd compulsive behavior. In the past, his compulsions or "'grooves" had been generally beneficial for him and his family. He was neat and orderly and careful with his grooming and appearance. He was also able to reliably complete self-care and work/school tasks because they were part of his daily routine. This changed as his grooves became more rigid and they began to interfere with his normal functioning. For example, he began to take the garbage out every hour and to hoard ever larger amounts of food in his room. He also became more and more extreme about the need to keep items in precisely the same spot. He had previously insisted on exact placement of items only in his bedroom, but as this need expanded to rooms in the rest of the house, it became a safety issue. The objects he moved now included massive items such as a piano, TV, couches, large glass objects, etc.

Perhaps most disturbing to Ben's family were his nightly tirades. Although he was not aggressive toward family members, he became increasingly angry and agitated as the night went on. The content of his tirades involved any negative or teasing comments directed toward him from others. Unfortunately, he would use his superb memory to draw on up to fifteen years of such comments. He tended also to repeat the same incidents over and over through self-talk every evening, with more and more intensity as the night wore on. To his family, Ben seemed to be carrying on conversations with imagined others (which is not uncommon; see Chapter 8), but they recognized most of these conversations as replays of past negative experiences. It appeared to Ben's family as if he was building a strong negative case against himself.

The diagnosis and treatment of Ben's problem began with a complete physical exam, which revealed hypothyroidism and impaired hearing. These issues no doubt had an effect on his current symptoms. However, his parents also reported that he had recently been a victim of abuse by a female student with a disability. This happened while Ben and the other student were participating in a special recreation group at a community center. The other student had serious problems of her own and had vented her anger on Ben, who was much smaller than she. On at least one occasion, the female student groped at Ben's genitals. His parents believed that the sexual groping was far more disturbing than the physical aggression to Ben.

Once we learned of the abuse, Ben's behavior became more understandable. His agitated self-talk was a clear example of the type of self-blame and self-recrimination that is common among victims of abuse. His exceptional ability to recall past negative events only added to his sense of shame and self-blame. On the positive side, his anger was a far better response to the abuse than withdrawal into a severe state of depression, which happens to many individuals who experience this type of abuse. His increase in more rigid compulsiveness is also a common response to stress, particularly for people with DS who have strong preexisting compulsive or groove-like tendencies.

Our treatment strategy was multifaceted, including medical treatment for his hypothyroid condition and a referral for a hearing evaluation. After careful consideration, Ben was also prescribed an antidepressant medication to help reduce the intensity of his compulsive behaviors and his upset mood. At the same time, we offered supportive counseling to Ben to raise his pride and self-esteem, which had been badly damaged by the abuse. We also counseled Ben's parents, who were very upset and concerned for Ben. In family meetings we praised Ben and his family for having great strength of character in their response to the crisis. This helped to reduce their sense of self-blame.

Additionally, in our work with Ben and his family, we used several counseling strategies which were discussed above. For example, at our suggestion, Ben's parents found many photographs and home movies of Ben involved in positive experiences. This served as a potent form of self-modeling, showing Ben as a strong, proud, and capable young man who enjoyed life. It also served as a substitute for his memory of negative comments and experiences that plagued his evenings. His parents were able to get him to focus on these positive memories in the "quiet time" after work when he was most susceptible to his memories of negative past events. They also commented positively on the pictures ("Look how good you looked….," how much fun you had…," or "how well you did that," etc.)

A modified version of a cognitive behavioral technique was also helpful to Ben. He agreed to use a simple but effective strategy of "turning the channel" whenever he had negative thoughts. One of Ben's parents described this technique as a "multi-media production." Ben would raise both hands up as if to turn the channel on an imaginary TV, while saying loudly and clearly "turn the channel." Ben's parents helped by reminding him to "turn the channel" whenever they noticed the negative self-talk. They also helped him to substitute negative comments with such positive statements as, "I am a good person ... and my family and friends love me." Although these were simple statements, they were very effective in helping him counteract the negative comments. He would then repeat these comments over and over, particularly in the evening when he was most susceptible to the negative self-talk.

After a number of practice runs and reminders, Ben was often able to use his positive self-talk and "turn the channel" technique fairly automatically. In time, he even was able to remind himself if he was aware of the negative self-talk. His parents also helped him to focus on something positive when he "changed the channel." They would either remind him of a favorite memory or show him a photograph of a favorite past event.

Over time, Ben showed a positive response to both the medical and counseling approaches. His mood improved, his obsessions and compulsions became less rigid and more productive (or groove-like), his anger dissipated, and he showed a renewed interest in doing all the activities that he had enjoyed before. After two years, he continues to do well in all areas of his life. He has even been able to work with the young woman who abused him. Fortunately, this woman had been treated and was watched closely by staff.

COUNSELING FOR PEOPLE WITH ACCEPTANCE ISSUES

One important reason for counseling is to help people better understand and accept who they are. At the Center, this often involves helping people accept the fact that they have Down syndrome. As discussed in Chapter 7, this is very important because acceptance increases the use and development of one's own skills and abilities and it encourages advocacy for one's own rights and needs.

Although there are relatively few people with Down syndrome who have acceptance issues, for those who do have them, these issues may have a profound effect on their lives. We see this in a number of key areas of life, including in the social arena and on the job.

Individuals with acceptance issues tend to have an aversion to socializing or associating with peers who have DS or other intellectual disabilities. For some people, this can be a minor problem. Some people prefer to socialize with staff, while others are selective about who they socialize with at social gatherings, preferring people who are more capable. In general, these individuals do not have an aversion to participate in activities with others with disabilities, and more importantly, they do not have a negative view of their own disability. Of course, we would not force these people to make friends they would not choose on their own any more than we would force someone without DS to be with people they do not choose. As long as they have good self-esteem and a positive view of their DS, their socialization habits are not a problem.

On the other hand, we have seen people who clearly do not want to associate with people with disabilities and who have a negative view of Down syndrome. Many view themselves as different from others with disabilities and they may actually say that they are "not like them" (referring to others with Down syndrome). A few even make negative comments about the others (calling them "retarded" or worse). What underlies this lack of acceptance is usually a type of rejection of self (some have even called this a self-hatred) which leads to poor self-esteem. How can it be otherwise when someone cannot accept a major part of himself? For people with DS, this lack of acceptance may have a disastrous effect on their lives.

Unfortunately, counseling is often difficult for individuals who have acceptance issues, because they are often very reluctant to discuss or acknowledge the fact that they have Down syndrome. For example, Patrick voiced his lack of acceptance by stating that he wanted a cure for "it" (the DS). This admission was actually a breakthrough in counseling because for months he wouldn't even admit that "it" existed. What harm comes from these negative feelings about Down syndrome? These individuals choose not to associate with people with DS and other intellectual disabilities, but often have at least some trouble being accepted by people in the general population. Consequently, they exist in a hellish limbo of loneliness and despair because they are cut off from the people they want to be with and choose to cut themselves off from the people with whom they could develop friendships (i.e., people with disabilities).

Additionally, because they do not understand or accept their own limitations, many of these individuals also have problems in the work place. For example, we have seen many people who lost good jobs (in offices, grocery stores, etc.) because they did not feel the job was up to par when compared to jobs siblings or others without disabilities have (as executives, lawyers, doctors, etc.). From this perspective, no job will be acceptable because no job will be good enough compared to what others have attained. The job failures that result from this attitude only add to the person's sense of despair and poor self-esteem.

Although acceptance is a difficult issue to treat, there are a few factors that may increase or decrease the success of counseling. One of the most important issues is whether the person's family accepts the Down syndrome. Lack of acceptance may be manifested in a myriad of ways, such as when the family avoids or makes negative comments about people with DS or when they keep the family member with DS from participating in social gatherings or community outings because of embarrassment, etc. If the family has these types of acceptance issues, then our job is far more difficult and we are less optimistic about the outcome of treatment. Often these families ask us to treat the symptoms (depression, despair, etc.) without discussing the real cause of the problem: the lack of acceptance of the person's Down syndrome.

Even in these situations, we have had some success in turning the tide of acceptance. This happens for two reasons. First, through counseling and exposure to other individuals with Down syndrome while at the Center, we are able to promote a positive view of DS. This may occur even if the issue of Down syndrome is not discussed directly, at least not in the early stages of counseling. Second, we have found that people may become more receptive to the message that it is OK to have Down syndrome as they age and mature. In these situations, patience and persistence will pay off. For example:

Judd has been followed in the Clinic from 1996 up to the present. Over this period, he has come in at various times with complaints of loneliness, depression, and problems keeping jobs, which were all related to his lack of acceptance of Down syndrome. Each time he came to the Center we listened and supported him, while we also promoted a positive view of DS and of his own unique talents and resources as a person with DS. We encouraged him to view his problems as solvable if he could accept himself.

After years of pain and hardships, Judd has finally begun to show signs of self-acceptance and pride. One thing that helped to turn the tide for him was a successful job experience, after a string of job failures. Interestingly, this job involved assisting people with physical disabilities in a rehab hospital. We recommended Judd for the job because we had found this to be a successful experience for a number of others who had acceptance issues. Like the others, Judd did surprisingly well in this job. This may have been due in part to the fact that the supervisors were familiar with people with physical and intellectual disabilities and were very patient and encouraging of him. In addition, the act of helping someone else was a transforming experience for Judd, just as it is for all of us. This is not an experience many people with DS have. They are taken care of but they are rarely given the opportunity to care for others, despite our findings in the clinic that people with DS are often very sensitive and responsive to others. Judd responded to this opportunity by working patiently and sensitively to help others in his job. For this, his supervisors gave him praise and acknowledgment which he sorely needed. Equally important, he developed a greater understanding of, and level of comfort with, the idea of disabilities, which he could use to view his own disability more positively.

Additionally, patience and persistence may pay off in our work with families who have acceptance issues. Families who are initially reluctant to accept DS may become more accepting over time with exposure to the Center and other families. In effect, the meetings at the Center become a type of family counseling related to acceptance issues even if not formally defined as such. This is very important because, if there is acceptance in the family, we are far more likely to resolve an issue of acceptance in the family member with DS. One reason is that these accepting families often encourage the family member with DS to participate in social and recreation activities with people with disabilities, despite whatever reluctance the person with DS has to do so. These individuals often learn to "tolerate" social events with peers with disabilities, and, over time, may actually develop friendships.

Our experience is that people may initially choose to stay to themselves when they attend social and recreation activities. Usually this does not last as other participants begin to talk to them and they cannot help but respond when this includes a team activity. For example, one young man was initially aloof with his softball team but when his group began to compete for Special Olympics medals, he was caught up in the team effort. Another adult became more social because he was courted by a very friendly and attractive young woman with Down syndrome. Similarly, Judd's boss encouraged him to attend Special Olympics, and he has become more and more involved in these types of activities as a result.

We have seen some adults with DS who have difficulty accepting that they cannot drive, go to college, get married, and have their own life like siblings or peers. For example:

> Bridget "made a mess" (as her family described her behavior) during her younger sister's wedding. She was a bridesmaid for the wedding but she was in a foul mood and would not participate in the dancing or other festivities at the reception, even though she loved parties and dancing. Her siblings and parents tried to talk to her and to bring her out of her bad mood, but she simply could not talk or change her mood for the wedding. Over six weeks later, Bridget was able to explain to her sister, Colleen, that she was upset that her sister would have a family, career, and independence, while she would not. Colleen was very sympathetic to her and she brought Bridget to discuss this further in counseling at the Center.

> Over a number of sessions, Bridget, Dr. McGuire, and Colleen discussed Bridget's dreams and her limitations. Eventually, she was able to understand that others also had dreams which were not going to be fulfilled. For example, her sister admitted that she did not marry her childhood sweetheart, that she was not able to go to medical school or to be a singer in a rock band as she had always hoped as a child and a teenager. Still she was able to find happiness in what she was able to do and become. Following from this, and over some time, the counseling shifted from what Bridget was unable to do to what was possible.

> Bridget decided that she had three key goals for her life: 1) to go to college, 2) to find a good job, and 3) to live independently. She, like her sister, found good enough solutions to these goals in time by: 1) attending courses at a community college, 2) finding an enjoyable and good paying job in a grocery store, and 3) moving to an apartment where she was given as much independence and support as she needed (by a good agency serving the needs of persons with disabilities). Bridget returned recently to the Center after several years' absence and admitted that she still sometimes wished she was able to have the life her sister had but that she was much more content and proud of what she was able to do.

In many respects the counseling that Bridget or others with DS receive at the Center is not different than the counseling people in the general population receive when trying to come to terms with their own dreams and the reality of their limitations. For people with DS, the counseling may simply be more focused on a different standard of attainment, but a standard nonetheless that challenges them to the skills and talents they have.

FAMILY COUNSELING

Because of the critical role families play in the lives of people with Down syndrome, we will have an extended discussion of family counseling approaches. We will describe how family counseling is conducted at the Adult Down Syndrome Center, in the hope that you will be able to find equivalent counseling in your area, if you think it would be useful for your family.

As with individual counseling, family counseling approaches include elements of support and insight. In general, families who come to the Center feel a great sense of support from the experience. They feel that they and their family member with DS are welcome, valued, and understood at the Center. Furthermore, the family's feelings and opinions are heard and their expertise as caregivers and advocates is greatly respected.

At the Center, the psychosocial interview with the caregivers and the person with DS (by Dr. McGuire) may explore substantive issues and concerns which may be very insightful to the family. This may include sensitive issues, as well as family concerns that may result in the person with DS feeling criticized or scrutinized. Often, what happens in the ensuing assessment process is a type of family counseling which is educational in nature.

In interviews with thousands of families since 1992, we have identified many issues of key importance in understanding people with DS. During the course of the assessment we can use this knowledge to help explain what is normal (or not so normal) to the family and other caregivers. We look at this process as a way to bring to the meeting the shared wisdom of all the families and caregivers that we have seen. We have heard so many times from so many families about these issues that we can talk with authority about them. Frequently, this brings an enormous sense of relief and understanding to both the person with Down syndrome and his family. For example, we ask whether the person with DS talks out loud to himself, and are able to state that this is a common and normal behavior in most instances. Similarly, we may be able to convey to the caregiver and person with DS that the need to follow certain set routines and patterns may have many benefits. In regard to these and other issues discussed in this book, we become a source of insight for the families and for the person with Down syndrome. Equally important, we can pass on to these families insights and strategies shared by thousands of other families which may solve problems resulting from such issues as self-talk, grooves, etc.

What transpires in these meetings, then, is a type of counseling that helps to normalize and educate people with DS and their families based on the wisdom and expertise of other families.

While not all families have access to a Center serving the needs of Adults with DS, there may be other ways of obtaining education and support. For example, you may gain a great deal from attending conferences offered by local or national DS parent groups. You may benefit from the educational workshops but perhaps benefit as much or more from the process of exchanging information and experiences with other parents and caregivers at the conference. We have found that when we offer group counseling sessions to people with DS, there are often spontaneous support group meetings between the parents of these participants. Often when we notice this is happening, parents agree to have their own counselor present to facilitate these meetings. We have also found that any time parents get together to meet and talk, there may be an exchange of useful information and support.

SUPPORTIVE FAMILY COUNSELING

When the person with DS has more serious problems, supportive family counseling may be essential to the success of the treatment process. For example, when an adult with DS has severe depression which includes a more severe form of withdrawal, family members often curtail their own social and work activities to care for the adult. In effect, the whole family is at risk for depression because of the problem. In these and other related situations we have learned that supporting the family is critically important. After all, family caregivers play a critical role in the person's life when there are no problems. They are even more important when there is a problem to support the treatment and recovery process. If the family is overwhelmed and stressed, then the person with DS will also be overwhelmed and stressed and the severe problems will continue.

In dealing with these issues, it is important to instill hope and confidence, but it is even more important to act as quickly as possible. The number one goal of treatment is to get the person with DS to return to his normal social and occupational schedule so that the family can do the same. Getting back to a more normal schedule allows the family to continue to be a strong base that supports the gains made by the depressed adult. The one snag we have encountered with this strategy is that some employers are reluctant to have people with DS return to work, particularly if there are more severe-appearing symptoms, such as agitated self-talk (yelling at people who are not there). We often advocate for the person to go back regardless of whether severe symptoms are still present. We try to convince staff that this behavior is not uncommon for people with DS who have depression and that it will go away with time. What we, and the agencies, have found is that once people are back in a regular routine, much of the "crazy behavior" dissipates as they become absorbed in their work and the social activities that surround them on the job.

Other types of problems in a family member with DS may be as challenging for families as depression, but for different reasons. For example, people with DS with more severe obsessive-compulsive behaviors may have rituals that control and upset the whole family's routines. In this case, counseling helps the family to learn the best ways to understand and respond to the compulsive behaviors. For example, they learn that anger or attempts to stop the behavior may actually make things worse, whereas gently diverting the behavior to something else may be far more productive. This process helps the family learn how to reduce the rigidity and intensity of the person's rituals, which helps them get back to normal. (See Chapter 16.)

The third reason for family counseling is to resolve conflicts between members of a family or group which affect the person with DS. The counseling approaches that deal with these problems look at a family as a system of relationships that have a mutual influence on each other. This influence is generally beneficial, such as in the case of caregivers who take care of the emotional and material needs of the person with DS. On the other hand, problems occur when there is conflict between parents or other caregivers. It seems that the greater the dependence of the child or adult on the caregivers, and the greater the intensity and duration of the conflict between caregivers, the greater the stress for the person with DS in their care. For example:

Andre, 28, was brought to the Center by his parents and several older siblings. He had become increasingly withdrawn and depressed and would often not get out of bed, even to go to work or to social activities he had previously enjoyed. It turned out that his parents had a bitter, long-standing conflict, but they would not divorce because of religious convictions. Andre's three older siblings had moved out of the family house to go to college and to establish their own homes, while Andre stayed at home with his parents.

After the last of Andre's siblings moved out, the conflict between his parents worsened. His father dealt with the conflict by spending more time at work, and his mother by focusing more of her attention on Andre. During the day, Andre's mother doted on him, doing more and more of the tasks that he was able to do for himself. At night, his parents got into frequent fights which were ostensibly about him. They blamed each other for Andre's depressive symptoms: Father accusing Mother of spoiling Andre, and Mother accusing father of abandoning Andre (and her).

As time went on, Andre became increasingly depressed by the conflict. His refusal to get out of his bed was an indication of the depths of his despair and perhaps it was also his way to send a message that the situation needed to be fixed.

At the first appointment at the Center, Andre's siblings explained how the problem had come about, and how they were trying to remedy the situation for Andre. Some time ago, they had put him on waiting lists for group homes in the hope that he could escape from the parental conflict (like they had). In fact, there was an opening available in a desirable group home, but his parents were both reluctant to have him proceed with the move. Andre's siblings were concerned that their parents were dragging their feet about the move because they wanted to keep Andre home as a buffer for their own conflicts.

After a number of family meetings at the Center, Andre's parents agreed to let him move out. Once he was in his new residence, his depression gradually lifted. Within several months he had adapted to his new residence, and in time he was back to his old self and was participating in important work and social activities.

The counseling freed Andre enough from the parental conflict to move to the new group home. This occurred because the ADSC counselor was able to channel a considerable amount of the parental conflict off of Andre (as the third party in the marriage) and onto the counselor him- or herself. To facilitate this, a number of marital sessions were held between the counselor and the parents without Andre being present. During these meetings, the couple agreed to follow through with a marriage therapist for intensive counseling of their own. Additionally, Andre's siblings kept him at their own houses when their parents met for marital counseling at the Center. They were extremely helpful in setting up and following through with the residential placement. This gave Andre some needed space from his parents, which helped to prevent the parents from pulling him back into the marital conflict. They also brought Andre to many individual counseling sessions to support the process of separating from his parents' conflict.

As explained above, family and marital counseling is a specialized approach to counseling. You cannot assume that counselors who do individual treatment are trained or experienced in family or marital counseling. One way to locate a counselor with this training is through a local chapter of the American Association for Marriage and Family Therapy. This is a national group with affiliates in every state. They have a referral service representing most of the counselors with this training and they may even have counselors in different locations who have experience working with the families of persons with DS or other disabilities.

THE NEED FOR GOALS AND OUTCOME MEASURES

As we discussed in the introduction of this chapter, counseling should have meaningful goals and a means to determine whether these goals are reached. Behavioral approaches are very clear about defining and evaluating change. Insight and supportive counseling approaches will often emphasize more subjective goals, such as "enhanced self-esteem" or "a better attitude," etc. Often, goals for these approaches may also include more objective behavioral measures, such as an increase in participation in beneficial activities, more smiling, etc. Outcome may also be measured as a decrease in negative emotions, such as angry outbursts.

Close family members or caregivers can often assess outcome, since they are often excellent observers of the person with DS in their care. If the counseling is helpful, caregivers will notice a definite change in some key areas of the person's mood, temperament, or behavior. The counselor should discuss outcome goals very clearly at the start of the counseling and progress toward them should be monitored throughout the course of the counseling.

Some counselors may also use standard assessment tools, which are normed for people with DS and other intellectual disabilities, to aid in the assessment of mental health symptoms and maladaptive behaviors. These tools may also be used at the end of treatment to assess improvement. The most widely used assessment tool for this purpose is the *Reiss Screen for Maladaptive Behavior.* Some counselors may also use maladaptive scales from the following assessment tools: *The Inventory of Client and Agency Planning (ICAP)*; the *American Association of Mental Retardation Adaptive Behavior Scales (AAMR ABS);* and the *Scales for Independent Behavior (SIB-R).* In our own practice at the Center we have begun to use the Reiss screen as an aid in diagnosis, to assess outcome, and as a means to compare our findings with other centers who also use this tool. These measures may be especially helpful to clinicians who have less experience with diagnosing and treating people with Down syndrome.

CAN LESS VERBAL PEOPLE BENEFIT FROM COUNSELING?

Some counselors question the benefits of counseling for people with DS who are less verbal. In our experience, counseling may be conducted very successfully with this group through the creative use of nonverbal mediums such as signing, pointing, and pantomime. This may also include the use of augmentative communication devices such as talking computers and lower tech devices such as picture books, written notes, etc. In other words, a counselor may use whatever medium someone customarily uses to communicate with others.

Parents and other caregivers often play an important role as intermediaries in this process. They may help to interpret nonverbal communication, particularly more idiosyncratic gestures and communications that the person uses. They may also give a description of relevant history and of the day-to-day events that transpire between sessions. For example:

> *Molly, a young woman with Down syndrome, had been hurt when her boyfriend chose another woman over her. Molly had relatively limited verbal skills, but her foster mother, Joan, told us Molly's story. As she explained, Molly was very sensitive to this type of loss. She had been put up for adoption at birth because her parents could not accept her Down syndrome. Molly was aware of this fact because she continued to see a grandmother, several siblings, and an aunt who were accepting and supportive of her. While her relationships with accepting family members and her adoptive family were very loving, her feelings of loss from her parents were still strong. This was particularly the case when she experienced a new loss, such as of her boyfriend.*
>
> *Although Molly had limited verbal skills, in counseling she was very expressive with her face and gestures and with written notes. Additionally, her foster mother helped explain the historical issues and the events that occurred during the two to three weeks between sessions. Molly's foster*

mother often sat in with her and the counselor for approximately ten or fifteen minutes prior to their individual meetings. This gave the counselor reference points which Molly and her counselor could discuss during the course of their sessions. For example, the counselor could ask Molly how she experienced an event and she would communicate her response through facial expressions or through a written message.

According to Molly's foster mother, the sessions were very helpful for her. Molly had her own unique sign to indicate she wanted to continue the counseling. She expressed this by moving her hands from her heart outward. She continued to use this sign for approximately three months until she felt she no longer needed the sessions.

Although parental input is usually helpful for people with limited speech, there are several circumstances in which parents should not be used as interpreters. First, parental input may be counterproductive if the person with DS wants to vent about his parents or if they are a part of the person's problem. Usually, this problem is very evident to the counselor when the person with DS responds to his parent's comments and interpretations with negative facial expressions and body language. When this happens, the counselor should look for alternative sources of information from other caregivers who are part of the person's daily life and activities. For example, there may be siblings living in the family home or nearby, teachers in school, or staff or supervisors in residential, work, or recreation settings. If these individuals cannot come to the Center, we try to go to them in order to get the information we need to better understand what the person with DS needs to communicate.

There is also another type of problem with having parents as interpreters. Some people with DS have no major problem or complaints about their parents, but they do want to speak for themselves. They often try to block their parents from speaking and try to communicate on their own. While this is laudable, this creates a problem for the counselor if the person's speech is incomprehensible. In these instances, the counselor will often find some excuse to talk to the parent or parents before and during the individual meeting to get relevant history and help with interpreting the person's speech. In most cases, the parents are very helpful in clarifying the person's comments because they usually involve some key issues or events that occurred in the recent past.

PHOTOGRAPHS AND MEMORY IN COUNSELING

We have found that photographs may be an especially rich medium to help people express thoughts and feelings in counseling. This is particularly the case for people with DS because they tend to have exceptional visual memories, whether or not they have good verbal skills. They may use pictures of past events to express a significant theme or issue. In addition, if the caregivers who accompany the person with DS to counseling have participated in the event shown in the photograph, or are aware of the particulars of the event, they can be helpful by describing more of the feelings and actions captured in the picture. In this way, as the expression goes, a picture truly is worth a thousand words.

For instance, in the above example of Molly, pictures from two different family gatherings helped her to talk about her feelings for her family. The first set of pictures were from her sister's wedding. Molly was not invited to the wedding because her parents were present. The wedding pictures were a poignant example of her parents' lack of acceptance of her and of the many family gatherings she could not attend. Up until she looked at the photographs, she had avoided talking about her feelings about her parents' lack of acceptance. It was much easier for her to talk about missing her boyfriend. The pictures helped her to see the real reason why she was so sad about her boyfriend.

Molly and the counselor also looked at a second set of pictures showing the baptism of her sister's baby. Molly was able to attend this event because her parents were out of the country. This set of pictures helped her appreciate the love she had from accepting family members and from her adopted family (who also attended this ceremony). This not only took the sting out of her parents' rejection of her, but also allowed her to accept her situation and to get on with her life.

As this example shows, pictures may be an excellent therapeutic tool for people with DS, with or without verbal limitations. They may help people to work through losses and problems, as well as to accept the positive resources and supports they have in their lives.

ART AND MUSIC THERAPY
· · · · · · · · · · · · · · · · · · · ·

There are other types of counseling that use other rich mediums to help people express themselves, whether or not they have verbal skills, such as art and music therapy. We have seen great benefit to people from having individual and group sessions with trained and sensitive art and music therapists. People who participate in these types of counseling do not have to be accomplished in either art or music to use these mediums therapeutically.

Art therapists teach people how to paint, create sculptures, or use other forms of art to express themselves in a nonjudgmental and supportive environment. They then help the person to identify the themes and feelings expressed through his art. Similarly, music therapists help people, in a supportive and nonjudgmental setting, to participate in the expression of music through a wide variety of different percussion and musical instruments. The therapist is often able to encourage the person to express some emotion through the music, from exhilaration and gladness to fear and sadness, and then to help the person to interpret what he is expressing through the music.

These therapies may be used effectively in individual or group therapy. In group meetings, the therapist helps people to communicate with each other as well as to the therapist.

Signs That a Counselor May Be Biased

In our experience, there is some bias in the counseling field that may make it difficult for people with Down syndrome to find knowledgeable counselors, committed to working respectfully with them to resolve their issues. When interviewing a counselor to determine whether he or she may be an appropriate counselor for a family member with Down syndrome, look for someone who does not express the following biased beliefs:

People with Down Syndrome Are Incapable of Insight

Some counselors mistakenly believe that people with Down syndrome are not capable of using insight to change their behavior. Practitioners with this bias assume that the reliance on concrete forms of thought may prevent people from understanding how and why they behave certain ways.

In fact, extensive research has shown that there are many different types of intelligence and understanding which may lead to many different forms of learning. For example, one of the ways people with DS may compensate for a lack of abstract thinking is by being very sensitive to the feelings and emotions of others (what we call "emotional radar"). They often interpret and respond to other people's behavior through this lens of understanding.

Even when people with DS show a blatant lack of understanding of the effects of their behavior, this does not mean that they are insensitive to others or that they cannot learn. For example, it may have appeared that Teresa (above) was unaware of her behavior because of her inappropriate questions to strangers about private sexual matters. However, she readily stopped her questions when she learned that they were offensive to others and harmful to herself. What may have prevented her from changing her behavior earlier was that the strangers may not have felt comfortable telling her that her behavior was inappropriate. Her mother may also have been unable to teach her because of an existing adolescent-like conflict with her daughter. Like any adolescent, Teresa tended to rebel against anything communicated by her mother.

Modifying Someone's Behavior without Involving Them in the Process Is OK

Some behavioral counselors underestimate the ability of people with DS to understand and participate in the counseling process. This may lead to an emphasis on modifying the person's behavior without their personal involvement in the process. The person with DS may then feel that they are "done to" rather than "participants in" the counseling. The counselor may not ask questions about what the person wants or needs, which may limit his personal interest and cooperation with the process. These types of problems can often be avoided if the counselor consults caregivers. Even if the counselor has a bias, caregivers may be able to bring the person's feelings, preferences, strengths, and human qualities to life in the process.

UNDERSTANDING THE MESSAGE BEHIND THE BEHAVIOR IS NOT ESSENTIAL

Another more serious problem may result if an inexperienced counselor looks only at a person's behavior and not at the reasons for the behavior. As we have stressed throughout this book, most people with DS cannot easily verbalize thoughts and feelings, so may sometimes rely on behavior as their primary means for communication. Unfortunately, inexperienced or uninformed counselors may not look for the message in the behavior. They may downplay the notion that the person with DS is aware of and responsive to his environment. Consequently, they may believe that all that is necessary is to identify a problem behavior and eliminate it. For example:

> Gina was refusing to go to work in the morning. Staff in her group home had attempted a variety of strategies, ranging from patient encouragement to forceful insistence, without success. An agency behaviorist then proposed that Gina be rewarded for returning to work with a sodapop and a token. If she earned 5 tokens, she was to be rewarded by an outing with her favorite staff person. Unfortunately this, too, did not seem to make any difference to her.
>
> The real reason for Gina's refusal was discovered when her sister accompanied her to an appointment at the ADSC. Unbeknownst to group home staff, Gina had had a bowel accident in her sister's car during a recent weekend visit. (Gina had a history of lactose intolerance which resulted in occasional diarrhea.) The accident in her sister's car was very upsetting to Gina because she was very meticulous with her hygiene. She began to fear that car rides would put her at risk for more embarrassing accidents. This was particularly the case on longer rides, such as between the group home and her workshop.
>
> Once we understood the reason for Gina's behavior, we developed a plan for Gina which included frequent stops at bathrooms on the route to work. Gina was even shown pictures of the route with the bathrooms at different sites highlighted (bathrooms were located at several fast food restaurants, a donut shop, and several other agency sites). The plan included a gradual increase in distance with each bathroom on the route representing a checkpoint. Interestingly, Gina never needed to use the bathrooms during the process. She merely wanted some assurance that she could if she needed to.
>
> Staff continued to stop at each bathroom on the route for many months to appease her sense of anxiety. Additionally, for any other outings into the community, staff made sure that Gina had a plan for

bathrooms on the way to allow her to feel comfortable with the outing. For two years, this overall plan has now worked well for Gina and the staff at her group home.

Clearly, behavior is frequently a nonverbal message which must be understood before any intervention is attempted. Otherwise, the results may be less than satisfactory.

PART 2: WHEN MEDICATION IS NECESSARY

Medications can also be a very important part of treatment for mental health conditions. Sometimes, however, parents or other caregivers are reluctant to consent to the use of "brain altering" medications or think of medications as a treatment of last resort. In reality, however, certain mental health conditions can alter brain chemistry, and using medications to restore brain chemistry to normal may be an essential part of treatment.

This part of the chapter will help you understand why medications may be medically necessary for people with mental health conditions in general, as well as why they may be helpful for people with Down syndrome in specific. In addition, this chapter discusses a number of issues that must also be addressed before prescribing a medication, including:

1. obtaining consent,
2. discussing the philosophy of the use of medication, particularly in a person who may have a limited ability to understand the implications of the treatment, and
3. developing a plan that includes medications as one part of an overall treatment strategy.

The specific medications used to treat specific mental health conditions are discussed in the chapters on those disorders (Chapters 14 to 23). Addendum 1 lists classes of medications, their use, their effects, and side effects.

BRAIN CHEMISTRY AND MENTAL HEALTH

Most medications that are prescribed for mental health conditions have an effect on the chemicals in the brain. For you to understand how these medications work, you need a basic understanding of how brain chemicals or *neurotransmitters* communicate with one another and the specific functions of some of the brain chemicals that play a role in certain mental health disorders.

NEUROTRANSMITTERS

Our central nervous system (brain and spinal cord) and peripheral nervous system (nerves outside the brain and spinal cord) contain millions of microscopic nerve cells called neurons. When a nerve cell is stimulated, a small electrical current is generated at one end. This current travels along the nerve cell. This current must be transferred to the next nerve cell (and then the next and the next) in order to send a signal from one part of the nervous system to another. The cells are separated by small gaps called synapses. The first cell must send the message to the next cell and this is done through chemicals. The electrical signal causes the release of a chemical that crosses the synapse and causes an electrical change in the next cell. The signal is carried along the next cell and then crosses the next synapse until it reaches its destination. For example, if you want to move your left arm, an electrical change occurs in the nerve cells in the part of the brain that controls left arm movement. The signal passes along cells and across synapses until it reaches the left arm, where the electrical signal has an effect on the muscles in the left arm, causing the appropriate, desired movement.

Neurotransmitters are the chemicals that the brain (and peripheral nervous system) uses to communicate from one nerve cell to another. A neurotransmitter is released from the sending (*efferent*) end of the first cell, crosses the microscopic space between the cells (the *synapse*), and then attaches or "binds" to the receiving (*afferent*) end of the next nerve cell. The neurotransmitter binds to a receptor on the second cell. The act of binding causes the small electrical change to occur. Depending on the cell, the receptor, and the neurotransmitter, the effect of the electrical charge may be:

1. **excitatory;** it excites the cell (increases activity in the cell) or
2. **inhibitory;** it inhibits the cell (decreases activity in the cell).

Again, depending on the cell, the receptor, and the neurotransmitter, the effect may be rapid or slow. After the neurotransmitter binds to the cell and causes the change in the cell's electrical activity, the neurotransmitter is broken down by other chemicals or reabsorbed. This stops the electrical change and the cell can prepare for another message from the adjoining cell(s).

After the neurotransmitter has been bound to the next cell for a short time, often the effect of the binding stops. Therefore, if the neurotransmitter is not broken down, the receiving cell cannot "reload" electrically to get ready to fire again when another molecule of the neurotransmitter binds to its receptor. If the neurotransmitter is not removed or broken down, additional neurotransmitter does not have any additional effect on the nerve cell.

Medications can be used to change this process at any of the steps or sites. Medications can affect the neurotransmitter level between the cells by increasing or decreasing the release of the neurotransmitter or the breakdown of the neurotransmitter. The sensitivity of the receptor of the cell receiving the message can also be affected. If the receptor is made more sensitive, then either less neurotransmitter is required to obtain the same effect in the cell or the same amount of neurotransmitter has greater effect. In addition, if the receptor binds the neurotransmitter more tightly, the neurotransmitter cannot be released. If it is not released, more neurotransmitter cannot bind or cause the electrical change. This reduces the passage of the next signal from the first cell.

TYPES OF NEUROTRANSMITTERS

There are several types of neurotransmitters in the brain. Each has one or more functions. The function is determined by the part of the brain the cell is in, the amount of the neurotransmitter in that area of the brain, the relationship to the other neurotransmitters in the brain, the type of receptors, and other factors. All these issues complicate the use of medications.

Below are the neurotransmitters that play a role in some of the most common mental health disorders. Although it is difficult to directly measure the level and activity of neurotransmitters in the brain, researchers have deduced that many mental health disorders are caused either by deficiencies or excesses of one or more of these brain chemicals.

Glutamic Acid. Glutamic acid (glutamate) is the most common neurotransmitter in the brain. It is excitatory. It appears to play a role in learning and memory. One glutamic receptor is called the NMDA (N-Methyl-D-Aspartate) receptor.

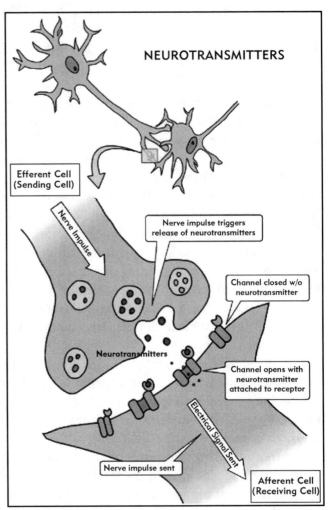

Excess glutamic acid binding to the NMDA receptor can cause toxicity and destruction of neurons (nerve cells) in such diseases as Alzheimer disease.

Gamma Amino Butyric Acid. Gamma amino butyric acid (GABA) is an inhibitory neurotransmitter. It is the second most common neurotransmitter and the most common inhibitory transmitter in the brain. It reduces signals in the brain and thus helps prevent overstimulation of the brain. It appears to have an anti-seizure effect and calming effect on the brain. Unlike many other neurotransmitters, GABA is not reabsorbed into the neuron that released it but instead is transported into specialized cells (*astrocytes*) that surround the neurons. Just as with other neurotransmitters, the effect is to remove GABA from the synapse, which prepares the cell to bind with another molecule of GABA.

Acetylcholine. Acetylcholine is the main neurotransmitter in the peripheral nervous system, but there are relatively few acetylcholine (cholinergic) receptors in the brain. It is usually an excitatory neurotransmitter. It is the main neurotransmitter controlling skeletal muscles, so it is needed for making most voluntary movements. It is also used by part of the nervous system (parasympathetic nervous system) that controls involuntary functions (bowel and bladder function, digestion, etc). (Norepinephrine is the other neurotransmitter used in the peripheral nervous system and is described below.) An enzyme called acetylcholinesterase breaks down acetylcholine. Blocking this enzyme with medications results in a greater effect of acetylcholine. Despite its presence in small amounts in the brain, the neurons with acetylcholine play an important role in Alzheimer disease. The destruction of these nerve cells in certain parts of the brain are instrumental in the development of some of the symptoms seen in AD.

Dopamine. Dopamine is an inhibitory neurotransmitter that, paradoxically, produces arousal. The reason that this inhibitory neurotransmitter causes arousal is because the receiving cells are inhibitory themselves. When dopamine inhibits an inhibitory cell, the net result is excitation or arousal. Depending on the location of the cells, dopamine facilitates the body's posture, the speed that muscles move, attention, and feelings of pleasure.

Norepinephrine. Norepinephrine is also known as noradrenaline. Like acetylcholine, it is found in both the peripheral nervous system and the brain. It is synthesized from dopamine, so levels of norepinephrine in the brain are directly linked to levels of dopamine. If dopamine is increased, norepinephrine will increase; if dopamine is decreased, norepinephrine will decrease. So, it's important to keep this in mind when prescribing a drug that increases dopamine. Like dopamine, norepinephrine is an inhibitory neurotransmitter that causes arousal. In the part of the brain where over 40 percent of the neurons that contain norepinephrine are found, electrical stimulation causes increased arousal and attention. This area of the brain has been identified as the pleasure center. Both norepinephrine and dopamine play a role in attention, arousal, and feelings of pleasure. With higher levels of norepinephrine, anxiety can result. Conversely, norepinephrine is lower during sleep.

Serotonin. Most of the serotonin in the body is found outside the brain, primarily in the blood. However, the small amount in the brain plays a large role in mental health. Serotonin is synthesized from the amino acid tryptophan. Serotonin can make a person drowsy. Eating a meal that contains a large amount of tryptophan can cause drowsiness because it is converted to serotonin in the brain. (This may be part of the reason we feel sleepy after eating turkey, which has a large amount of tryptophan.) Serotonin is used to synthesize melatonin in the part of the brain called the pineal gland. Melatonin, in turn, plays an important role in regulating diurnal patterns of sleep. Serotonin also plays a role in pain perception and in mood.

Low serotonin levels play a role in anxiety, impulsive (and violent) behavior, and depression. Aggressive behavior has also been linked to low serotonin levels.

Endorphins. Endorphins are inhibitory neurotransmitters that reduce pain and can give a sense of euphoria. This sense of euphoria may be what leads some people to seek out self-injury. Because when you hurt yourself, endorphins increase to reduce the pain, the increased endorphins can be pleasurable to some people. Opiate drugs such as morphine, codeine, and other narcotics work by binding to these receptor sites.

BRAIN CHEMISTRY IN PEOPLE WITH DOWN SYNDROME

There are differences in neurotransmitters and brain structure in people with Down syndrome. Some of these differences mean that people with Down syndrome may be at increased risk for mental health conditions linked to particular neurotransmitter abnormalities. That is, there are biochemical reasons for some of the cognitive, emotional, and behavioral difficulties that can be issues for people with Down syndrome. In addition, people with DS have fewer nerve cells in their brain than usual, as well as fewer connections between the nerve cells in their brain. This means there are fewer nerve cells to produce neurotransmitters, and fewer places for the brain chemicals that are produced to bind. This is more evident in some parts of the brain than others; therefore, the amounts of some neurotransmitters are affected more than others.

For example, researchers have found that aspartate, glutamate (glutamic acid), norepinephrine, and dopamine are all decreased in the parahippocampal gyrus (temporal lobe) of adults with DS. The temporal lobe plays an important part in processing auditory and visual stimuli and in memory. However, these neurotransmitters are not decreased in the frontal lobe. The frontal lobes are considered the emotional control center and the center of our personality. The frontal lobes are also involved in motor function and problem solving. Memory, language, impulse control, and sexual behavior are all controlled by the frontal lobes (Risser et al., 1997). Furthermore, adults with Down syndrome have been found to have increased SERT (serotonin transporter) in their brains. SERT is part of the serotonin system that regulates the level of serotonin in the brain. This could contribute to serotonin dysfunction/deficit (Engidawork and Lubec, 2001). It is clear from these findings that the brain is a very complicated system. In addition, there are a number of differences in the brains of people with Down syndrome that are being studied on an ongoing basis.

Imbalances of neurotransmitters are involved in a number of mental health conditions. We say "involved" rather than "the cause" because more than one factor is thought to be involved in causing most of these disorders. For example, depression is believed to be connected with deficiencies in serotonin and the sensitivity of serotonin receptors. We also know that it can be related to life events. So, if a person with Down syndrome has reduced levels of certain neurotransmitters as a result of having DS, he may be more susceptible to disorders that are linked to deficiencies of those neurotransmitters or imbalances between those and other neurotransmitters.

In addition, people with Down syndrome have differences in the neurotransmitter receptor proteins. The receptor proteins are the parts of the receptor where the neurotransmitter attaches. The different receptors may be more or less able to bind to the different neurotransmitters in people with DS. For example, later in life there is a decrease in cholineacetyl transferase. This may be related to cholinergic impairment seen in later life associated with Alzheimer disease. However, there is also an increase of metabotropic glutamate receptor 5, which may have a protective role for the brains of people with Down syndrome. There is a complex interaction between neurotransmitters, receptors, and other enzymes that promote mental health or contribute to mental illness.

The next section briefly reviews how neurotransmitter abnormalities play a role in several common mental health disorders, with special reference to the neurotransmitters that are known or believed to be affected by Down syndrome.

NEUROTRANSMITTERS IN DISEASES AND CONDITIONS

DEPRESSION

The role of neurotransmitters in depression has not been completely delineated. It has been hypothesized that an imbalance of serotonin, norepinephrine, and dopamine plays a role. This is based largely on the fact that changing the level of these neurotransmitters with medications can successfully treat depression. Another clue is that contraceptives with high levels of estrogen can cause depression, apparently by lowering serotonin levels in the brain.

As discussed in Chapter 14, depression is one of the most common mental health concerns among the adolescents and adults we see at the Adult Down Syndrome Center. The reasons are complex, as explained in the chapter, but reduced levels of these neurotransmitters in the brain probably play a role for at least some individuals with DS and depression.

One class of medications that can effectively treat depression is the tricyclic antidepressants. Some medications in this class increase norepinephrine by inhibiting its reuptake. Others affect both norepinephrine and serotonin. It is interesting to note that while the medications immediately increase the neurotransmitters, it may take several weeks for the person to become less depressed. The antidepressant effect may actually come from a modification of the receptors that occurs over time, rather than the more immediate effect on the level of the neurotransmitter.

A newer class of medications, the selective serotonin reuptake inhibitors (SSRIs), can be part of a successful treatment plan for depression. The SSRIs reduce the reuptake of serotonin back into the first (efferent) cell. The net effect is to increase the serotonin in the synapse. Similar to the tricyclic antidepressants, the effect on the level of serotonin is rather immediate, but the effect on depression can be delayed. This suggests a possible role of the medications in modifying the receptors. We sometimes see a brief (and unexpected) improvement in the first few days, followed by a return of the symptoms. Then a few weeks later, the expected improvement occurs. This may reflect the initial effect on the level of serotonin and later the effect on the receptors.

The atypical antidepressants such as bupropion (Wellbutrin) affect serotonin, norepinephrine, and/or dopamine levels. In some individuals, the effect on multiple neurotransmitters causes more benefit than the effect on one alone. However, sometimes it also brings greater side effects. Some of the SSRIs also appear to affect norepinephrine.

See Chapter 14 for more information about medical treatments for depression. In addition, the Addendum at the back of the book categorizes all the medications discussed in this book according to class, action on brain chemicals, uses, etc.

ANXIETY

People with anxiety disorders are thought to have imbalances of the neurotransmitters norepinephrine, serotonin, and GABA. Cholecystokinin may also play a role. Since people with Down syndrome tend to have abnormal levels of norepinephrine and serotonin in their brains, it makes sense that anxiety disorders are fairly common in people with DS.

As discussed in Chapter 15, there are several types/classes of medications that can help normalize the levels of these neurotransmitters, often reducing anxiety. The benzodiazepines, such as diazepam (Valium), work to increase the inhibitory effect of GABA, which decreases neuron activity (reducing anxiety) and also reduces the release of norepinephrine. The selective serotonin reuptake inhibitors (SSRIs) such as paroxetine (Paxil) increase serotonin, which can also reduce anxiety.

ALZHEIMER DISEASE

Alzheimer disease results in changes in a number of neurotransmitters, as well as other changes. Although we still do not understand completely what causes the disease, research indicates that excess glutamic acid overexcites the NMDA receptors and can lead to toxicity and neuron destruction. There is also a reduction in neurons that use norepinephrine and serotonin. In addition, cells that use the neurotransmitter acetylcholine are also affected. Agents that block the effect of acetylcholine in the brain result in memory loss for normal individuals. In people with Alzheimer disease, there is a reduction in neurons in an area of the brain called Meynert's nucleus. The reduction of these cells, which use acetylcholine, may play a role in memory loss in

Alzheimer disease. Clearly, Alzheimer disease has a complicated effect on the brain and we still have a limited understanding of its causes.

The medications donepezil (Aricept), tacrine (Cognex), galantamine (Reminyl), and rivastigmine (Exelon) are cholinesterase inhibitors. They block the enzyme that breaks down acetylcholine. By blocking this enzyme, the acetylcholine remains active longer, which improves the function of the cells that use acetylcholine. This does not cure or change the course of Alzheimer disease, but it can temporarily improve the cognitive function of some people with AD.

Memantine (Namenda) blocks NMDA receptors. This reduces the overexcitation of the cells and may also slow cell destruction.

Research into Alzheimer Medications and Down Syndrome

Why is there interest in trying Alzheimer's drugs in Down syndrome?

Donepezil (Aricept) has been assessed in a few small studies in people with Down syndrome who don't have Alzheimer disease. Speech skills improved in some of these people. In our small study, donepezil seemed to increase the amount of speaking that the person was capable of, but didn't help articulation. In other words, a few people who ordinarily did not speak much, talked more on the donepezil. Although their articulation did not improve, their increased speech helped them interact with others, make their interests and wants known, etc.

After our study was completed, some of the subjects chose to continue the donepezil. However, we did not notice any clinical benefit for those who had not experienced benefits during the study. For those who had benefited during the study, the benefit faded over several weeks to months, and their speech returned to the level it had been before starting the medication. Further study is being done at this time on a greater number of people with Down syndrome; over time, this study should help determine any possible benefit for people with Down syndrome.

MEDICATIONS FOR PEOPLE WITH DOWN SYNDROME: THE ART AND SCIENCE

Understanding the science of medications, neurotransmitters, brain chemistry, and the particular issues in people with Down syndrome is crucial when prescribing medications for people with Down syndrome who have mental health or behavioral issues. However, the practice of medicine has long been described as both an art and a science. The art of medicine comes into play for a number of reasons: each person is different; medications work differently in different people; different situations demand alternative approaches; and sometimes the expected result is not what occurs.

Some of the questions that need to be answered have more to do with clinical nuances or idiosyncrasies of the patient. Issues we consider include:

1. Whether it is a good idea to try medication;
2. How to involve the patient in the decision as to whether to use medication;
3. Which medication to use and at what dose (which may depend on administration issues, side effects, need for trial and error);
4. How best to monitor medication use and make decisions based on the patient's response (watching for paradoxical effects, deciding when to change or discontinue the medication).

DECIDING WHETHER TO TRY MEDICATION

Once a mental health condition is diagnosed and we recommend considering medication, there are still additional issues to be addressed. In fact, there is a step even before the medication is recommended. The first question is, "Is a medication the correct approach?" Is the behavior part of "normal" or "characteristic" behavior for a person with Down syndrome who is not in need of any treatment but rather just education and/or reassurance? If treatment is needed, is a medication needed at all? Counseling and behavioral approaches are addressed above. Often these approaches can be used in place of medications.

However, sometimes counseling and/or behavior therapy are not enough by themselves. This may be because the condition is "beyond the person's control" or "beyond the control of therapy." For example, the drive to perform an obsessional behavior can be so strong that no amount of counseling or behavioral therapy may be able to overcome it. Counseling may help the person cope with the problem, avoid situations that trigger the obsession, use an alternative behavior to avoid doing the behavior, etc. However, the drive may still be there, and without reducing the drive, the person may not be able to avoid the obsessional behavior. Other times, an adult has a condition that will require medications because of the nature of the problem or the severity of the symptoms. For example, when someone is severely depressed, counseling and behavior therapy may help (and may actually be enough treatment). However, often it is not and medication is required. Also, the severity of the symptoms often necessitates use of medications to get to a healthier place more rapidly and to ease the suffering more quickly.

We generally look at medications as therapy used in addition to counseling and/ or behavioral approaches. Many times we view the medication as helping the person reach a point where he will be able to respond to counseling or behavioral therapy. There are a number of issues that must be addressed once the practitioner reaches the decision to recommend a medication.

INVOLVING THE PATIENT IN THE DECISION TO USE MEDICATION

The first issue to consider before starting an adult with Down syndrome on medication is whether he will consent to treatment with the medication. Addendum

2 is a sample of the consent form that we use. Our approach is to recommend therapy, explain the risks and benefits, and help the person, family, or guardian make a choice that is best for them.

Sometimes people with intellectual disabilities are not able to fully participate in the decision. We make a concerted effort to make the person part of the process, though. If a patient is his own guardian, we obtain the consent from him. In addition, we ask his permission to discuss it with his family. If the patient is not his own guardian, we obtain consent from the family/guardian. We also obtain "assent" when we can from the patient who is not his own guardian. Assent is agreement on the part of the person (with DS) who is not his own guardian and, therefore, cannot legally consent to the medication. While not a legal agreement to take the medication, assent includes the person in the decision and makes him part of the process. He agrees that he understands why we are recommending the medication and he agrees to take it.

Having the person with DS be part of the process is not only (in our opinion) "the right thing to do," but is also critical in achieving clinical success. Although observers can give some indication of benefit and side effects, no one else can give feedback about how the adult feels on the medication. Not all adults with Down syndrome can give this feedback, but it is important to obtain it whenever possible.

Another consideration is whether the person can manage his own medications. There are a number of questions to consider:

1. Has he been able to learn other important tasks that involve regimens that must be followed for potentially dangerous activities (if done incorrectly)?
2. Has he demonstrated that he can do these activities repeatedly?
3. Is he willing and interested in managing his own medications?
4. If he lives in a residential facility, are there policies that would allow or prevent him from managing his own medications?
5. Does he understand why he is taking the medications, the potential for side effects and the need to report them, and the importance of taking them on the prescribed schedule?

If the answer to these questions is yes, the adult may be successful in managing his own medications.

If a patient is resistant to swallowing any medication, we try to avoid "hiding" the medication as much as possible. Again, we want to make the person a partner in the treatment as much as possible. Hiding medication may hinder the relationship between the patient and physician or between the patient and the family (or care provider) who is giving the medication. This may have a deleterious effect on treatment. In addition, we have seen patients become reluctant to eat certain foods (that the medication was put in) or even to eat at all. However, if the problem requires a medication and the guardian consents but the patient doesn't assent, it may be necessary to hide the medication or use other methods to get the person to take the medication.

Legal Guardianship

In most states in the United States, a person is considered legally competent to make his own decisions once he reaches the age of 18. While a family may provide support in a variety of ways, the person is legally able to make independent decisions for himself. This includes making decisions regarding medications. Adults with Down syndrome are considered legally competent, just like anyone else, unless a guardian is appointed for them.

Should we get legal guardianship for our son/daughter? We are frequently asked this question. We are not attorneys and don't provide legal advice, but do discuss some of the issues that families can consider and then direct them to an attorney. The decision to obtain guardianship is technically a legal decision that a judge makes (using information provided by medical professionals) after determining that a person is not legally competent.

We have patients who live very independent lives, have their own bank accounts, pay their bills, and have jobs that provide a livable income. We also have patients who are very dependent on others for much of their care. Many of our patients fit somewhere in between.

In the ideal world, none of our patients would need legal guardianship. Society would recognize that some people need more assistance and would provide it. Unfortunately, there are unscrupulous people who, instead, try to take advantage of adults with Down syndrome—sometimes in financial matters and sometimes in medical situations. We have seen some adults who were put on a medication for a behavioral or mental health condition without their family's knowledge. This may be appropriate if the person with Down syndrome has the ability to understand the issues of concern and the potential benefits and side effects. However, often the person with Down syndrome really had very little, if any, input into the decision.

Having a legal guardian provides a legal safety net to help prevent the person from being treated inappropriately. *However, it may also mean that the adult loses the right to vote or do other things.* There may be alternative approaches to guardianship, including power of attorney for health, or other legal protections.

We recommend exploring issues of independence, safety concerns, and the family situation. There is no one answer that fits all, and an attorney can help the family make the appropriate decision for their situation.

CHOOSING A MEDICATION AND DOSAGE

As discussed in the chapters on specific mental or behavioral disorders, there are often many choices of medications for a given disorder. Sometimes, there are considerations that can help us narrow down which one might be best to try first; other times, there is no way to know for sure which medication will work the best for this person with this condition. In a sense, we must use a trial and error approach to find the best choice(s) for this individual.

For adults with Down syndrome, one important consideration is often whether they can swallow pills and if not, which of the available medications can be used. For example, sometimes we must use pills that can be crushed, capsules that can be opened and sprinkled on food, or medications that come in liquid forms. This may limit or alter the choice.

Another consideration is whether any of the possible medications have side effects that may be especially advantageous for a given patient. For example, sedation can be an unwanted side effect of some medications. However, for people who are having sleep disturbance as part of their symptoms, this side effect can be an advantage. For instance:

> *Thanh, 26, lives at home with her father. Her mother died a year earlier and in the last several months she has displayed symptoms of depression. In addition to waking during the night, she was having trouble falling asleep. When we prescribed an antidepressant for her, we chose sertraline (Zoloft), which has caused sedation in some of our patients, and had her take it in the evening. Within a few days, Thanh began to fall asleep more readily. As the full antidepressant effect was realized over the next few weeks, her other symptoms improved, including her waking during the night.*

Further discussion regarding using side effects to advantage is included in the chapters on specific conditions.

Finally, as unscientific and as bothersome as it may seem at times, there may be a certain amount of trial and error in prescribing medications for individuals. While there are guidelines for adults with DS, because different people respond differently, what works for the majority may not be what works for the particular individual. Although a solitary medication works for most, a combination may be necessary for the individual who is being treated. One medication in a class of medications may not work for an individual but another in the same class that is very similar may work very well.

> *Warren, a 42-year-old with bipolar illness, responded very well to a combination of ziprasidone (Geodon) and carbamazepine (Tegretol). This combination was reached only after a number of unsuccessful treatments. He had a reaction of tardive dyskinesia (abnormal facial movement) to multiple other similar anti-psychotic medications. Once on ziprasidone (Geodon), he had an increase (although not to the previous level) of agitation. The addition of carbamazepine (Tegretol) helped tremendously.*

Finding the right dose of the medication is also critical. If there is a general rule we follow, it is "start low and go slow." By that we mean start at a low dose and work slowly to higher doses. A number of other factors, however, also guide dosing the medication, including severity of symptoms, age of the patient, size of the patient, other health problems, previous reaction to medications, family history of medication effects, and others. Some medications have standards for appropriate blood levels and, therefore, blood tests can guide dosing.

Another rule is to increase a medication to maximum dose (if additional benefit is being gained with increasing the dose) or until intolerable side effects occur before adding additional medications. We generally try to avoid using multiple medications at lower doses because this often increases side effects without getting clear therapeutic benefit from any of the medications. Occasionally, however, we find that a person with DS cannot tolerate a larger dose of any medication but will respond to a certain combination of medications at lower doses. Dosing specifics will be addressed as medications are addressed in the following chapters about specific conditions.

It is important to assess the use and the dose of the medication on an ongoing basis. Is the medication still needed? Is it a condition that, once adequately treated, is unlikely to recur when the medication is stopped? For example, someone who develops depression in response to a traumatic event and who has never had depression before might be successfully weaned off the medication after a period of time.

In addition, as people get older, go through puberty, through menopause, lose weight, gain weight, take other medications, and other changes, the needed dose may change. Sometimes symptoms increase. Other times an increase in side effects will be the indicator that the dose needs to be changed.

Another reason to assess the dosage on an ongoing basis is to ensure that we are maximizing benefit and minimizing side effects. Decisions to change the dosage in this case are made in discussion with the person with DS and his family. For example, if the patient is 95 percent improved, we will consider increasing the medication but only after we discuss the potential for greater side effects that may impede the patent's recovery (and potentially reduce the net effectiveness of the medication) versus the potential for continued improvement in the condition.

MONITORING MEDICATION EFFECTS AND USAGE

Because some people with Down syndrome have difficulty accurately reporting how a medication makes them feel, it is important to plan at the outset how to monitor the medication's effects. For example, monitoring might be done by tracking behaviors before and after the medication is started through a checklist or by writing symptoms down, or by observing the patient for ourselves, in the office or at home, work, or school (see Chapter 12).

When first beginning a medication, it is important to watch for "paradoxical reactions"—or reactions that are the opposite of what is expected. For example, sometimes people become more depressed when they take an antidepressant. Some people become more agitated and anxious when taking one of the anti-anxiety benzodiazepine medications. It can be very difficult at times to determine whether the problem is that the condition or behavior is worsening or that it is a side effect of the medication. At times, the only choice is to discontinue the medication. We will sometimes later reintroduce the medication to see if it appears more likely that the change is a side effect of the medication.

Monitoring is also vital if any changes are made in dose, time of administration, etc. In a sense, we have found that "any change is a change." Another way to say this is that "even a good change is a change." We have seen a number of patients who had an initial negative reaction to changing the dose, time of day taken, or adding or subtracting another medication. For these patients, the behavior or condition may temporarily worsen for a few days, a week, or sometimes more. After this initial phase passes, however, the change is positive. Whether we have the time to "wait out" the change depends on the medication, the severity of the symptoms, and the effect it is having on others.

For some patients, it is necessary to confirm that the medication has been swallowed:

Kyle, 24, was doing very well with his treatment regimen for several months. Then his original symptoms unexpectedly returned. After a few medication changes failed to improve his symptoms, his mother solved the problem with a watchful eye when vacuuming. She looked into the heating vent in the floor of their living room and discovered a pile of Kyle's medication. The medication showed signs of being slightly dissolved (from a brief stay in Kyle's mouth) but was essentially intact. The previously successful treatment regimen was restarted, with Kyle's mother now confirming the pills were swallowed, and Kyle returned to good health.

Finally, it is important to monitor for potential long-term side effects. It is especially important to monitor for:

1. *Downregulation*—in which the neurotransmitter receptors adapt to the medication so that their sensitivity or number is reduced. This results in "tolerance" and the need for a larger dose to produce the same clinical effect.
2. *Upregulation*—in which the receptors become more sensitive to the medication so that a smaller dose is needed to produce the same effect.

When upregulation or downregulation have occurred, there may also be effects when the medication is discontinued. This is because when the medication is removed (particularly suddenly), the receptors don't immediately return to their previous number or sensitivity. So, for example, if a benzodiazepine has caused downregulation, the brain has fewer or less sensitive receptors for GABA, which ordinarily inhibits anxiety. If the medication is stopped, increased anxiety can occur until the receptors regain their usual sensitivity to GABA. The increased anxiety and other symptoms that occur are withdrawal. The effects of tolerance and withdrawal demonstrate dependence on the medication.

While not generally considered withdrawal in the standard sense (as noted above), when some people stop taking SSRIs they have a withdrawal-like reaction. These medications should be weaned instead of stopped "cold turkey."

QUESTIONS TO ASK THE DOCTOR

If you are a parent or caregiver of an adolescent or adult with Down syndrome, make sure you understand what to watch for *before* a medication is started. Ask the doctor:

1. What the common side effects are;
2. Whether you should call him/her immediately if any particular effect occurs;
3. Whether it is OK to discontinue the medication if an adverse reaction occurs;
4. Whether the medication should be taken at a certain time of day, spaced apart from other doses in a specific timeframe, taken with or apart from other medications, or taken with or apart from food or drink.

CONCLUSION

In subsequent chapters, the principles outlined in this chapter are discussed as to how they are applied to specific mental health problems. For each problem, assessment (and often reassessment), the use of specific medications, counseling, and other therapies, and an assessment for contributing (or causative) physical problems are described. Wherever possible, we provide examples of ways in which medications benefited patients with Down syndrome we have treated.

Chapter 14

Mood Disorders

* * * * * * * * * * * * * *

Mood disorders are very common in our society in general. Depression, the most frequently diagnosed mood disorder, affects about 9.5 percent of American adults per year and about 20 percent at some time in their lives (Yapko, 1997). Not surprisingly, mood disorders are also common in adults with Down syndrome. In fact, depression is the most commonly diagnosed mental illness at the Adult Down Syndrome Center. In the 13 years of the Center's existence, approximately 18 percent of our patients have been diagnosed with depression. As we track our patients over their lifetimes, that number is expected to exceed the lifetime rate of 20 percent for the general population. Because of the frequency of this condition, this chapter will discuss in some detail the various causes and manifestations of depression in people with Down syndrome.

Bipolar disorder and mania are two other types of mood disorders that occur far less frequently than depression in people with Down syndrome. Bipolar disorder is characterized by periods of depression alternating with periods of mania. This chapter will discuss bipolar disorder at some length because the symptoms can be very severe and debilitating. It also takes a look at mania, which may also be severe, but is fairly rare in adults with Down syndrome.

WHAT IS DEPRESSION?

* * * * * * * * * * * * * * * * *

Depression is a primary mood disorder that is characterized by a sad mood and/or a decreased interest in things the person previously enjoyed. As described below, there may be several accompanying symptoms. These symptoms, as well as the persistent nature of the problem, differentiate depression from merely feeling blue or sad. A major depressive episode lasts at least two weeks. A related diagnosis is dysthymic disorder, which is characterized by at least two years of depressed mood for more days than not, but the change in mood and effect on the individual is less than with depression.

WHAT ARE THE SYMPTOMS OF DEPRESSION?

In the United States, depression is usually diagnosed by comparing a person's symptoms against the diagnostic criteria for depression listed in the *Diagnostic and Statistical Manual of Mental Disorders, Fourth Edition, Text Revision* (DSM-IV-TR) of the American Psychiatric Association. This manual lists the "official" criteria used for diagnosing all "mental disorders." DSM-IV-TR includes conditions traditionally considered mental illnesses, such as depression, obsessive-compulsive disorder, schizophrenia, and others. It also includes criteria for other conditions, including mental retardation, learning disorders, substance abuse, dementia, tic disorders, and others.

The diagnostic criteria listed in the DSM-IV-TR rely heavily on the self-report of subjective feelings. For instance, feeling sad or worthless (and articulating those feelings) are considered important symptoms of depression according to the DSM-IV-TR. Only rarely, however, do we hear these complaints from adults with Down syndrome who actually *are* depressed.

Table 14-1: Symptoms of Major Depression in Adults with Down Syndrome

DSM-IV Symptoms of Depression	Percentage
Sadness or unhappiness (also described as loss of liveliness, humor, or spontaneity)	100%
Apathy, loss of interest/participation in activities, including withdrawal from family and friends	100%
Psychomotor retardation (activity slowdown)	83%
Loss of energy or overly fatigued	78%
Increase in irritated mood or moodiness	78%
Loss of focus, concentration, or task completion	74%
Loss of self-care or independent skills	71%
Noticeable change in sleeping habits; less/more	71%
Noticeable change in eating habits; less/more	65%
Psychomotor agitation (for example, aggressive behavior or difficulty with sitting calmly)	63%
Self-absorbed, inattentive, or unresponsive (to people/things)	63%
Psychotic features (extreme withdrawal, hallucinatory self-talk, etc.)	57%
Inappropriate fears or avoidances of people/things	47%

The most common symptoms in 98 people with Down syndrome diagnosed with major depression at the Adult Center are outlined in Table 14-1. This sample included people in their 20s to people in their 60s.

If the symptoms described in Table 14-1 last more than a few weeks, further assessment is recommended.

In addition, other disorders may occur concurrently with depression. These are called "co-morbid" disorders. For example, an anxiety and obsessive compulsive disorder may occur along with depression. Many medical conditions may also be considered co-morbid (see Chapter 2 and below for more on this). Behavior disorders (Chapter 19) and psychotic features (Chapter 17) can also accompany depression.

Psychotic features are fairly common and involve symptoms which may appear very odd and may make the person appear to be out of touch with reality. These symptoms may include agitated or hallucinatory-like self-talk, extreme withdrawal, and self-absorption. These symptoms are rarely an indication of a true psychosis, which is why they are called psychotic "features." Not surprisingly, these types of symptoms are also more common in children in the general population who have depression. For both groups, the line between fact and fantasy is often blurred, which may result in more odd-appearing symptoms. Additionally, depression may be more debilitating for people with DS and for children. This explains why they are more likely to demonstrate severe withdrawal and self-absorption. This often serves as a protective mechanism so as to conserve their own life and energy.

In a sample of 130 people diagnosed with symptoms of major depression at the Adult Down Syndrome Center, co-morbid disorders were present for 93 people representing 77 percent of the total sample. See Table 14-2 for data.

Table 14-2: Major Depression and Co-morbid Disorders

	Number	Percent
Major Depression (MD), no co-morbid disorder	27 people	21% of sample
MD and medical conditions	33	25%
MD and obsessive-compulsive disorder	24	18.5%
MD and anxiety disorder	22	17%
MD and psychotic-features	19	14.5%
MD and behavior disorder	5	4%
Total MD and all co-morbid disorder	130	100%

DIAGNOSIS

In people without cognitive disabilities, depression is primarily diagnosed through a face-to-face interview with a mental health professional. A physical exam, laboratory tests, and history from others may provide additional information.

The diagnosis of depression may be more complicated for people with Down syndrome. As described in Chapter 12, the impairment of verbal skills, conceptual thinking, and overall cognitive functioning presents challenges in obtaining the appropriate history from the patient. Thus, there is a greater reliance on the report of family and/or care providers. This adds a level of interpretation of symptoms and can lead to under- and over-reporting of symptoms. Added to this, people with DS may have some symptoms that appear more severe than they are. Like children, they may have some difficulty with distinguishing between fact and fantasy, particularly when they are experiencing other symptoms of depression. For example, as mentioned above, hallucinatory-like self-talk, skill loss, or extreme withdrawal can be symptoms of depression for people with Down syndrome. If these symptoms are overemphasized, while other symptoms are missed or underemphasized, the person may be misdiagnosed with a primary psychotic disorder. This may result in the inappropriate use of a medication for psychosis.

As discussed in Chapter 12, these limitations often make it necessary for the person making the diagnosis to do some observation of his own. Sometimes there is no better information than what we obtain by viewing and/or being with the person in her home or work setting. In addition, having the person draw how she is feeling may reveal important information. Through a trial of counseling, the person may also learn how to articulate feelings better.

CAUSES OF DEPRESSION

In people with Down syndrome, as in everyone else, three general factors can contribute to the development of depression:
1. social and environmental stress;
2. physical differences or changes within the brain;
3. medical problems.

STRESS

Examples of stress that can lead to depression include:
- personal losses (such as the death of a parent, or the loss of a sibling's company when she moves out of state);
- environmental stress (such as a problem at work that the person finds stressful);
- changes in care providers.

Previous chapters address many issues that are important for mental health promotion. A change in, or loss of, any of these positive, healthy aspects of a person's life may contribute to depression.

Understanding how social and environmental stress can lead to depression can be useful in reaching a diagnosis. Looking for potential contributing social factors not only helps put the problem in context, but can be very beneficial in developing a treatment plan.

Some people respond with anger and aggressive behavior to stress or loss, but most people with DS respond more passively with depression. They often withdraw from family and friends and from participation in activities they formerly enjoyed. We believe that this more passive response is due to a sense of helplessness that comes with having little control of their lives and relatively few opportunities for solving problems for themselves. Depression may also be a protective mechanism to conserve life and energy, especially if the person feels overwhelmed.

DIFFERENCES WITHIN THE BRAIN

Biochemistry also appears to play a role in depression, at least some of the time. The brain functions much like an electrical system, with the gaps between brain cells bridged by the release of chemicals called neurotransmitters. Depression is thought to be related to a decrease in the neurotransmitter serotonin. In addition, the sensitivity of the receptors of the cells to which serotonin binds also plays a role in depression. What causes the change in the amount of serotonin or sensitivity of the receptors is still being investigated. The neurotransmitters norepinephrine and dopamine may also play a role. The role of genetics, environmental stress, social factors, and other issues may all contribute to these changes.

Studies have suggested that there may be a relative decrease in serotonin in the brains of people with Down syndrome. The role of serotonin and other neurotransmitters, the receptors, and other factors related to neurotransmitters in people with and without Down syndrome are all areas that are still being investigated.

MEDICAL PROBLEMS

Many medical conditions, particularly those that last a long time or are severe, can contribute to depression. The frustration of not feeling well, the changes in routine, the inability to participate in activities, and the discomfort and inconvenience of procedures and tests can all contribute to depression.

Persistent or chronic pain can also be a significant contributor. First, being in pain can be depressing. Second, being frustrated at not being able to communicate one's pain can also contribute to depression. This cycle is further discussed in Chapter 2. However, an issue that bears repeating here is that treating the painful condition and/or the pain is an important aspect of treating the depression. As the pain persists and the depression increases, it can become a chicken and egg situation. Which came first or which is causing or exacerbating the other can be confusing. In truth, deciding on cause and effect is much less important than evaluating and treating both conditions.

In Chapter 2 we discuss in detail the medical problems that most commonly contribute to mental health problems in adults with Down syndrome. Of those disorders, the conditions most likely to cause depression include:

Hypothyroidism (Under-active Thyroid): More than 40 percent of the patients seen at the Adult Down Syndrome Center have hypothyroidism. It is often associated with lethargy, decreased interest in activities, and depressed mood. At times, it can cause a full-blown depression. Hypothyroidism is diagnosed through a blood test.

Treating the hypothyroidism generally has benefit in treating the depression. Sometimes the only treatment needed for the depression is treating the hypothyroidism. If a person is depressed and the hypothyroidism is not treated, treatment for the depression will likely not be completely successful. Conversely, sometimes treatment with thyroid medication is not all that is necessary. In that situation, it may be that the hypothyroidism is not the cause of the depression but only contributing. It is also possible that the hypothyroidism was the initial cause, but now other factors have developed. In either case, additional treatment is needed. This may include counseling, antidepressant medications, and other interventions.

> *Lyle, 35, was seen in his home because he refused to go outside. For the several months preceding the visit, he had refused to get out of bed, even to go to the kitchen to eat or to the bathroom to use the toilet. He was found to have hypothyroidism and was started on appropriate therapy. He became more animated and began to get out of bed. A number of other issues needed to be addressed before further improvement was achieved, but treating his hypothyroidism was a successful first step in his treatment.*

Sleep Apnea: Sleep apnea is defined as a complete cessation of breathing from any cause during sleep, resulting in decreased oxygen in the blood or increased carbon dioxide (a greater increase than would be seen in normal sleep). Sleep apnea can cause depression. It probably has an indirect effect related to persistent fatigue and a direct effect on the brain due to inadequate sleep cycles and oxygen deprivation. The depression may even have psychotic features of hallucinations and delusions. Diagnosis and treatment of apnea are discussed in Chapter 2. Treatment may include weight loss, changing the position of sleep, a mouth appliance, a CPAP or BIPAP machine, or surgery.

Celiac Disease: Celiac disease is caused by sensitivity to gluten, a protein found in wheat, barley, and oats. This sensitivity results in an inflammation in the small intestine, leading to poor absorption of food, vitamins, and minerals. Symptoms may include weight loss, diarrhea, fatigue, and a sense of ill health. Particularly when experienced on a chronic basis, these symptoms can contribute to depression. In addition, the vitamin and mineral deficiencies caused by celiac disease can contribute to depression.

Celiac disease is thought to be more common in people with Down syndrome, perhaps as much as 100 times more common. Particularly since the symptoms can be subtle and people with Down syndrome may have difficulty describing their sense of poor health, celiac disease should be considered when a person is depressed.

> *Alberto, 27, came to the ADSC with chronic dysthymia (sadness). While he did not have full-blown depression, he seemed unhappy, fatigued, and reluctant to participate in activities. He was also known to need iron supplementation to treat and prevent iron deficiency anemia. In addition, he had a history of recurrent, crampy abdominal pain. After the diagnosis of celiac disease was made and a gluten-free diet was started, Alberto's abdominal pain decreased, he no longer needed iron supplementation, and his mood remarkably improved. His fatigue and reluctance to participate in activities gradually improved as well. He required no further treatment and "returned to his previous self."*

Vitamin B12 Deficiency: Vitamin B12 deficiency can contribute to depression. It seems to be more common in people with Down syndrome, perhaps due in part to celiac disease. A blood test for Vitamin B12 deficiency is recommended when a person has depression. Treatment may consist of increasing B12 in the diet (through vitamins or dietary changes), treatment of the cause of poor absorption of B12 (such as celiac disease), or regular B12 injections.

Vision or Hearing Impairment: Impaired senses can also cause depression. Impaired hearing and impaired sight can be significant challenges for anyone. If someone has a reduced intellectual ability to compensate for the loss, it can be particularly problematic. The challenge may be more than some people can manage, and this can lead to depression. If the problem is correctable, direct treatment of the impaired sense is clearly part of the treatment of the depression. When not correctable, treatment consists of optimizing the function of the sense as well as teaching compensatory mechanisms. Often antidepressant medications are also necessary.

TREATMENT

In addition to pinpointing possible medical problems that cause depression and providing medical treatment for them, a variety of other strategies are also used to treat depression. They include:
1. counseling (see Chapter 13);
2. identifying and reducing stress (discussed throughout the book, and especially in Chapter 11);
3. medication (see below); and
4. encouraging participation in affirming activities and exercise.

MEDICATIONS

We have found that medications can be useful in treating depression in adolescents and adults with Down syndrome. The goal of prescribing medications is not only to improve the depression but also to help the person be more responsive to the other treatments. Generally, the other treatment methods described above are also beneficial.

In choosing an antidepressant medication, both the effects and potential side effects must be considered. If several medications are equally effective, generally, the medication with the lowest potential for side effects will be chosen. However, in some situations, a potential side effect may be an asset and, therefore, the medication with that side effect might be chosen. For example, a medication that is sometimes sedating might be helpful for someone who is having difficulty getting to sleep.

The antidepressant medications can be quite effective. It often takes several weeks, though, to see the effect of starting the medication or increasing the dose.

Antidepressants can basically be separated into three classes:

1. tri-cyclic antidepressants,
2. selective serotonin reuptake inhibitors, and
3. antidepressants not specified.

TRI-CYCLIC ANTIDEPRESSANTS

Tri-cyclic antidepressants were the first medications specifically developed to treat depression. Examples include amitriptyline and nortriptyline.

These medications are often quite effective. However, their side effects can be problematic. Particularly of note are the anti-cholinergic side effects. Anti-cholinergic side effects are caused when the effects of choline, a neurotransmitter, are blocked in the peripheral nervous system or the brain. Choline plays a large role in the autonomic nervous system (control of body functions that do not require conscious thought such as heart rate) and skeletal muscles. Anti-cholinergic side effects include dry mouth, constipation, urinary problems, dizziness, low blood pressure, and others. People with Down syndrome tend to be particularly sensitive to these side effects. Therefore, we use these medications less frequently.

Some tri-cyclic antidepressants tend to be sedating. This side effect can be used to an advantage if difficulty sleeping is one of the symptoms of the depression. Using these medications in the evening or at bedtime can promote improved sleep. We have found doxepin (Sinequan®) and amitriptyline (Elavil®) to be particularly sedating and potentially helpful. However, the anti-cholinergic side effects often outweigh the benefit, so we do not use them frequently.

SELECTIVE SEROTONIN REUPTAKE INHIBITORS (SSRIs)

As discussed in Chapter 13, selective serotonin reuptake inhibitors (SSRIs) work by slowing down or blocking the re-uptake (recycling) of the neurotransmitter serotonin in the brain. Since depressed people are thought to have insufficient serotonin, using these medications to increase the availability of serotonin in the brain can be effective in reducing symptoms of depression.

In our experience, the SSRIs citalopram (Celexa®), escitalopram (Lexapro®), paroxetine (Paxil®), fluoxetine (Prozac®), and sertraline (Zoloft®) are all effective in improving the symptoms of depression. Fluvoxamine (Luvox®), another SSRI, does not have an FDA indication for depression (it is indicated for obsessive-compulsive disorder) and we have not found it to be particularly helpful for depression. As explained in Chapter 13, the choice of medication is determined by the expected benefit, the side effect profile (using side effects as an advantage or avoiding medications that tend to have certain side effects), and by individual issues (for example, a liquid is preferable if the person cannot swallow pills).

We have found that SSRIs tend to have fewer side effects for our patients than the tri-cyclic antidepressants. They are not without side effects, however. Common side effects are listed in Addendum 1 at the back of this book.

Some of our patients with DS have developed agitation apparently as a side effect to these medications. It seems to be most common with fluoxetine (Prozac), and, therefore, we tend to use it less frequently. With fluoxetine, the agitation is often delayed several weeks or even a few months. We have also seen agitation with paroxetine (Paxil®), but it tends to occur earlier, within a few weeks of starting the medication or of increasing the dose. In our experience, agitation occurs less frequently with citalopram (Celexa®), escitalopram (Lexapro®), and sertraline (Zoloft®).

Sedation can be a side effect with these medications. Alternatively, these medications may make some people more awake. There doesn't seem to be any clear pattern as to who will have which side effect or which medication causes which side effect in any given individual. A trial of the medication seems to be the only way to determine whether someone will have either of these side effects. Interestingly, despite the similarity of the medications, a person may not tolerate one of the medications because of these side effects but may tolerate another one.

Weight gain and increased appetite can also be side effects of SSRIs. Paroxetine (Paxil®) is the SSRI that most often seems to have this effect on our patients with Down syndrome. While this can be a detriment for some patients, for those who have a decreased appetite as part of their depression, the weight gain side effect can be a huge benefit.

In the general population, increased suicide risk has been described as a potential side effect of these medications. We have not observed this side effect in people with Down syndrome. In fact, while we have occasionally heard patients discuss thoughts of suicide, actual suicide attempts are not common in people with Down syndrome.

Another aspect of treatment with SSRIs is the need to wean the medications when they are discontinued instead of abruptly stopping them. For some individuals, there appears to be a withdrawal-type phenomenon when discontinuing the medications.

OTHER ANTIDEPRESSANTS

In addition to SSRIs and tri-cyclic antidepressants, other medications are sometimes used to treat depression. They do not fit neatly into one category because they act on a variety of neurotransmitters. We have found medication in this third category of antidepressants to also be effective for adults with DS. Often they have contributed to improvement when there were additional issues besides depression to be addressed.

Bupropion (Wellbutrin®) is an antidepressant that increases serotonin, norephinephrine, and dopamine. It can be a good antidepressant and seems to help some people lose weight. When an increased appetite or weight gain are part of the depression, Wellbutrin can be of particular benefit.

Venlafaxine (Effexor®) is believed to work by increasing norephinephrine, serotonin, and dopamine. We have found it to have benefit particularly when the person has a reduced activity level (psychomotor retardation). The effect of venlafaxine on norepinephrine reuptake seems to give some patients a "boost" in their activity or motivation. This effect usually requires higher doses of the medication.

Trazodone (Desyrel®) is an antidepressant that also has an FDA indication for insomnia. We have not found it to be particularly beneficial for treating depression in adults with Down syndrome. However, we have found it to be a useful additional medication when there is difficulty sleeping. Trazodone has a nice sedation side effect that can be used to advantage by prescribing at bedtime only. As the depression improves with other treatment, the trazodone can often be weaned.

Mirtazapine (Remeron®) and duloxetine (Cymbalta®) are other drugs in this class that are approved for treating depression. We have not used these medications often enough to comment on them.

TREATMENT DURATION

We generally treat depression with medications for six to twelve months beyond the time the symptoms resolve. If the symptoms were severe before treatment (for example, aggressive behavior accompanied the depressive symptoms) or there were other difficult circumstances (such as the person refusing to take medication when she is depressed), we consider treating longer or perhaps indefinitely. If depression recurs after the medication is weaned, we also recommend considering treating subsequent episodes longer or indefinitely. Each time a person has a recurrence of symptoms, she is more likely to have another recurrence when the medications are discontinued.

WHEN DEPRESSION ISN'T THE ONLY PROBLEM

As mentioned above, other mental illnesses sometimes accompany depression (so-called "co-morbid conditions.") In these instances, it is often helpful to prescribe a medication to treat the co-morbid condition, in addition to an antidepressant.

ANXIETY

Anxiety often occurs with depression. Several of the antidepressants can also be helpful in treating anxiety (*although only paroxetine and escitalopram have FDA ap-*

proval). However, it may take several weeks to see the anxiety-reducing benefit, just as the antidepressant effect of the medication may take time. Often an individual who has both depression and anxiety is most disturbed by the anxiety. Therefore, it can be beneficial to start an anti-anxiety medication along with the antidepressant. Then, once the person starts to feel the effect of the antidepressant medication, the anti-anxiety medication can be weaned.

In this situation, we generally use a short- or mid-acting benzodiazepine. A benzodiazepine is a medication that reduces anxiety, and, perhaps the most recognized name in the category is Valium® (diazepam). Alprazolam (Xanax®) and lorazepam (Ativan®) have both proven beneficial. Short- and mid-acting benzodiazepines act relatively quickly after they are taken and their effect is relatively short-lived (several hours). These medications reduce anxiety very quickly and the dose can be adjusted every few days. Since these medications cause sedation, the goal is to find the dose that gives the maximum benefit with the least sedation. See Chapter 15 for more information on treating anxiety.

> Drew, a 34-year-old man with Down syndrome, was noted to be withdrawn. He was declining to go to work, having difficulty sleeping, and would get agitated when his mother suggested leaving the house. He could get aggressive against his mother at times. When we met him, these symptoms had been increasing over the previous four to five months. No underlying medical conditions were found.
>
> We treated Drew with sertraline (Zoloft) and alprazolam (Xanax). His anxiety and agitation improved within a few days. Over the next several weeks, his mood also began to improve. The alprazolam was weaned so that his mother only needed to give it to him periodically, if he became agitated or if they were going someplace that tended to make him anxious. The dose of the sertraline was gradually increased over several months until most of Drew's symptoms were gone and he returned almost to his previous level of function. Over the next year, he resumed more of his previous activities and his symptoms continued to improve.

SLEEP DISTURBANCE

Sleep disturbance can also be a part of depression. Antidepressant medications often benefit sleep disturbance, although once again, this benefit may not be seen immediately. As mentioned above, choosing an antidepressant that is more sedating can be helpful. However, sometimes it is beneficial to start a medication that benefits sleep more directly and quickly.

A short-acting benzodiazepine such as alprazolam can be a beneficial sleep aid. Using a shorter-acting benzodiazepine makes it less likely that the person will be sedated or have difficulty arising the next day. As mentioned above, trazodone has been beneficial to a number of our patients as a sleep aid. Another category of sleep agents that have been helpful is those that interact with the GABA-benzodiazepine system. GABA is an inhibitory neurotransmitter and it tends to reduce excitation in the brain. In our experience, zolpidem (Ambien®), zaleplon (Sonata®), and eszopiclone (Lunesta) can be helpful.

In addition, melatonin is beneficial to many of our patients with sleep difficulties. Melatonin is a hormone that is commonly used by travelers to help improve sleep problems associated with travel across time zones (jet lag). We have found melatonin to be a helpful sleep aid both for people with and without depression, although caution is recommended when using it in a person with depression. We generally start with 2 mg at bedtime and increase to 4 mg at bedtime a week or two later if 2 mg is not enough. Further research is needed regarding long-term use, however, before we would recommend using melatonin indefinitely.

PSYCHOTIC SYMPTOMS

Psychotic symptoms are symptoms of hallucinations and delusions. Some people develop psychotic symptoms as part of their depression. In some individuals, it can be difficult to determine which are truly psychotic features and which are features that are commonly seen in people with Down syndrome who have developed depression. For instance, self-talk often increases in people with Down syndrome who are depressed. So, too, can talking to imaginary friends. These can be strategies that help the person with Down syndrome cope or work through her problems. However, they can also be signs of a psychotic process. In addition, symptoms of extreme withdrawal and abnormal thought processes can occur. Often these symptoms will improve with the treatments for depression discussed above.

Sometimes, however, an anti-psychotic medication can be helpful. We have found the newer "atypical" anti-psychotics to be of particular benefit. In addition to treating the psychotic symptoms, they also can improve the depressive symptoms. Risperdone (Risperdal®), olanzapine (Zyprexa®), quetiapine (Seroquel®), and ziprasidone (Geodon®) have all proved beneficial for adults with Down syndrome. Similarly, aripiprazole (Abilify®), which is classified as an "antipsychotic, other," is effective. Unfortunately, though, side effects of these medications such as weight gain, sedation, and elevated blood sugar have been particularly problematic for a number of people we have treated. When side effects occur, careful assessment of the side effects and the benefits for the individual is essential to determine the best course of action.

The older anti-psychotics such as thioridazine (Mellaril®) and haloperidol (Haldol®) can also be beneficial, but we have found that the side effects are even more problematic. Furthermore, these medications don't have the additional benefit of treating the depressive symptoms. A potential side effect of particular concern is tardive dyskinesia (TD), which can also occur with the newer anti-psychotics but seems to be more common with the older ones. Tardive dyskinesia is a neurological syndrome characterized by involuntary and abnormal movements. It can be permanent, even after discontinuing the medication.

In our experience, using an anti-psychotic medication is frequently not necessary, even if an adult has apparent psychotic symptoms. Particularly when the symptoms are self-talk and use of imaginary friends, an antidepressant can often successfully treat the condition. Again, these symptoms may be more coping strategies used by the patient rather than psychotic symptoms.

> *Sally, a 29-year-old woman with Down syndrome, had been talking to herself in an agitated manner for several months. She had previously talked to herself, but in a calm manner in her own room. Now she was talking to herself in many locations. She was waking during the night, had no change in her appetite, declined to participate in the activities at her group home, and had lost her sense of humor. A staff member Sally had especially liked had left the group home a few months prior to the onset of her symptoms and the company she was working for had gone out of business a month before that.*
>
> *We found no underlying medical causes for Sally's behavior changes. We discussed the treatment options with Sally and her mother. The psychotic-like symptoms of agitated self-talk were particularly disturbing to Sally and her mother. However, the prospect of weight gain with the anti-psychotic medications concerned them, since Sally already weighed 183 pounds at 5'1". We decided to try an SSRI, since the chance of significant weight gain is usually less than with anti-psychotic medications. We also thought there was a good chance that Sally's symptoms would respond to antidepressants alone. Sally was started on sertraline (Zoloft) and her dose was adjusted over the next few months. With the assistance of Sally's family and supportive staff who encouraged her back into activities, Sally's mood, sleep patterns, and willingness to participate in activities all improved. As Sally began to feel better and she was able to verbalize her concerns, her self-talk decreased and she began to self-talk only in her bedroom again. Her mother excitedly said, "Sally is back."*

> *Frank, on the other hand, required anti-psychotic medications. For several months, Frank, 36, had been severely withdrawn. He had lost interest in activities, was often agitated, awoke during the night, had a decreased appetite, and was doing more self-talk. Frank has limited verbal skills so it is very difficult to delineate the content of his thought processes or his self-talk. Frank was found to have hypothyroidism and appropriate treatment was provided. However, in light of the severity of his symptoms, we also prescribed an antidepressant. When there was little improvement in Frank's symptoms, risperdone (Risperdal) was added at bedtime. His sleep and agitation improved fairly rapidly. With time and dose adjustments, his other symptoms also improved. In addition, Frank was regaining a sense of pleasure from activities that he previously enjoyed.*

Mania

* * * * * * * * * * * * * * *

As discussed in the previous section, depression is one of the mood disorders in the DSM-IV-TR. Mood disorders may also include an opposite state of emotion called mania. Mania may include feelings of wellbeing or euphoria, and, at the extreme, a manic-like state which may include agitation, sleeplessness, hyperactivity, angry rages, and even self-destructive behavior. Fortunately, mania does not appear to be common in adults with DS. We have seen just a handful of people with mania alone (not associated with depression) at the Center.

> *Penny, 24, was brought to the Center in November by her concerned parents. Penny's parents had begun to notice a change in her in January when she lost a valued job as a result of her company moving out of state. She became increasingly more restless and preoccupied over the course of the year. She had not been able to find a new job and had therefore spent some time alone at her home doing hobbies and things of interest to keep her busy. Despite losing her job, she continued to attend many social or recreational activities every week. However, her parents began to observe that she seemed distracted and had difficulty focusing on the activities and socializing with her peers as the year wore on. During this time, her parents were watching her closely and did not observe any evidence of a sad or depressed mood or any other evidence of depression. For example, Penny did not withdraw, show a lack of interest in doing activities she enjoyed, or have any change in her appetite.*
>
> *In September and October, Penny's parents noticed new disturbing changes in her behavior. First, she seemed to focus more intently on playing the piano, for which she had considerable talent. Her parents were initially pleased because they wanted to support her talent. Their pleasure quickly turned into alarm, however, as Penny's piano playing seemed to turn into an obsession. She played day and night as if she could not stop. She became more frantic in her playing until one day she suddenly stopped and did not play again.*
>
> *Afterwards, her parents noted other disturbing changes. As her father noted, Penny's anxiety seemed "to have gone through the roof." Although she had restless sleep earlier in the year, during this period she did not appear to sleep at all. Even though Penny appeared tired in the day she did not seem to take any naps. Despite her excellent speech, she began to speak nonstop in an extremely fast and pressured form of speech which was garbled and very difficult to understand. When her parents could understand what she was saying, the content of her speech was disturbing to them. She was repeating statements about petty worries or concerns which she appeared to have blown out of proportion. For example, she*

was worried that she had offended a neighbor by not waving to her. In the daytime, when not occupied or moving about, Penny would often pick at her skin or fingernails. At the appointment, she grimaced constantly and seemed irritated and uncomfortable with herself. She could not seem to relax or stop her constant movement.

In her initial evaluation at the Center, the physical exam showed a hyperthyroid condition which could result in manic-like symptoms. After treating this condition, her mania continued. The decision was then made to treat Penny with psychotropic medication. After a trial of several different types and classes of medications, Penny responded well to a combination of an anti-psychotic and an anti-convulsant medication. To support the gains made from the medications, we encouraged Penny's parents to get her back into beneficial social, recreational, and vocational activities whenever possible. As her mania began to recede, she became more social, attentive, and engaged in the activities. Equally important, her parents and Penny's job coach agency were able to find a new job that was similar to her previous position. As her symptoms began to dissipate and she resumed her normal activities, she regained her sense of wellbeing and eventually her pride and self-esteem. In time, she even began to play the piano in a more normal and enjoyable way.

See the section on Treatment below for more on medications and other means of treating both mania and bipolar disorder.

BIPOLAR DISORDER

As discussed in this chapter, depressive disorders are the most common type of mental health disorder found in people with DS and mania is one of the least common. What we have seen slightly more often than mania at the Center is a condition called bipolar disorder in which people fluctuate between manic and depressive mood states. (This condition used to be called manic depression.)

To explain this condition in people with DS, it may be helpful to first look at bipolar disorder in the general population. People with this condition who are in an "up" or manic state often have feelings of exhilaration and euphoria. They may have boundless energy to work day and night on projects and activities of interest. Unfortunately, as the mania increases, people often "go over the top" and become more extreme and unreasonable in their grandiosity and their behavior. For example, they may buy extravagant items on a whim, gamble away life savings, or engage in risky sexual behavior. Mania may also lead to agitation, restlessness, sleeping problems, and anxiety.

What goes up invariably comes down in this disorder. At some point, the pendulum moves back toward the other pole and the person begins a descent into depression. In this depressed state, people often shut themselves off from the world for weeks or even months at a time before the pendulum once again moves toward the other (manic) pole. Like all mental health disorders, bipolar disorder varies in intensity or severity for each individual, but the pattern of fluctuation in mood states remains a hallmark of the condition.

Although it has been known for many years that bipolar disorder occurs in adults, practitioners have only recently found that a significant number of children in the general population have this condition (Papolos & Papolos, 1999). It may have taken some time to discover this because children often have a very different pattern of symptoms compared to adults. Similarly, it may have taken time to confirm that people with DS may also have bipolar disorder because they have a symptom pattern which is very similar to that of children in the general population. In fact, because the pattern was different from adults without DS it was only recently realized that adults with DS do get bipolar disorder.

What are these differences compared to adults in the general population? First, children and people with DS are more likely to cycle rapidly between up and down mood states. They may cycle back and forth in as short a period as a day or even over several hours, compared to adults in the general population who typically cycle between mood states after weeks or even months. Also, symptom presentation is different. In the down or depressive state, children and people with DS are far less likely to verbalize feelings of sadness, worthlessness, or guilt. However, they do show such observable changes as an irritable mood, withdrawal, loss of interest in activities formerly enjoyed. (See above section on depression for more on this.) Similarly, mania in children and people with DS may not include the out-of-control spending or sexual behavior displayed by adults in the general population. Nevertheless, the pattern of over-stimulation, agitation, restlessness, angry rages, and hyperactive behavior occurs, and these changes are unmistakable symptoms of mania to parents or other caregivers, once they are educated on this condition. For example:

> Jaqui, a 19-year-old with DS, began showing symptoms of the disorder six months before her parents brought her to the Center. She exhibited a pattern of cycling back and forth from mania to depression and back to mania over the course of just one day. Prior to the onset of symptoms, Jaqui and her family had been proud about how capable and independent she was. She was also meticulous about her grooming and her appearance. This changed once the symptoms started, particularly in the morning. Every task was a challenge and a struggle between her and both her parents. Invariably as the morning routine progressed, things would become more and more tense as Jaqui resisted her parents' urgings to get ready for work. She would eventually "lose it" and unleash a barrage of screams, yells, and foul language, and she would often become physically aggressive with them.
>
> This was all behavior that Jaqui's parents had never seen before and they were horrified by it. Perhaps most upsetting to them was the cold look

in her eye when she would rage at them. As her mother stated, this was "not her." She appeared as if "possessed." Although Jaqui weighed only 100 pounds, her father, who was a big, muscular man, was intimidated by her during these rages.

By the time her parents finally got Jaqui on the van to work, they were physically and emotionally exhausted. Jaqui's supervisor reported that upon arriving at work and throughout the morning she was lethargic and listless, doing little of her work, although she had previously been a good worker. She was also quite often in a foul mood. By mid-afternoon, she would begin to perk up and would often cooperate with work tasks for several hours. Then, as the afternoon wore on, she became first silly, and then would seem to become anxious and agitated. In this state, she would fight any attempt by her supervisor to get her to do her normal tasks and she began having angry outbursts, just as at home. Although the work site staff had been tolerant or her behavior, as her angry outbursts became louder and more threatening, her parents worried about whether she would be able to continue at her job.

When Jaqui returned home from her work, at around 4:00, she would often withdraw to her room until after 7:00 or 8:00 in the evening. She sometimes took short naps during this period, but much of the time she would just lie on her bed staring at the ceiling. When she would finally come out of her room she was "like a different person." She would often begin by laughing and joking with her parent, but this could turn into seemingly uncontrollably laughter. As her up mood seemed to escalate, she would often become more irritable and unreasonable. Her parents tried to walk around her very gingerly, but she could respond with shouts of anger if she became upset about anything, including the simplest of requests.

Later, as her exhausted parents prepared for bed, they were shocked to find that Jaqui actually seemed to become more alert and agitated. In this state she simply could not settle down. Finally, by 1:00 or 1:30 am, she would seem to settle down or, rather, "crash in her bed," but even this did not end the ordeal for her parents. They would often hear her waking up several times in the night and one of her weary parents would try to settle her down once again. In the morning, Jaqui's parents would get up and try to get her ready for her job all over again. Every day as this went on, they became more exhausted and Jaqui's symptoms seemed to get even worse.

When Jaqui's parents brought her to the Center, they explained her behavior to our staff and they also reported one additional issue that was disturbing to them: during her more active or manic periods, Jaqui displayed certain odd ritualistic behavior consisting of rubbing her hands together and making a loud "raspberry-like sound" with her mouth. This was particularly upsetting to her parents who were already on edge from her behavior, and from sleep deprivation. They were also *concerned about her doing this in public, believing that it would draw negative attention to her and to the family. As a result, they had stopped sending her to social and recreation programs. This cut Jaqui off from her friends and from physical activities which may have helped her to run off some of her manic energy. Equally importantly, they had stopped going out as a family, which essentially made them feel like they were prisoners in their own house and of the situation.*

TREATMENT OF BIPOLAR DISORDER

The essential first step in successfully treating this condition is to make an accurate diagnosis. Practitioners must be careful to take a very complete and detailed history of the symptoms. If they are too hasty, they may only hear about one mood state, which may lead to inappropriate or ineffective treatments. For example, if they only hear about the depressive symptoms, they may use an anti-depressant medication that may actually worsen the problem by increasing agitation or other symptoms of mania. Once bipolar disorder is identified, the goal of a treatment is to stabilize the extreme mood fluctuations.

MEDICATIONS

There are a number of choices of medications to treat mania and bipolar illness. The medications include lithium, anti-psychotics, and anti-seizure medications. Some people benefit from one medication alone, while others need a combination of medications.

Lithium is a medication that has been used for a long time but is still a very effective choice. It affects the transport of sodium into nerve cells. Although how that action affects mania or bipolar illness is not clear, lithium does stabilize mood. However, lithium has a number of side effects. Care must be taken to make sure the person is drinking enough fluids. Anything that reduces the output of urine, including dehydration or kidney problems, can raise the level of lithium in the bloodstream to dangerous levels. Lithium can affect kidney function, cause hypothyroidism (underactive thyroid), and cause disturbances in the heart rhythm. Drowsiness, tremor, and frequent urination are more common side effects.

Anti-psychotic medications can also be an effective treatment for mania and bipolar illness. Ziprasidone (Geodon), risperdone (Risperdal), quetiapine (Seroquel), olanzapine (Zyprexa), and aripiprazole (Abilify) are all approved for treatment of bipolar illness and acute mania. They can very effectively improve the symptoms. We have found them to be particularly effective in reducing agitation and aggressive behavior. Some of the side effects include weight gain, sedation, hyperglycemia (elevated blood sugar), diabetes mellitus, and swallowing dysfunction. We regularly monitor blood sugar tests for our patients on these medications. In addition, we monitor for tardive dyskinesia (TD). TD is a potentially permanent movement disorder that appears to be much less common with these newer medications than it was with the older anti-psychotic medications.

Anti-seizure medications can also stabilize mood for people with mania or bipolar disorder. Valproic acid (Depakote) is approved for mania. Carbamazepine (Tegretol) is also frequently effective. Lamotrigine (Lamictal) is approved for maintenance therapy once the person has been stabilized.

Antidepressants, as discussed in detail earlier in this chapter, can be very helpful for the depressive symptoms of bipolar disorder. However, care must be taken because they can also cause mania, particularly in people with mania or bipolar illness.

Counseling and Support

Although it is critically important to stabilize bipolar disorder and mania through treatment with medications, practitioners also need to be extremely sensitive to the emotional havoc the disorders play in people lives. Bipolar disorder is one of the most trying and stressful disorders experienced by individuals with the disorder and, of course, by their families and caregivers. It is difficult to understand how stressful and demoralizing this disorder is unless one has had a similar experience.

One of the first steps in helping people cope is to educate them on the cause and nature of the condition. Like many medical conditions, such as asthma or type 2 diabetes, the condition may be aggravated by stress, but it is clearly not something that the person (or caregivers) has caused. This may help to greatly reduce people's sense of self-blame. Additionally, many parents or caregivers often feel demoralized and like failures when, no matter what they do, the person's behavior seems to worsen. Educating people about the neurological basis of the condition helped Jaqui's parents to regain a sense of confidence. For her part, Jaqui was also very upset by her behavior. She did not feel she had control over herself and yet she felt very bad about "hurting" her parents and her supervisor at her worksite. She needed much time in individual and family meetings to understand that this was not her fault. Her parents were especially helpful in explaining to her that they did not blame her or feel angry at her for something that was not her fault.

Getting on with Life

Once the treatment helps to even out the person's moods, it is important for others whose lives were disrupted to begin to resume their normal patterns of life. For Jaqui's parents, the first step was to finally get some rest at night. They also needed to go back to work or to other important outlets that they may have suspended during the crisis. Both of Jaqui's parents, who had each stopped going to work in the morning to cajole Jaqui to go to work, were able to go back to work once her behavior moderated. This allowed them both to connect with friends and colleagues at work and to think and worry about something other than Jaqui.

For approximately three to four weeks during the peak of her symptoms, Jaqui stayed home on leave from her job. As soon as her mood fluctuations began to diminish, we strongly encouraged her family and her worksite staff to let her go back to her work.

To facilitate this, we scheduled a meeting at her worksite with her parents, worksite staff, and our ADSC staff to work out the details of her return. This helped to appease any fears the staff had about her displaying more extreme behavior and gave her parents a plan for making this happen. In this meeting, the worksite staff requested a simple behavior plan to help encourage Jaqui into a positive work routine again. She was to earn a sticker for each day that she stayed on task with her job and had no outbursts. After three weeks the behavior plan was suspended, because it was not necessary. Jaqui was motivated to do her job on her own. Additionally, as Jaqui's symptoms began to dissipate, especially her raspberry-like noise and hand wringing, her parents felt more comfortable allowing her to return to her social and recreational activities. This allowed her to reconnect with her many friends. It also allowed her to get some exercise which was very helpful in reducing whatever manic-like symptoms remained.

As Jaqui's mood fluctuations were reduced, the entire family began to get back to normal. One area that had been a problem was the lack of opportunity for the family to go out together because of Jaqui's noises and hand wringing. As this became less of a problem, they once again were able to go out. This helped to free them from their self-imposed imprisonment in the house.

BIPOLAR DISORDER AS A LIFELONG CONDITION

It is important to recognize that bipolar disorder is a chronic, lifelong medical condition which will require ongoing monitoring and attention throughout the person's lifetime. Finding the right medication to treat the condition at the onset of the disorder (often in the teen years) is essential, such as in the case of Jaqui. In addition, symptoms need to be monitored closely by caregivers and treating professionals. After the person is stable, we see our patients at least every three months. Of course, if active symptoms reemerge, caregivers should return to the treating practitioner immediately.

During the course of treatment, there may be some periodic fluctuations in the disorder which may adversely affect the effectiveness of the medications. This may relate to stressors in the person's life or to physiological or neurological changes that may occur in the person. When this happens, practitioners who are treating this condition may need to look for different medications or different levels of prescribed medications to once again treat the condition effectively. For example, Jaqui has had a number of medication changes during the three years she has been followed at the Center.

Another important issue relates to compliance with taking the prescribed medication. In the general population, one of the well-known problems with treatment is that people may go off the medications when they are feeling up because they like the feeling of euphoria and concentrated energy the disorder may give them when in the manic state. This may be somewhat less likely to occur with people with DS because family members and other guardians usually have a say in their treatment. Still, this may be a problem if the caregiver or guardian believes the person is doing better and appears to no longer need the medication. This may occur if they are not aware that the bipolar is a lifelong condition requiring a continuation on medications. In these instances, we often have crisis calls from these caregivers once the symptoms begin to get out of hand again. We try to prevent this by actively including caregivers in the treatment process and by educating them about the condition.

In summary, mania and bipolar illness are less common in people with DS than depression. However, bipolar disorder in particular appears to be more common than previously suspected. The reason, again, is that in people with DS, bipolar disorder looks more like the conditions seen in children than in adults in the general population. With that appreciation and assessing for symptoms of mania in acute mania and for symptoms of depression and mania in bipolar illness, the diagnosis can be effectively made. Effective treatment depends on the correct diagnosis.

CONCLUSION

Attention to psychological, social, biological, and medical issues are all important aspects in the diagnosis and treatment of mood disorders in people with Down syndrome. Therapy needs to be tailored to meet the unique aspects of the person's personality and environment as well as the symptoms. If depression is suspected, it is imperative that the people diagnosing and treating the condition understand characteristics often seen in adults with Down syndrome, such as self-talk, strong visual memory, and others previously addressed.

Additionally, it is important to recognize that depressive symptoms may also be part of bipolar disorder. In adults with Down syndrome, this typically includes a rapid fluctuation between depressed and manic mood states. The manic state may be characterized by agitation, over-activity, and angry outbursts, which is similar to how this would be expressed in a child, rather than an adult in the general population. Moreover, mania, like depression, may be a separate mood disorder, or it may be part of a bipolar pattern. Understanding how mood disorders in adults with Down syndrome may differ from the textbook definitions may significantly improve the diagnosis and treatment of depression, mania, and bipolar disorder.

Chapter 15

Anxiety

Disorders

Essentially all people would admit to feeling anxious at one time or another. That is, they feel worried or apprehensive, and may experience physical symptoms such as a pounding heart, shortness of breath, or "butterflies" in the stomach.

Depending on the circumstances, anxiety is often a normal reaction and not an indication of mental illness at all. For example, it is normal for a student to feel some anxiety about taking an important test, or for an adult with Down syndrome to feel anxious about moving to a new residence. This sort of normal anxiety usually has a clearly identifiable cause and is short lived. Once the test (or whatever) is over, the person no longer feels anxious.

When anxiety interferes with someone's day-to-day life on a long-term basis, however, an anxiety disorder may be diagnosed. The *Diagnostic and Statistical Manual of Mental Disorders (DSM-IV-TR)* defines a number of types of anxiety disorders. We will discuss the types that are the most common among adolescents and adults with Down syndrome:

1. generalized anxiety disorder,
2. agoraphobia, and
3. panic disorder.

Obsessive-Compulsive Disorder is also a type of anxiety disorder and is described in detail in Chapter 16.

GENERALIZED ANXIETY DISORDER

To be diagnosed with a generalized anxiety disorder, the DSM-IV-TR manual requires:

    A. Excessive anxiety and worry occurring more days than not for at least 6 months, about a number of events or activities.

    B. Difficulty controlling the worry.

    C. The anxiety and worry are associated with three (or more) of the following six symptoms (with at least some of the symptoms present for more days than not for the past 6 months):

        1. restlessness or feeling keyed up or on edge

        2. being easily fatigued

        3. difficulty concentrating or mind going blank

        4. irritability

        5. muscle tension

        6. sleep disturbance (difficulty falling or staying asleep, or restless unsatisfying sleep)

    D. The worry is not confined to features of another disorder (e.g., not about having a panic attack, as in Panic Disorder).

    E. The anxiety, worry, or physical symptoms cause clinically significant distress or impairment in social, occupational, or other important areas of functioning.

    F. The disturbance is not due to a substance (e.g., drug abuse), a medical condition (e.g., hyperthyroidism), or does not occur exclusively during a Mood Disorder, a Psychotic Disorder, or a Pervasive Developmental Disorder.

[Reprinted with permission from the *Diagnostic and Statistical Manual of Mental Disorders, Fourth Edition, Text Revision* (Copyright 2000). American Psychiatric Association.]

Like many people, people with DS have worries and concerns, but this does not mean they have a disorder. For some, these worries may be fairly strong and yet still not debilitating. However, anxiety and worry may become a disorder when it begins to interfere in essential activities. For example, this may occur when someone refuses to go outside because of the presence or possibility of a thunderstorm or another type of feared weather condition. Sometimes this fear is a little more complicated. We have seen a number of people who are afraid of certain weather conditions because they had fallen when there was rain, ice, or snow on the sidewalk. If the fear of these conditions is strong and the particular weather condition occurs often, a major problem may result, such as refusing to leave the house to work or to participate in recreational activities. The anxiety becomes *generalized* when it extends beyond the weather condition and other situations or events cause anxiety.

Symptoms of Generalized Anxiety Disorder (GAD)

As with other mental illnesses, the diagnosis of GAD is usually made on the basis of subjective reports. That is, the individual complains of feeling anxious, or is able to articulate what happens to his body when he is worrying. People with DS may not verbalize subjective feelings of anxiety or anxiousness. Nevertheless, for experienced caregivers, the changes in behavior of a person with anxiety are unmistakable. Additionally, and as discussed in the section on expressive language (Chapter 6), people with DS are not good at hiding their feelings. Facial grimaces, body tension, and pacing can all be clear indications of anxiety and agitation. Some people show their anxiety through mild self-injurious or habitual behavior such as hand rubbing or wringing, picking at sores or at parts of the body, hand chewing, or excessive nail biting, etc. These behaviors often seem to be out of the person's conscious awareness.

Many people with Down syndrome also develop a sleep disturbance when they are keyed up or worried. The sleeping problem may or may not be detected by caregivers, especially if the person has minimal supervision in the evening. However, whenever other symptoms of anxiety are present, sleeping habits should be looked at very closely, such as through nighttime observations, etc. (see section on sleeping problems in Chapter 2). Anxiety may also result in irritability and loss of concentration, but this may also be associated with depression or other types of disorders and thus is not as readily identifiable as anxiety.

Excessive worry is also a common symptom of an anxiety disorder. People who are verbal may express worry directly, but for those who are less verbal, their behavior is often a clear indication of worry. For example, many "weather watchers" closely monitor TV and radio weather reports on storms. When a dreaded weather change is forecast, families or caregivers often observe the telltale signs of anxiety listed above. This pattern is often repeated over and over, so that the association of anxiety with the weather or some other concern becomes obvious in time. Anxiety about the weather alone can be classified as a phobia. However, we have also seen this "triggering" event develop into a generalized anxiety disorder with other triggers also causing anxiety.

> Colin, 28, was brought to the Adult Down Syndrome Center because of suicidal statements. This was very unusual for Colin. Although his parents had been deceased for some time, he had a strong, positive relation with his two sisters, who were actively involved in his life. He was well liked and supported by his family and friends, active in sports and recreation activities, and was a talented artist. One evening, however, he was noticeably upset. When questioned by staff members at his group home, he reported wanting to hurt himself.
>
> At first, Colin could not give an explanation for his suicidal thoughts. Over the course of the meeting at the ADSC, the mystery began to unravel. The first clue came from the staff person who shared with us the agency's concerns that Colin might be psychotic as well as suicidal. This concern

was based on the observation that he made odd statements to staff (in the present tense) about people and events of which they had no knowledge. In the meeting, we were able to explain that many people with DS confuse past and present tense and have a tendency to relive past traumatic events.

Colin's sisters were then helpful in recognizing that his comments reflected times in the past when he was very frightened by severe thunderstorms. When he visited his sisters for overnight stays, he would usually hide in the bathroom during storms, so he could not hear the thunder. This led to a discussion of his worry about storms and his need to monitor the weather closely. The staff person offered that Colin was often reluctant to go out of the house on stormy days. This then lead to the discovery that his roommate had been gone for several weeks on vacation. During this time, there had been frequent and severe thunderstorms. Apparently, Colin's roommate's presence typically gave him a sense of comfort during storms.

Unfortunately, Colin could not easily discuss his worries or concerns with others. Thus, over the two-week period that his roommate was gone, his fears and worries escalated until he could no longer tolerate the situation. This resulted in his suicidal comments and the meeting at the Center.

For the remainder of the meeting, we determined that there was no real threat of suicide and then developed a plan to deal with Colin's concerns. His roommate was to return from vacation that day, which would help with his fears in the evening. Beyond this, staff in his group home would meet with him daily to assess his degree of weather fear. On days he was more worried and especially on stormy days and evenings, he would have special attention from staff to help him. Finally, he benefited from a relaxation therapy incorporating pictures of favorite people and past events. This helped him to substitute comforting pictures for the picture of frightening experiences related to past storms. One year later, Colin continues to have worries and concerns, but they are far more manageable now because of the awareness and assistance of staff and his family.

AGORAPHOBIA

We have found that worry among adults with Down syndrome is often also associated with another type of anxiety condition, agoraphobia. Agoraphobia is a fear of being in certain places or situations. We have seen a number of people at the Center who are terrified of going to a medical clinic, no doubt because of some painful experience in the past. We have heard that for others a negative experience at a store, shopping mall, work, or recreation site may create a similar fear and refusal to leave home. This is because the person worries that the feared place will be visited during the outing. The original experience may have occurred quite some time in the past, but the fear may still be very intense. Recall from Chapter 5 the story of the woman who had been molested by another resident in a group home at the age of 21. At the age of 38, she had lived successfully in a foster home arrangement for 15 years. However, she still was very fearful of leaving her sister's house after visiting her sister for fear of being taken back to the group home she had left 17 years ago.

As discussed in Chapter 5, people with DS may be more susceptible to traumatic experiences that may live on in their memory to terrorize them over and over. For example, it is easy to imagine how weather-related fears may be based on a previous traumatic experience. The fear of the original event may be re-experienced every time the person hears a weather forecast that predicts the feared weather condition is coming. He may become overwhelmed with worry and express his fear by refusing to leave the house—hence the agoraphobia.

TREATMENT OF AGORAPHOBIA

Treatment of agoraphobia and other anxiety conditions may take a great deal of time, patience, and detective work. People with an overwhelming fear need to regain some sense of control in these situations. Medications may be helpful to "take the edge off the fear." (See below on medications.)

The next step is to help the person identify situations that are legitimately fear-producing. It may take some careful assessment to understand why the person doesn't want to leave the house. Sometimes families or other caregivers may not know what specific place or event is feared. In these situations, someone in the person's environment often holds the key to the problem. For example, in Chapter 6, Bruce refused to leave his house. When staff from his workshop were contacted, they gave the critical piece of information, that he was being bullied at his workshop. This information marked the turning point in treatment.

Often, the person's behavior gives clues about the source of his fear. For example, we assume that people who are terrified of coming to the Center had a negative experience in a previous hospital or medical clinic visit.

Once the source of anxiety has been identified or surmised, family members and other caregivers may need to spend a great deal of time explaining that the feared place will not be visited. This may allow the person to go about his normal business in all but the feared place. As discussed in Chapter 5, pictures may help to reduce fear because so many people with DS have a strong bent toward visual images. For example, the woman who was afraid to leave her sister's house was shown pictures of her real destination (her current foster home). This destination was a safe place for her and not the place where she encountered the previous trauma. With the continued use of pictures, a brief period of anti-anxiety medication, and the patience and encouragement of her sister and staff in her foster home, she regained the confidence to leave without experiencing debilitating fear. For her and for others, the ability to do what was feared provides an enormous sense of relief and confidence, which is therapeutic in and of itself.

If the source of anxiety cannot be pinpointed, sometimes the best solution is to change the person's environment or routine in hopes of distancing him from the source of anxiety. As in the example below, if you are fairly sure his home life is OK, you change his work situation.

> Anthony, a 34-year-old man who was nonverbal, refused to go to his work at a community pool, even though he had been in the job for five years and was very enthusiastic about this position. After repeated attempts to get him to go back to the pool, he was transferred back to his previous workshop program, where he seemed to function without fear. Only later was it learned that a supervisor at the pool had been fondling another employee. Anthony's dramatic change in behavior coincided with the presence of this supervisor. Unfortunately, if this supervisor victimized him, he could not communicate it to others.

DESENSITIZATION

Desensitization can be an important part of the treatment strategy for any type of phobia or agoraphobia. Some of the steps in desensitization were touched on above, but not formally explained. Desensitization is a means of gradually reducing a person's fear by incrementally helping him tolerate being around the thing he fears.

Ideally, a step-by-step plan for desensitizing the person should be written down. You start by determining the maximum exposure to the feared item that the person can tolerate (e.g., perhaps just a picture or a model of the thing that he fears viewed across the room). The next step might be actually holding the picture or the model. Over time, he is increasingly exposed to the item until his fear and anxiety are decreased.

For example, we have learned to be very patient with people who are afraid to come into the Clinic for a physical exam. We often recommend that the person go through a gradual process of exposure to the Center. This may start with a drive by the Center on one day, a drive into the parking lot on another, and then a walk up to the front door, etc.

As discussed previously, medication may help in this process by reducing the level of anxiety. Medication may be particularly important at the place of greatest fear, such as the point where the person enters the Clinic building or the exam room, takes a needle, etc. Sometimes the desensitization process takes months, but the need for a medical exam or procedure is so great that it is all worth it. For example, one man with Down syndrome finally allowed a blood draw after practicing with staff for nine months to have everything but the needle in his skin. This man turned out to have hypothyroidism that needed to be treated and was not diagnosed until the blood was successfully drawn.

One fairly common and particularly difficult version of agoraphobia occurs when people refuse to leave the house and get into a vehicle. The same process of gradual exposure to the feared condition applies as in the above medical situations. Again, medication may greatly help to reduce the level of anxiety, allowing people to be more receptive to the desensitization process. Family members or other caregivers will then very gradually and patiently expose the person to the feared object by a daily process of moving him farther and farther from the home and into the car. In extreme cases, a beginning step might be for the person just to stick one arm outside the door or to stand on the porch for ten seconds before returning inside. Eventually, the person will work up to standing next to the car, then briefly touching the car, etc.

Having desensitized the person to riding in the vehicle, caregivers are often able to get him to ride to most daily events. It is important, however, to watch closely to see if any particular environment seems to generate more anxiety. This may help in pinpointing the specific place that triggers anxiety, even if it does not provide insight into what occurred in this place. This place may then be avoided. If this is impossible, then desensitizing the person to the place by gradual exposure is the best option.

PANIC DISORDER

One of the most common types of anxiety disorders and also a cause of agoraphobia in the general population is a panic disorder. The DSM-IV-TR describes this as a condition that has discrete periods of intense fear and discomfort and at least four of the following:

- palpitations,
- pounding heart, or accelerated heart rate,
- sweating; trembling or shaking,
- sensations of shortness of breath or smothering,
- feelings of choking; chest pain or discomfort,
- nausea or abdominal distress,
- feeling dizzy, unsteady, or faint,
- derealization (feeling of unreality),
- fear of losing control or of going crazy,
- fear of dying,
- paresthesias (numbness or tingling sensations),
- chills or hot flashes.

[Reprinted with permission from the *Diagnostic and Statistical Manual of Mental Disorders, Fourth Edition, Text Revision* (Copyright 2000). American Psychiatric Association.]

These reactions can be spontaneous or can occur in response to a trigger—whether or not the person recognizes it as a trigger (Landon and Barlow, 2004).

We have seen panic disorder in patients at the Center, although it appears not to be as common in people with Down syndrome as some of the other anxiety disorders. It may, however, be more common than has been observed. The diagnosis may not be clear cut because people with DS are less likely to verbalize more subjective feelings because of verbal and articulation limitations. Nevertheless, some of the symptoms are definitely observable by sensitive caregivers. For example:

> *Sean, 24, was brought to us because of repeated problems at work. He would become very agitated and sometimes strike others. His mother told us that on two recent family trips, he had become similarly agitated on the plane, sweating, breathing heavily, and having a difficult time sitting still. We went back to the staff at his workshop and asked further questions. They observed him more closely and discovered similar symptoms before episodes of agitation.*
>
> *We diagnosed Sean with a panic disorder. He responded very well to a combination of sertraline (Zoloft) and sustained release alprazolam (Xanax) (an anti-anxiety) medication. We also gave his family short-acting alprazolam to use if he developed the symptoms. Sean has done very well with this combination. His ability to go to work regularly without difficulties has been therapeutic in itself. Doing well at his job and not losing control of himself is a very positive experience for him and quite rewarding. The better he feels about himself, the better is his self-esteem and the less anxious he is in many situations.*

Desensitization may also be beneficial for panic attacks. However, sometimes avoidance of the situation may also be necessary. Medications, including antidepressants and anti-anxiety medications, may be beneficial. We most commonly use the selective serotonin reuptake inhibitor antidepressant medications (see below).

DISTINGUISHING MEDICAL CONDITIONS FROM ANXIETY DISORDERS

When diagnosing an anxiety disorder or panic attack, it is important to rule out possible medical problems that can contribute to or mimic these problems. Ideally, the doctor will evaluate for the presence of these problems when first considering an anxiety diagnosis, as treating these medical problems, if present, may make it unnecessary to treat for anxiety.

The first consideration is hyperthyroidism (overactive thyroid). In the general population, nervousness is a very common symptom of hyperthyroidism. Studies suggest that 85 percent of people with hyperthyroidism experience anxiety (Reid and Wheeler, 2005; Katerndahl and Vande Creek, 1983). In people with Down syndrome, nervousness also seems to be a common symptom. Often when hyperthyroidism is medically treated, the anxiety disappears as well.

Another medical problem that can contribute to anxiety is sleep apnea. The chronic sleep deprivation associated with sleep apnea may be manifested as anxiety.

Sleep apnea may also cause hypoxemia (low oxygen in the blood) while sleeping. Hypoxemia can cause a person to feel anxious or even have a sense of panic. At night, he may awake in a panic or anxious when he experiences the low oxygen. During the day, there may also be a persistent sense of anxiety.

Anything that causes hypoxemia can contribute to anxiety. For instance, adults with Down syndrome who have congenital heart disease that was not surgically corrected and has led to chronic hypoxemia and cyanosis may develop anxiety. Particularly as the hypoxemia progresses, the sense of difficulty breathing or "air hunger" may lead to anxiety. When the person is more active, his oxygen level may fall even further, causing increased anxiety. Some of our patients with this problem have required anti-anxiety medications, but often oxygen therapy can be very beneficial physically and also reduce psychological stress.

Unfortunately, however, sometimes the recommendation of oxygen may be stress inducing. For example:

> Leah, a 37-year-old woman with cyanotic congenital heart disease, was slowly but progressively declining. Her heart function was decreasing and she was becoming short of breath with less and less activity. However, when we discussed the possibility of oxygen, she was very fearful. She adamantly refused to even consider oxygen therapy.
>
> After several discussions at home between Leah and her family, they discovered the source of her fears. Leah's grandfather had had severe emphysema. Shortly before he died, he had required oxygen therapy. Leah equated starting oxygen therapy with her grandfather's death. She thought that if she started oxygen therapy she would also die in the near future. Over time, we were able to reassure Leah and she began the therapy. As she experienced the benefits of oxygen, she became even less anxious and began to readily use it.

Another possible cause of anxiety symptoms is alcohol withdrawal. Alcohol withdrawal is experienced when a person's body becomes accustomed to drinking a lot over a long time and then the alcohol is stopped. While this has been extremely rare in our practice, it is something to consider. In the two people we have seen with alcoholism, making the alcohol unavailable was enough to solve the problem. Interestingly, both individuals did not later express craving for alcohol and either "forgot" or denied they ever drank heavily.

Illegal drug ingestion is even rarer among adults with DS (we have not seen it) but is theoretically a possibility. Much more likely is the consumption of too many caffeine-containing beverages. Caffeine can cause anxiety symptoms. It can also disrupt sleep, leading to anxiety. We recommend slowly weaning the caffeine-containing beverages and replacing with beverages that are well-liked but do not contain caffeine.

Finally, it is important to rule out illness as a cause of anxiety. Just as illnesses can lead to depression, they can also be anxiety provoking. This is particularly true if there is uncertainty about the diagnosis or treatment. In addition, if an adult has a limited ability to communicate his concerns, pain, or other symptoms, that can be anxiety provoking. And, as with anyone else, the person may feel stressed if he knows from previous experience, or is told, that there are potential bad outcomes or suffering associated with his illness.

TREATMENT

In the case histories in this chapter, we have already alluded to some of the treatments for anxiety disorders, including treating underlying physical problems, counseling, and medications. Considerations in treating underlying physical problems are mentioned above. In this section we will focus on medications and counseling for anxiety.

MEDICATIONS

The medications for anxiety generally fall into three categories:
1. azapirones,
2. benzodiazepines, and
3. antidepressants.

Buspirone (Buspar™) is the only azaperone presently available. Its mechanism of action (how it affects brain chemicals) is not known. It does not generally have an immediate impact on anxiety. It may take several days to weeks to see the effect. However, the advantage over the more quickly acting benzodiazepines is that it does not have an addictive potential. We have had some, but limited success in treating anxiety with buspirone.

The benzodiazepines such as diazepam (Valium) and lorazepam (Ativan) act relatively quickly. There is usually some effect with the first dose. With increasing regular doses, the effect often increases. These medications can also be used on a short-term basis while starting other medications that take longer for the onset of their effect. One downside to benzodiazepines is that they can be addictive.

Antidepressants can also be used to treat anxiety. We have found the selective serotonin reuptake inhibitors (SSRIs) and venlafaxine (Effexor) to be beneficial for most adults with DS who are experiencing anxiety. (However, only paroxetine and escitalopram have FDA approval for generalized anxiety disorder and only paroxetine, sertraline, and fluoxetine are approved for panic disorder.) We have recently also used bupropion (Wellbutrin™) with some success. It may take several weeks to see the full effect of these medications and, therefore, we often temporarily use a benzodiazepine while we are waiting for the SSRI to take effect. Some people require long-term use of antidepressants because their symptoms recur if the medication is discontinued. Antidepressants are further discussed in Chapters 13 and 14.

Steve, 34, was heavily sedated when we first met him. He was on a high dose of thiothixene (Navane) (an antipsychotic medication). He had become aggressive in his group home and struck one of the staff. Further investigation revealed that he would become agitated and tremble in certain situations, particularly when other people in the home were agitated. Steve was very sensitive to activity going on around him. We diagnosed him with a generalized anxiety disorder. After starting him on buspirone (Buspar), we were able to wean him off his thiothixene. Subsequently, he was much calmer and much more tolerant when other residents became agitated.

COUNSELING

Many of our patients with anxiety have benefited not only from treatment with medication, when warranted, but also from counseling. Counseling not only provides the person with an opportunity to express his concerns, but also helps the practitioner to determine if and how the environment needs to be adjusted to decrease anxiety. For example:

Edward, age 30, and Gabe, 39, were both brought to the Center by their respective mothers because of similar symptoms of a generalized anxiety disorder. Their symptoms consisted of agitation, body tension, pacing, and difficulty sleeping. Both also had mild self-injurious behavior. Gabe chewed on his hands. Edward picked at sores on his arms and legs. Both had lost their fathers some time ago and their mothers were struggling with some of their own issues of loss, having lost many family members and friends as they aged. Both Edward and Gabe were sensitive to their mothers' feelings of loss and this definitely created some anxiety for them. But what seemed to have precipitated a dramatic increase in their anxiety was job-related stress.

Edward worked in a cavernous worksite which became more and more onerous to him as the level of noise and conflicts between others increased. Making matters worse, several men at his worksite teased him unmercifully once they learned that he was upset by their teasing.

Gabe had a different problem. The agency managing his worksite changed from a workshop setting to a program that found and placed people in community jobs. Although this was a laudable goal, they actually closed the workshop before they had found community jobs for most of the program participants. As a result, most people came to the inactive workshop for community jobs but instead sat idle for hours on end. This was extremely difficult for Gabe, who needed to work and be productive. After approximately six months of sitting doing nothing, Gabe's mother noticed that his level of anxiety and hand biting were increasing dramatically.

Following the observed increase in anxiety by both their mothers, Edward and Gabe were brought to the Center within several months of each other. After ruling out any significant health problems, a diagnosis of generalized anxiety disorder was given to each and a treatment plan was developed. Anti-anxiety medications were prescribed for both to help reduce the intensity of their anxiety and to aid them with sleep. Counseling was also recommended and started for both families.

Edward and his mother had both joint and individual counseling sessions to discuss their feelings and issues. Edward was quite verbal and was able to discuss many of his concerns openly and honestly. Sessions with Edward's mother focused on her own needs for more friends and beneficial activities (which she found through greater participation in her church and a local social club).

Counseling for Gabe and his mother was different, in part because his mother's family viewed counseling as an admission of failure. As a result, she was less able to verbalize her own issues and concerns for herself. Therefore, we did not offer and she did not ask for individual meetings for herself. Nevertheless, she was very concerned with helping us find a solution to Gabe's problem and was extremely helpful in teaching us what we needed to know about Gabe to help him. For example, she told us how important Gabe's work was to his sense of wellbeing. Gabe met for several short sessions of individual counseling (approximately 15 to 25 minutes in length). These meetings seemed to be productive for him, even though he was not as verbal or articulate as Edward. (See Chapter 13 for more on counseling adults who are less verbal.)

Despite some differences there were several key similarities in our counseling strategies for both Edward and Gabe. This involved meetings with the staff at their respective worksites regarding problems at these sites. Additionally, sessions were held with both men and their mothers to introduce relaxation techniques to help them deal with their own anxiety.

Both families went with us to meet with the respective worksite staff and administrators to try to negotiate a solution to the problems at these sites. We were successful in negotiating a positive change for Edward, who was allowed to move to a smaller and quieter work space. We were less successful with Gabe, at least initially. His worksite staff were unwilling or unable to find suitable work for him either at his worksite or in the community. Fortunately, through the combined efforts of Gabe, his mother, counseling staff from the Center, and a local case management agency, Gabe was able to move to a new worksite that was near his home and had plenty of work for him.

As another important part of our counseling strategy, both Gabe and Edward were taught to use relaxation techniques. These are planned and practiced activities which give people some sense of control over their own anxiety by allowing them to relax in the face of an anxiety-provoking situation. In developing the right relaxation activities for this, we often try *to capitalize on a person's interests and strengths. For example, for Linda (above), who was terrified of thunderstorms, we used her superb memory and interest in pictures of past experiences to help her focus her attention on these positive experiences. She has learned to use this technique when she either experiences or is concerned about the possibility of a thunderstorm. (See more on the use of visual memory techniques in Chapter 13.)*

For Gabe we found that he, like many individuals with DS, had certain set routines or grooves he would do every day. One of these repetitious activities was copying letters or words in notepads. He would do this for hours at a time, particularly in the evening. This was extremely relaxing for him. Unfortunately, he was so anxious as a result of his worksite problems that he stopped doing this activity. In individual and joint meetings with his mother, we had him begin to do this activity again. We then had him progress to using this activity to relax when he was in a stressful situation. At first, his mother or another caregiver needed to remind him to do this activity when he was stressed, but in time he became skilled at identifying when to start it himself. For example, Gabe had some stress and anxiety at his new workshop program when there was some down time. His new supervisor reminded him just once or twice, and then he began to do this task routinely any time he had down time or stress at work or anywhere for that matter.

For Edward, we used modifications of two well-known strategies in the general counseling field for relaxation. One strategy is called progressive muscle relaxation. This technique involves tightening and then relaxing different muscles of the body. The second strategy is to control one's breathing, such as through deep breathing and exhaling exercises, to induce relaxation. We use versions of these techniques adapted to the ability of the person with DS.

For example, for Edward and many others, we usually depend on a simple isometric exercise which may be combined with a breathing exercise. Isometric exercise employs muscle resistance created by the person himself. For instance, the person pushes the palms of his hands together. Like progressive relaxation, this exercise may include different muscles and different parts of the body. People may push or pull their hands, push down or pull up their legs, etc. Typically, we teach the person to do each exercise for five seconds while he or another person says "Go," then counts "1001, 1002, 1003…. Stop." When someone else counts aloud, some people may also be able to add a breathing exercise. This involves taking in a deep breath when doing the exercise and letting go of the breath when the exercise is complete.

Some people simply do not like or are not able to use these techniques, but many others, like Edward, can. We have had some success with other types of relaxation techniques, again modified to meet the needs of the person with DS. Some people have been able to use smooth stones, called rubbing stones, which they rub with their thumb as a more healthy and socially appropriate means to express some tension or anxiety. In public, people are often able to keep these stones in their pockets and rub them unbeknownst to others. A number of different items may be used besides rubbing stones, such as stress balls or rabbits' feet, to allow people to keep their hands busy on more acceptable means for expressing tension.

To summarize the treatment and counseling strategies for Edward and Gabe who both were diagnosed with generalized anxiety disorder, the treatment consisted of a multi-pronged approach including:

- A complete physical to rule out health problems;
- Medications to reduce the intensity of the anxiety symptoms and promote better sleep;
- Counseling (which allowed both individuals and at least one family member to express their feelings and concerns and helped to promote beneficial social activities for at least one parent);
- Interventions at the respective worksites to promote healthy, less stressful work environments;
- Relaxation techniques tailored to each individual's needs, skill level, and interests to help them relax in the face of anxiety-provoking situations.

Although both men in the above example had a generalized anxiety disorder, we have found that counseling may be an essential component to the successful treatment of any type of anxiety disorder in people with Down syndrome. For example, people who require desensitization training may benefit greatly from counseling to help them better tolerate the process of being gradually exposed to a feared thing or activity. Counseling helps the person to express his fears and concerns more fully. Counselors are then able to help develop a plan that is better attuned to the person's issues and fears. Whether or not the training manuals for these types of treatments specify the need for counseling, in real life with real people, there is nothing more important to the success of these endeavors than to develop a therapeutic alliance through the counseling process. We find, too, that different types of counseling involving different numbers or groups of people, including the individual, family, and staff from worksite or residence, may all be necessary and beneficial to help resolve different types of anxiety disorders.

CONCLUSION

Anxiety can be a very debilitating illness. As with other mental illnesses, assessment and treatment must be directed toward underlying medical conditions, psychological issues, social issues, and the use of medications. After treatment is completed, anxiety may recur, so continued observation for symptoms is important.

Chapter 16

Obsessive-
Compulsive
Disorder

A s discussed in the chapter on "The Groove," many people with Down syndrome have a tendency toward sameness and repetition. Grooves may be very beneficial; for example, if they enable people to reliably complete routine self-care and work tasks. Grooves may become problematic, however, if thoughts or actions become stuck or rigid. Sometimes this tendency may lead to problems that are diagnosed as obsessive-compulsive disorder. Sometimes, however, the development of obsessive-compulsive disorder has no connection to previous grooves.

WHAT IS OBSESSIVE-COMPULSIVE DISORDER?

Obsessions are thoughts that preoccupy the mind. Compulsions are acts that one feels compelled to perform. In "classic" obsessive-compulsive disorder (OCD), these compulsions are linked to a desire to lessen the anxiety arising from the obsessions. For example, someone who is obsessed with the idea that she is going to accidentally burn down the house might constantly be compelled to check and recheck that the stove is turned off. When she sees that the stove is off, her anxiety is temporarily reduced until she starts worrying about burning the house down again.

Ordinarily, people with OCD realize that their obsessions and compulsions are abnormal or excessive, and would like to be rid of them so they will also be rid of the anxiety. In contrast, people with DS often don't have the desire to be rid of the obsessions and compulsions.

An example of an adult with DS who had a major problem with an obsession was Jill, age 25. She enjoyed working with Carmen, a young staff person at her job. She became obsessed with Carmen and started drawing pictures of her, following her around at work, calling her repeatedly, and putting notes on her car. Jill even cut and saved magazine pictures of the model of Carmen's car. This obsession interfered significantly with Jill's ability to function when she became so preoccupied with her obsession that she was unable to sleep, work, and participate in recreational activities.

Compulsive behaviors that interfere in people's lives are equally problematic. For people with DS, and in the general population, compulsions may be odd or nonsensical. For example, Sam, a 36-year-old man with Down syndrome, had a compulsion to turn around glass and other breakable objects and hang them off the edge of shelves in his apartment. He seemed compelled to do this activity over and over. His compulsion resulted in many broken items and it interfered in essential work and recreational activities of the people he lived with.

OCD occurs in about 1.5 to 2.3 percent of the general adult population in a given year and 2.5 percent during the lifetime (Kessler et al., 2005). Obsessive-compulsive disorder seems to be more common in people with Down syndrome. About 6 percent of our patients have been diagnosed with OCD in the 13 years our Center has been open.

SYMPTOMS

Obsessions are characterized by recurrent and persistent thoughts that are more than just excessive worry. Compulsive behavior includes repetitive actions or speech that the person is driven to perform. The symptoms become problematic when they interfere with the activities of daily life. For example, if a woman is compelled to make sure that the staff at her group home are doing their jobs and stays up all night to check on them, this would definitely interfere with her daily activities. The symptoms also need further evaluation when the person becomes very agitated, upset, or angry when someone interferes with the routine. For example, an adult may be compelled to turn the lights on and then become very angry when asked to stop because it is time to go to sleep (with the lights off).

CAUSES

People with OCD are thought to have an abnormality in the serotonin system (a reduction in serotonin or abnormality in serotonin receptors). People with Down syndrome are thought to have a greater incidence of abnormalities in serotonin and, therefore, are more susceptible to OCD. In addition, stress, support from family, and other precipitants to mental illness (as discussed in Chapter 11) can contribute to development or nondevelopment of OCD tendencies.

DIAGNOSIS

In diagnosing OCD in adults with Down syndrome, it is often necessary to deviate somewhat from the diagnostic criteria for OCD listed in the DSM-IV-TR. In the general population, OCD may be diagnosed for people who have either obsessions or compulsions that are debilitating. In many cases, clinicians find that compulsive behaviors are linked to obsessions. This is because people will engage in compulsive behavior in an attempt to ward off a disturbing thought or fear that has become an obsession. However, given the expressive language limitations of many people with Down syndrome, it can be difficult to determine whether or not their compulsive behavior is linked to obsessive thoughts. Additionally, as mentioned above, OCD is not typically diagnosed unless the person recognizes her symptoms as being abnormal or undesirable. With people with Down syndrome, however, we may diagnose OCD even if the person seems to take pleasure in her obsessions or compulsions.

On the other hand, it is important not to attach too much importance to the presence of compulsive-appearing behavior alone. The presence of grooves in people with DS can be over-diagnosed as OCD. Careful assessment of the symptoms with knowledge that people with DS do tend to have grooves is essential to making an accurate diagnosis. Attention must be given to those who interact with the person with DS. If those around her do not appreciate the normalcy of grooves, they may contribute to the situation becoming problematic. For example:

> Lynn, 43, really liked to sweep the floor in her residence. She was compelled to sweep and was very good at it. The staff had set up a system in which each of the four after-dinner jobs were divided among the four people who lived there. However, on the nights Lynn was assigned to do a job other than sweeping, she took the broom from the person assigned to sweep, causing confusion and frustration on the part of her housemates. The staff became frustrated with Lynn's behavior and were concerned that she had OCD. In fact, however, this was a case of a groove that was not being appreciated. The other people living with Lynn did not care if they

swept or not. Lynn was a good sweeper. Letting her sweep every night did not eliminate her groove but it did eliminate the problem.

Keeping a record of your son's or daughter's behaviors and reporting these to the practitioner who is assessing him or her for OCD can help prevent a misdiagnosis. A record of her typical groove, how this has been managed in the past, changes in the pattern of behavior, and stressors that may have contributed to a change can provide valuable information. In addition, remember that for a diagnosis of OCD to be made, the behavior must significantly interfere with the person's ability to complete day-to-day activities. It is therefore very useful in diagnosing OCD if parents or other caregivers can keep track of the amount of time the person spends performing her obsessions and/or compulsions and how it interrupts her life.

TREATMENT

Sometimes, no treatment of OCD is necessary. This might be the case, for instance, if a compulsion or obsession is somewhat annoying but does not interfere significantly with daily activities. For example:

> *Daniel, 58, had a compulsion to touch Kleenex boxes. Whenever he came into our office, he would stand up about every 5 minutes or so, walk over to the Kleenex box and touch it, and then sit back down. He did similar activities at his home. Although his compulsion was odd, it did not interfere in essential activities of his life. However, after a period of stressful losses and the development of hypothyroidism, his compulsion did become a problem. He was not sleeping at night because he was getting up repeatedly to touch a Kleenex box. He was treated for hypothyroidism and given a mild sleep aid. Once he was able to sleep, he continued to touch Kleenex boxes, but, as before the onset of his sleeping difficulties, this did not interfere in his daily work and home activities.*

Treatment is necessary if the OCD interferes with the person's life activities; is a major cause of strife within the family; and/or the obsessions or compulsions distress the person.

Treatment of OCD is multi-faceted. As described in Chapter 13, treatment includes attention to psychological, social, and biological issues.

REDIRECTION

For obsessive-compulsive disorder, redirection is an important aspect of the psychological and social approaches. By redirection, we mean trying to interest the person in another activity either just before or just after she begins a compulsive or obsessive activity. Keys to successfully redirecting someone include:

1. Select an interesting or preferred alternative activity in advance.
2. Do not get angry when trying to redirect.
3. Suggest rather than insist that the person try the other activity. Try this over the course of days; expect gradual, not instantaneous changes.
4. Offer rewards to do an alternative activity; this may help the person get started on the alternative activity.
5. Only select one obsession/compulsion at a time to reduce.
6. Remember that physical prompts may cause the person to become agitated.

Working with the person and others in her environment to redirect her away from the object, person, or activity that makes up the obsession or compulsion helps reduce the obsession or compulsion and encourages her to participate in other activities. In the above examples, both Jill and Sam benefited from staff attempts to redirect them toward more beneficial thoughts and activities.

MEDICATION

Medications can be of tremendous benefit in treating obsessive-compulsive disorder. Medications often reduce the strength and intensity of an obsession or compulsion enough to allow redirection to work more effectively. This was certainly the case for Jill in the above case example. She was prescribed an antidepressant medication (SSRI) that also treats OCD. As a result, Jill was more amenable to staff attempts to shift her obsession with Carmen to more normal work and recreation activities.

At the Adult DS Center, we have had the best success with the selective serotonin reuptake inhibitor (SSRI) medications. We most commonly use sertraline (Zoloft®) because of its effectiveness and a low incidence of side effects. We have also found paroxetine (Paxil®) to be beneficial, especially for patients who have a decreased appetite as part of the OCD symptoms. This is because weight gain is a fairly common side effect of paroxetine. We have also found citalopram (Celexa®), escitalopram (Lexapro®), venlafaxine (Effexor®), and buproplon (Wellbutrin®) to be of benefit in some patients, although none of these are approved for this indication by the FDA. It is often necessary to treat people with OCD for a prolonged period of time (and sometimes indefinitely) with the medications.

For some adults with DS, obsessive-compulsive disorder seems to take on a psychotic nature. The obsessions or compulsions go beyond the usual level, with a greater degree of self-absorption, detachment, and inability to participate in activities of daily life. For these individuals, a small dose of an anti-psychotic medication (in addition to or in place of the SSRI) may be of great benefit. Risperidone (Risperdal®), olanzapine (Zyprexa®), quetiapine (Seroquel®), ziprasidone (Geodon®), and aripiprazole

(Abilify®) have all been found to be beneficial. However, when the inability to sleep is a problem, we select olanzapine because it is usually more sedating than the other choices. These medications are FDA approved for psychoses but not for OCD.

Unfortunately, weight gain is a potential problem with all of these anti-psychotic medications. This concern must be addressed through good nutrition and increased activity. We have seen the greatest weight gain with olanzapine. Sometimes this can be used in a positive way for patients who have weight loss and/or decreased appetite as part of their symptoms. Ziprasidone and aripiprazole seem to cause the least weight gain in our patients. However, ziprasidone can cause cardiac rhythm disturbances, so periodic EKG monitoring is recommended. In addition, tardive dyskinesia is a potential side effect of each of these anti-psychotic medications. Tardive dyskinesia most commonly occurs after long-term use of a medication and causes the person to have involuntary movements, grimacing, or similar problems. We have only seen tardive dyskinesia in a few adults with Down syndrome out of the few hundred who have been prescribed these drugs.

COMBINING TREATMENTS

Sometimes when compulsions or obsessions are more difficult to resolve, they require both creative approaches to redirection and the use of psychotropic medication. The first step in treating these more complicated obsessions and compulsions is always to look for possible causes or precipitants. We try to pinpoint possible health and environmental stressors through the evaluation process described in Chapter 12. We also talk with the adult, family members, or others who know her well to get some history of her previous groove-like tendencies. This gives us a sense of the relative strength of this tendency for each individual.

In addition, we find out how family members and other caregivers have been responding to the person's grooves. Caregivers' response to grooves may play a critical role in either the development or reduction of a problem, as in the following example:

> Charles had lived with his parents all of his life. When he was 43, his last parent died and he moved in with his married sister's family, which included young, school-aged children. Although his sister, Zoe, had always been actively involved in Charles's and her parents' lives, the transition to her household was difficult. Zoe reported that Charles had always had a strong tendency for following set routines. She found that both he and his parents became more "set in their ways" as they got older and assumed a more sedentary lifestyle.
>
> When he moved to Zoe's house, Charles's habits and routines did not always fit in with her family's routines. For example, Charles demanded ice cream at 9:00 in the evening, which disrupted his sister's attempts to get the children to bed. After several weeks, Charles was able to adjust to an earlier time for ice cream and was even able to substitute healthier snacks. He also

had a habit of bringing his dirty clothing to the basement every night after he changed into his pajamas. His mother had dutifully washed and returned the items to him the next day. This was impractical for his sister. After repeated practice and much encouragement, he was able to put his clothing in a hamper, which was brought to the basement once a week to be washed.

There were other issues as well. For example, one of Charles's favorite activities was buying toiletry and other personal items at the store. While living with his parents, he had developed a habit of buying duplicates of items he already had at home. Zoe found out about this habit the first time they went shopping and Charles refused to leave the store unless he got the items he wanted. To prevent this problem from recurring, Zoe helped him develop a new routine before going to the store. The first step involved looking in his bathroom cabinet to see what items he truly needed. Zoe would then help him find a picture or make a drawing of the item, which he would take with him to the store to locate and buy. Charles was very pleased with this alternative because it gave him a routine and also a sense of independence and purpose. Equally important, it allowed him to cooperate with his sister's needs and wishes.

Later on, Zoe discovered a similar problem with movie rentals. Charles often wanted to rent movies that he already had at home. Following the tried and true parental strategy of picking one's battles carefully, Zoe wisely chose to let him do this activity. This practice did not cost much money, and, perhaps more importantly, it did not result in the accumulation of unnecessary items. Numerous situations like this occurred over the course of a year, but were solved effectively (and often very creatively). In time, Charles developed routines that fit into those of his sister's family.

After two years with his sister, Charles moved into a nearby group home. He had difficulty adjusting to this new living situation over the course of the first year. Fortunately, the house manager and key staff members were experienced and understood Charles's need for routines. Staff wisely chose to listen to suggestions from Zoe, whose knowledge and experience was an invaluable aid during this process of adjustment.

Unfortunately, toward the end of Charles's second year in the group home, this situation changed dramatically due to turnover of the house-manager and most of the direct care staff. The new house-manager ignored Zoe's offers of assistance because she viewed Charles's behavior as oppositional, rather than related to his need for routines. Over the next few months, Zoe watched with growing concern as problem rituals and routines that had been dealt with effectively in the past reemerged. For example, Charles once again began to take his laundry directly to the basement to be washed. He began to refuse to go to bed until he had his evening ice cream, even though previous staff had successfully substituted a healthier snack at an earlier time. Most problematic, however, was the staff members' refusal to follow Zoe's proven strategy of providing Charles with a picture of needed items before going shopping. As a result, Charles once again refused to leave the store unless he had his desired item.

Unfortunately, when the staff attempted to force Charles to comply, he had "aggressive outbursts" which he had never shown toward any previous caregiver (family or staff). One of these outbursts occurred on a Friday evening when Charles was with an inexperienced staff person. The police were called to the store, and Charles was transported to a local hospital emergency room for a psychiatric evaluation. There he was given an anti-anxiety medication and recommendations for follow-up for psychiatric treatment. This was the last straw for his sister, who called an emergency meeting at the ADSC to help resolve the problem. Unfortunately, the "aggressive incidents" only seemed to solidify the house manager's belief that this was oppositional behavior and that Charles was a danger to her staff and other residents.

This situation was resolved only after Charles moved to a new group home. Predictably, his response to the stress of the move was to become even more rigid in his routines, and on several occasions he was aggressive toward staff and other residents. During this transition period, he was started on an antidepressant medication that helped reduce his anxiety and the rigidity of his compulsive behaviors. Fortunately, the new staff were patient and took a positive view of routines and collaborated with the family and the ADSC to ease his transition. In time, Charles became comfortable with his new home. He is now in his second year of this residence and doing extremely well.

COMMON COMPULSIONS

Among the most common types of compulsions we have seen among our patients with Down syndrome at the ADSC are:
   ◆ ordering,
   ◆ hoarding, and
   ◆ excessive rigidity in completing a routine.

ORDERING

Putting objects in order, or "ordering" is a common and, often, beneficial groove among people with Down syndrome. Many people order pictures or collected items in their bedrooms. Similarly, some people have a need for a sense of "order" when it comes to lights. They are only in "order" when they are turned on (or off, depending on the individual). Closing or opening doors is another behavior that establishes a sense of order for certain individuals. However, maladaptive ordering occurs when someone's life increasingly revolves around the need to put items in order. This was clearly seen in the example of Sam at the beginning of this chapter. He had a compulsion to put breakable objects in a certain set place. Ordering becomes a problem, as it did for Sam, when people begin to miss work, social gatherings, or previously desired activities to continue to arrange certain items "just so."

Ordering may be a form of compulsion that reduces the anxiety the person feels if things are not "just so." It may also reduce stress that is being experienced from other causes. For example, after a rough day at school, one preteen girl gets extremely irritable and out of sorts if she is not allowed to put her things just how she wants them. She is obsessed with keeping the top of her dresser tidy, for instance, and feels compelled to put things back right where they were if someone moves them. She may insist on having the blue pillowcase on her pillow because the yellow one does not look "right" with her bedspread (and she will hunt all around the house for the missing pillowcase and hound her mom mercilessly until the "right" pillowcase is found).

In addition, ordering things can be related to the person wanting to assert control over her life. The ordering appears to give the person a sense of control.

HOARDING

Hoarding items is another compulsive behavior we frequently see. Hoarding may work hand-in-hand with ordering objects. Sometimes adults with Down syndrome collect and store excessive quantities of specific items; unnecessary items (pens, excessive amounts of soap); useless or other nonsensical items (trash, ripped paper); or food (including perishable items). In the above example, Charles had a tendency to save soaps and other grooming items. Hoarding can be a problem if the individual cannot participate in her usual activities because she is so focused on hoarding items. It can also become a public health concern if the person hoards perishable food items, trash, or other items that make for unsafe conditions.

It can be difficult to redirect hoarding. The first objective is to help the person avoid hoarding items that create an unsafe situation. Replacing the item(s) with something that does not create an unsafe situation is recommended. The next step is to help the person put some limits on the hoarding. As with Charles, helping him develop an understanding of what is needed by depicting it in pictures and giving him control of the purchasing can be helpful. Making available other fun and interesting activities may also be beneficial.

RIGID ROUTINES

Perhaps the most common type of maladaptive compulsion we see at the Center is being overly rigid in completing some routine activity. This was clearly a problem for Charles (above example), as well as for the woman in Chapter 9 who refused to change her bath time to go out with residents of her new group home. These types of rigid routines seem to occur most often when people are asked to make a dramatic and difficult change in their lives.

At the ADSC, we frequently hear of maladaptive bathing routines. This occurs when people take baths or showers repeatedly and for extended periods of time. Such bathing routines are no longer productive when they begin to interfere in work or social activities. Often, parents or other caregivers have no idea what led to the development of these maladaptive routines. However, they frequently report that there has been stress in the person's life, such as a move, and that the person had a preexisting tendency to take longer baths or showers. We have not heard reports that this appears to be caused by an obsession with germs (a common compulsion in the general population), but it may be related to concerns about cleanliness.

The compulsion to do things in a certain order during the day or through the week is also fairly common, and can be considered a form of ordering. For many people, this is part of their healthy groove discussed in Chapter 9. However, this tendency can be problematic and consistent with OCD if it significantly disrupts daily life. Care must be taken, however, to avoid over-diagnosing OCD on the basis of this behavior, because this tendency is so common and part of the typical behavior for many people with DS.

In addition to stress, other common precipitants to overly rigid routines are underlying health problems. When an adult with Down syndrome is diagnosed with OCD, it is imperative to look for a physical problem that could have triggered the problem. Sometimes a health issue that creates sensitivity to a specific area of the body can lead to rigid routines. For example:

> Janine, 32, had a surgery that required an incision across her lower abdomen. During her recovery, she had quite a lot of bleeding and needed a frequent change of bandages. After leaving the hospital, Janine began to shower morning and night for excessive amounts of time. She also developed a habit of fixing her underwear until "just right." Her family believed that these rituals were an attempt to manage a feeling of uncleanness or contamination linked to the excessive bleeding in the hospital.

> As a result of her extended showers and "fixing" behavior, Janine was getting to work later and later in the morning. She also began to spend increasing amounts of time in the bathroom at work fixing her underwear, which began to interfere in her work activities. In the evening, her shower and fixing behavior interfered with social and recreational activities.

> For Janine, treatment included the use of an SSRI medication and behavior management to take the edge off her compulsive routines. The resolution of her problem also took a great deal of patience and persistence from her family. To limit her time in the bathroom, she agreed to use a timer which would signal an end of her shower and then be reset to signal the end of her fixing behavior. As an incentive, she was given cards representing a specified amount of money to buy her beloved music CDs. Gradually, the timer was set to shorter times. After approximately three

weeks, Janine was back to a more normal pattern of showering and fixing of underwear. This then became her regular routine and the incentive was no longer necessary.

Interestingly, Janine's family noted that as her time arranging her underwear became more reasonable, she began to substitute a new ritual of arranging certain personal items in her room "just so." Fortunately, she was far less rigid about the time spent on this activity and was able to continue her daily tasks without getting sidetracked on this activity.

At the same time that Janine's family was giving her incentives to alter her bathroom routines, staff at her job provided her with incentives to return to work more quickly after visiting the bathroom to fix her underwear. These incentives included time and attention from her favorite staff person and also a prized job of delivering mail if she returned from the bathroom after lunch in a timely manner. In time, these incentives helped her regain a more normal work pattern. As with the routines at home, this new behavior then became her routine and she no longer required incentives.

There are many other compulsions resulting from health issues. For example, for some people, chronic sinusitis may lead to compulsive nose blowing or wiping, coughing, or throat clearing. For others, excessive hand washing may interfere with social and work activities and lead to serious problems with dry skin. For example, Allen began to wash his hands excessively after an extended period of persistent diarrhea. Even after he recovered from the diarrhea, he continued to wash his hands often, for prolonged periods of time.

Do's and Don'ts in Dealing with Compulsive Routines

For people like Allen and others who develop compulsive routines, we recommend first determining whether the behavior really interferes in the person's life. If it doesn't, it may not be worth the effort of pushing to change the behavior. If it does interfere with some key area of functioning, or is a problem because it occurs in a public setting, we suggest these steps:

1. *Try to keep the person busy with physical activities or activities that require some attention or concentration.* At home, involving the individual in sports and recreation activities or even playing video games can reduce the time she spends doing compulsive routines. On the job, ensuring that she has meaningful work to occupy her time can do the same. In our experience, people with DS are much more likely to engage in compulsive activities when they have nothing else to do.
2. *Limit sedentary activities such as watching TV.*
3. *Consider substituting the problem behavior with a more appropriate alternative behavior.* This strategy often involves trial and error and creativity to find the right alternative behavior. Sometimes the alternative

may be fairly simple. For example, some people with sinus problems may simply need to use a Kleenex (instead of their hand) when repeatedly blowing or wiping their nose. Sometimes the substitute behavior requires more thought. We have found that a worry stone, rabbit's foot, or foam- or sand-filled stress balls may keep people's hands busy enough to begin to reduce the repetitious habit. With encouragement, the behavior may become a more appropriate regular habit. If encouragement alone doesn't help, a concrete reward may help some people.

It is usually best *not* to try to forcibly stop a compulsive behavior. As the psychologist Milton H. Erickson observed, it is far easier to swim in the same direction of a stream to help redirect it from within rather than to try to stop the stream.

OBSESSIONS

As previously defined, an obsession is an idea or issue that preoccupies the mind to the extent that it interferes with the ability to focus on other ideas or issues. It is more than just daydreaming. The person is limited in her ability to control the thought process.

In contrast to compulsions, obsessions can be harder to detect in a person with Down syndrome. That is, you can observe a compulsion, but an obsession takes place in the mind. Therefore, if the person is not very verbal or does not talk about her obsession, it may require some detective work to discover that she is obsessing about something. If the person is not verbal, she may repeatedly show a desire to see the source of her obsession (either the actual person or item or a pictures of them).

Adolescents and adults with DS can develop obsessions about anything that particularly interests them. Some of the more common obsessions we've seen include:

- Obsessions about fictional people (movie or TV characters) or people the person does not associate with in real life (celebrities),
- Obsessions with people the person knows,
- Obsessions with food.

PEOPLE AS OBJECTS OF OBSESSION

We have found that obsessions with people may be either negative or positive, and they are some of the most intense and persistent of obsessions. We believe this is due to the complex and provocative nature of human relationships, which may be fertile ground for the development and maintenance of intense obsessions. Sometimes the object of an obsession is an imaginary person or a celebrity. Sometimes the object of an obsession may either look like or act like someone else in the person's life. This person may be gone (due to a move or death) or it may be someone whom it would not be possible or advisable for the adult to talk to directly.

We are rarely able to understand the real cause of an obsession. This is true for people in the general population, who usually cannot communicate why they have an obsession. It is even more likely for people with DS to have difficulty expressing the underlying cause of such an obsession. We do know, however, that as with other types of grooves, stress may play a major role in the development of an unproductive obsession.

Preoccupations with Imagined Others

We have seen a number of people who are intensely preoccupied with an imaginary person or a celebrity whose movie role or persona is the object of the obsession. Sometimes the adult has had fleeting contact, such as at a concert, but in general there is little contact with the person who is the object of the obsession.

Many parents of preteens and teenagers in the general population have reported celebrity obsessions as a phase of adolescent development. (Remember: adolescence often occurs at an older age for people with DS; see Chapter 10.) This type of obsession usually subsides as people with Down syndrome age. However, in some instances the obsession continues and begins to interfere with normal functioning. For example:

> Sheri had a number of intense stresses, including the untimely loss of her beloved stepfather, who died of a massive heart attack. After this loss, Sheri developed an obsession with members of a favorite rock band. (She had previously had a harmless interest in the band.) She created an imaginary family of these band members. Other individuals were also added to this imagined family, including a fireman who had been discussed in the news as a local hero. Sheri's mother believed this officer took on a role of a protector in her imagined family.
>
> Sheri became more and more obsessed with her imaginary family, to the detriment of her normal life activities. She would listen to the band's music, or talk incessantly about her imagined "family members" to others and through her self-talk. Her interest in the fireman developed into an obsession with anything in the news about the fire department. Over time, her imagined friends became more and more of an interference in her life. Even though Sheri loved her job and was a conscientious worker, her work suffered as she spent most of her time in her fantasy world. A previously willing participant in social and recreation activities, she began to withdraw to her room and her imagined world.
>
> Treatment for Sheri included an SSRI, sertraline, coupled with an intensive strategy to get her to return to her real-life work and social interest. After several months with no change, a small dose of an antipsychotic medication, risperidone, was added to the antidepressant medication and she began to respond favorably to this treatment. This helped to reduce the intensity of her obsessions, and, perhaps more importantly, also helped to reduce her resistance to participate in real world activities.

The first step in reawakening Sheri's interest in activities was to tweak her strong interest in managing her weight. With a little encouragement, she agreed to maintain an exercise chart of daily walking and stationary bike riding. This helped to focus her in the here-and-now and bring her out of her room. Over several months, she was bolstered by the successful loss of 11 pounds. She also agreed to keep a journal of her thoughts for discussion at ongoing counseling sessions. This served a number of important purposes. It saved her family from some of the frustration of hearing her repeated and relentless comments about her imagined family. If her comments went on for any length of time, they could direct her to her journal to write out her thoughts, which she did. Counseling gave her someone other than family members who would listen to her, although in a time-limited format (which is the nature of counseling).

Although the counseling may have seemed to encourage her attention to her imagined family, writing her thoughts actually reduced the obsession. Writing her thoughts down on paper gave them concrete form and structure, which somehow reduced the need for her to verbalize these thoughts over and over. It may have also been enough of a real activity to help her come out of her fantasy world. The counselor also gave her homework assignments, such as to list some of her favorite activities to further encourage her attention on real-life events and activities. In time, she also began again to attend social and recreational activities in the community. This allowed her to reestablish her friendships and to get additional exercise, as well as to move more into the real world and out of fantasy.

PREOCCUPATIONS WITH REAL PEOPLE

We have also seen quite a few people with Down syndrome who have had positive or negative obsessions with real people in their lives. Positive obsessions mean having pleasant, enjoyable thoughts about the person; negative obsessions mean having bothersome, upsetting thoughts about the person. An example of a negative obsession:

Jennifer, age 32, lived in a cottage in a larger residential facility. She was seen at the Center with her brother, who lived nearby, and staff from her residence. Jennifer's brother reported that she had a history of negative obsessions, often occurring at stressful points in her life. The object of her present obsession was another resident in her cottage. As in the past, this obsession took the form of constant complaints about this other person, expressed most often through bouts of angry self-talk. Jennifer also complained to staff or to her brother about the woman. Her brother noted that the obsession was typically accompanied by other compulsive behaviors such as a tendency to be more "stuck" or rigid with her routines. Additionally, she had been very meticulous with her self-

care and reliable with work routines but now was so absorbed with her obsession that she required more reminders to do these tasks. Despite repeated attempts by her brother and staff to distract her from her obsession, it persisted and worsened.

Aside from Jennifer's obsessions and compulsions, she was also depressed, as evidenced by her irritable mood, restless sleep, loss of appetite, and a loss of interest in the things she had formerly enjoyed, such as music and dancing. She tended to stay by herself in her room, complaining about the object of her obsession.

For Jennifer, successful treatment was similar to the treatment offered to Sheri, discussed above, although she did not need an antipsychotic medication. An SSRI medication was the only medication needed. The staff made an intensive effort to get her out of her room and back to normal activities. In time, she became less obsessed and depressed and she was back on track with her life. In this case, there was no need to change her contacts with the woman she was obsessed with. Observation of their interactions had not revealed reasons for Jennifer to complain about her so much. However, if a problem had been found, addressing this with Jennifer and the other person would have been essential, and, if no resolution could be found, separation of the two may have been necessary.

Approximately three years later, Jennifer began complaining about a different person in her group home. Not surprisingly, Jennifer was under stress from a construction project in her group home, from turnover in staff, and the loss of a close friend who had left the group home. Additionally, Jennifer was diagnosed and treated for hypothyroidism, which undoubtedly was another source of stress for her.

Jennifer was immediately scheduled for an evaluation at the ADSC. Treatment was started quickly and within a short time she was back on track. For her family and staff, the message from all this was to look for early signs of an obsession and to seek treatment as soon as possible. Of equal importance, they learned to reduce stress whenever possible and to predict the likelihood that an obsession would happen based on the presence of unpredictable or uncontrollable stress in her life.

As noted above, obsessions with people may also be "positive." For example, when Elizabeth began her new job, she seemed to develop an obsession with the husband of one of her coworkers. She would flirt with him, send him love notes, talk about him as being her "honey," etc. For Elizabeth, explaining to her that her behavior is problematic would be the first step in treatment. If the object of her obsession was willing to gently discuss with her why her obsession with him was not appropriate, it might also be helpful. Sometimes, however, the only way for the person who is the object to deal with an obsession is by not having any contact with the person with Down syndrome. Redirection, counseling, and medication may also be necessary.

"The Pace" and Obsessional Slowness

Obsessional slowness is an apparent form of obsessive-compulsive disorder that appears to be more common in people with Down syndrome. At this point, much more needs to be learned about obsessional slowness. However, we have seen it in a dozen or so people.

The pace of life in our society always seems to be increasing. The persistent stress of the rapidly moving environment can lead to anxiety, depression, or other psychological problems in some people. People with Down syndrome can also perceive the stress of the fast-paced world. One particularly difficult response to this stress is obsessional slowness, which we have also labeled "The Pace."

For some of our patients, the world seems to move too fast. High expectations (whether real or perceived by the person with DS) may play a role in the development of this problem. They may sense a need to perform at a level or pace that they can't keep up with. They may feel as if they don't have control of their lives.

When they cannot keep up with the pace of the world, some adults with Down syndrome (consciously or unconsciously) slow down. We have seen people who eat slowly, walk slowly, and take an inordinate amount of time to do daily tasks. They seem to slow down or even shut down when they can't live up to the expectations of the pace of society. This slowing down may be a direct "benefit" to them—for example, because they move so slowly, they miss the bus and don't get to their stressful job. For others, there doesn't seem to be a direct avoidance. These people have a more global avoidance of activity. They are not avoiding something specific but have slowed down in all (or nearly all) activities.

Until recently, we had to speculate that our patients perceived that the world was going too fast. However, recently one patient who is moving very slowly confirmed our suspicions when he reported that he feels that "the world is too fast."

Obsessional slowness often (but not always) occurs fairly abruptly. We have found that usually there is not one triggering event. Instead, it seems more likely that a chronic build-up of frustration or desperation causes the problem.

Treatment must start with an acknowledgement that for these individuals, part of the acceptance of their disability (Down syndrome) must include an acceptance of the need to move at a slower pace. They will probably not move at the pace that society sets. They will probably not be able to function at their previous pace because that rate eventually led to their decline.

While acceptance of a slower pace is a large part of the therapy, there are some additional helpful approaches. Giving an allotted time for some activities and then moving on or discontinuing the activity at the end of the time can be helpful. For example, some people who eat very slowly will suddenly start eating more rapidly as they see the clock reach the final minutes of the allotted time for eating. Occasionally the person may become aggressive or very angry if you take away her food, turn off her shower, etc.

Telling the person to hurry up is usually not effective, but may contribute to agitation. We don't recommend physically forcing the person to hurry up. However, it might be beneficial to help her do tasks in some situations. For example, if she is in danger of losing her job because of tardiness, assisting her get her shoes on might be helpful to get her to work on time. However, it is also important to assess whether the job is appropriate for the person or is a cause of stress that could be contributing to the problem with obsessional slowness.

Counseling may provide some limited benefit in giving the person an opportunity to share her concerns. A change of environment—such as having the person switch to a job where the pace is slower, or to a residence where the other people are more sedentary—may also provide benefit.

We have not had tremendous success with medications. In some patients, we have seen some improvement with the use of medications for obsessive-compulsive disorder (see the section on SSRIs above). One patient seemed to have some benefit from L-tryptophan, an amino acid supplement.

A common response to the rapid pace of our society is to race to keep up. However, occasionally this can be overwhelming to the point where people with Down syndrome cannot or will not keep up, and may actually move very slowly as a defense against this stress. "The Pace" at which they function can be described as obsessional slowness and requires a degree of acceptance as well as some intervention.

Chapter 17

Psychotic

❖ ❖ ❖ ❖ ❖ ❖ ❖ ❖ ❖ ❖ ❖ ❖

Disorders

❖ ❖ ❖

Many more adults with Down syndrome are initially suspected of having a psychotic disorder than actually turn out to have one. This is especially likely to occur when people with Down syndrome are seen by mental health professionals who have little experience with Down syndrome. In reality, adults with Down syndrome do not commonly have psychoses.

Psychosis is a psychiatric disorder in which the individual experiences delusions or hallucinations, and these symptoms interfere with the ability to function in daily life. In the general population, the types of psychoses include schizophrenia, schizoaffective disorder, brief psychotic disorder, substance-induced psychotic disorder, psychotic disorder secondary to a medical condition, and others. These specific diagnoses seem to be less common in people with Down syndrome. However, occasionally adults with Down syndrome have psychotic symptoms, as discussed below.

WHAT IS PSYCHOSIS?

❖ ❖ ❖ ❖ ❖ ❖ ❖ ❖ ❖ ❖ ❖ ❖ ❖ ❖ ❖ ❖ ❖ ❖

Psychosis is a disorder that includes:
- ◆ delusions (a false or irrational belief);
- ◆ hallucinations (seeing, hearing, or sensing something that is not present);

- ◆ withdrawal from reality (for example, an intense preoccupation with hallucinations in place of reality);
- ◆ paranoia (an irrational fear or distrust; for example being afraid that someone is out to get you when it is not true);
- ◆ flat affect (lack of emotional responsiveness);
- ◆ altered thought process and disorganized thinking and speech (for example, stringing thoughts together that have no connection to each other).

The diagnosis of the different types of psychotic disorders is based on the symptoms and the duration. It is also important to evaluate for other causes of psychoses such as a substance (a drug or medication) or a medical condition (such as sleep apnea).

DIAGNOSIS

Psychoses can be quite difficult to diagnose in people with Down syndrome. In order to determine that a thought process is abnormal or psychotic, it is necessary to understand what the normal thought process of the person was prior to the change. This can be a challenge in adults with Down syndrome, particularly those who have limited verbal skills. In addition, there are a number of issues to consider in people with Down syndrome that we have previously discussed. These include the issues of self-talk, imaginary friends, and other behaviors that have been described as "psychotoform" behavior (Sovner & Hurley, 1993). When taken out of context, these behaviors can be misinterpreted as psychotic. However, when taken in the context of a person with an intellectual disability, they are usually not psychotic, but consistent with the function of a person at that developmental level. For example:

> Leonard, 29, was brought to us because of a concern that he had developed a psychotic disorder. He had a long history of self-talk but it had recently increased. He was also isolating himself more in his room. At work, he was refusing to go out to the parking lot to gather the grocery carts. A psychologist told his family that Leonard was psychotic, and they came to us for a second opinion.
>
> We encouraged Leonard's mother to listen outside his door to try to hear what he was saying to himself. He kept repeating a phrase about no one helping him get up. Discussions with the family and with a counselor eventually led to a better understanding of the problem. Leonard had been struck by a car while working in the grocery store parking lot. He had been knocked down, the driver had not stopped, and no one had helped him up. He never told anyone. He was afraid to tell his boss because it took him so long to get back into the store with the carts and the boss had been angry.

Leonard's family discussed the situation with him and then arranged a meeting with his manager. The manager agreed to let Leonard continue bagging the groceries but no longer asked him to gather the carts in the parking lot. In addition, Leonard underwent regular counseling. His self-talk returned to the previous level, he became more involved in activities again, and he did well at work. Leonard was not psychotic. However, he continues to have a fear of parking lots and prefers to walk close to someone when walking through one. He also continues to periodically express concern that no one helped him up. When he mentions this concern, he is reassured that people care for him and that the person who struck him did not act appropriately.

Further complicating the diagnosis, the emotional and psychological response to an underlying physical problem may sometimes result in symptoms that appear psychotic. One particular physical health problem to consider when assessing a person with psychotic symptoms is sleep apnea. Both the chronic sleep deprivation and the oxygen deprivation can cause significant psychological symptoms, including psychotic symptoms.

To diagnose an adult with DS with a psychotic disorder, it is generally necessary to carefully observe him in a variety of settings. Observation in the physician's and mental health professional's office is helpful, but direct observation and/or talking to others about their observations is often required to make the diagnosis. Sometimes the diagnosis is made by excluding other diagnoses that don't fit the symptoms and "reading into" the behavior that the person is displaying. An example of the value of observations in reaching a diagnosis follows:

Jonathan, 47, had a long history of self-talk and interaction with imaginary friends. At first, his family was able to redirect him when necessary to help him function in his daily activities, he participated in his work program, and he was active with his family. However, his family noticed a change in his behavior over time. His self-talk became more intense, it was more difficult to redirect him when he talked to himself, and he was spending more and more time interacting with his imaginary friends to the exclusion of his family, coworkers, and friends. The diagnosis of psychosis became clear when he began reporting seeing monkeys swinging through his home. He responded well to risperdone (Risperdal), an anti-psychotic medication, as well as to his family's efforts to redirect him into his usual daily activities.

TREATMENT

• • • • • • • • • • • • • • • • • •

Treatment of psychoses includes:

    1. emotional support for the person and the family or care providers,

2. attention to medical issues that may be contributing to the psychotic symptoms or that may have been a result of the person being less able to care for himself, and
3. medications.

Chapter 13 discusses the importance of counseling and evaluation of, and intervention in, the environment. These are necessary to assess whether the situation is clearly one of psychoses and to give clues as to how best to intervene.

Medications seem to always be an essential piece of treating psychoses in our patients with Down syndrome. Doctors have two types of anti-psychotic medications in their arsenals: the older anti-psychotic medications, and newer, atypical anti-psychotic medications.

The older anti-psychotic medications include drugs such as haloperidol (Haldol), thioridazine (Mellaril), and thiothixene (Navane). Although these medications work well, our experience has been that people with Down syndrome have more side effects from these medications. The anti-cholinergic side effects are particularly common and problematic. These include constipation, urinary retention, difficulty urinating, dizziness, and others.

The newer, atypical anti-psychotic medications are often a better choice. (These are often called second generation anti-psychotics, as compared to the older, typical anti-psychotic medications.) These include: risperdone (Risperdal), olanzapine (Zyprexa), queitapine (Seroquel), ziprasidone (Geodon), and aripiprazole (Abilify). Clozapine (Clozaril) also belongs to this class, but we don't use it because of the possible effect on the white blood cell count. These medications work well and seem to have fewer side effects than the older medications. In addition, these newer medications can help with the depressed mood that often occurs with psychoses.

We have found that olanzapine (Zyprexa) generally causes greater sedation. This can be used as an advantage when sleep disturbance is part of the problem. It also tends to cause the most weight gain, which, again, can be an advantage if poor appetite is a symptom.

Elevated blood sugar is a possible side effect of the atypical anti-psychotics, and this can lead to diabetes mellitus. We have seen this to a greater degree with risperdone (Risperdal) and olanzapine (Zyprexa) than with queitapine (Seroquel), ziprasidone (Geodon), or aripiprazole (Abilify). We regularly monitor blood sugar in our patients on these medications through blood draws. In addition, monitoring for the development of cataracts is recommended when using quetiapine (Seroquel).

When using any anti-psychotic it is important to monitor for tardive dyskinesia (TD). TD is a neurological syndrome characterized by involuntary and abnormal movements. This most commonly affects the muscles of the mouth or face but may affect any muscle. It most often occurs after long-term use of an anti-psychotic medication, particularly when used in high doses. TD seems to be less common with the atypical anti-psychotic medications. Discontinuing the medication is often enough to eliminate the symptoms, but sometimes they continue indefinitely even after the medication is stopped.

CONCLUSION

Psychotic disorders are relatively uncommon in people with Down syndrome compared to people without Down syndrome. They are also less common than other mental health problems in people with Down syndrome. Careful assessment is necessary to delineate true psychosis from "psychotoform" features or characteristics. Fortunately, psychosis in adults with Down syndrome does usually respond to counseling, environmental intervention, and medications.

Chapter 18

Eating Refusal

• • • • • • • • • • • • • • •

Refusing to eat is not considered a mental illness per se. But in adults with Down syndrome, it can be a symptom of so many mental health and physical problems that we have chosen to devote a separate chapter to eating refusal. It is also a difficult-to-treat example of the interaction between mental and physical health problems.

WHAT IS EATING REFUSAL?
• • • • • • • • • • • • • • • • • • • •

By eating refusal, we mean a significant change in the eating or drinking pattern of an individual that produces significant weight loss or other health risks. This may include:
- ◆ stopping eating and drinking altogether,
- ◆ refusing to eat all but a small, select group of foods,
- ◆ refusing to eat certain textures (for example, the person will drink but not eat solid foods), or
- ◆ eating small, inadequate amounts of food.

We have seen a number of patients with Down syndrome who have declined to eat and had significant weight loss. The problem generally seemed to be a symptom of a physical problem or to have started as a complication of a physical health problem. Often the person stopped eating in response to pain related to the health problem but then continued to refuse food after she was no longer in physical pain. In these cases, eating refusal appears to have become a learned behavior, a compulsion, or part of depressive or anxiety symptoms. Depression can also be a trigger for a significant change in appetite.

When eating refusal accompanies the onset of symptoms of a mental health disorder such as depression, we consider the eating problem as part of the symptoms of that disorder. However, often this is not what occurs. Most often, the most significant and challenging eating problems start after the development (or apparent development) of a medical problem. Frequently, the symptoms of a mental health disorder come later. However, the mental health condition seems to be a secondary condition that occurs in response to the stress of the initial medical condition and the eating refusal. For example:

> *Jim, 38, had a long history of a mild swallowing problem. However, as long as he ate slowly and his food was well cut, he did well. Then, at a local carnival, he ate a hot dog and choked. He developed a fear of eating and would only drink fluids. He became distraught over his fear, as well as the attempts of others to try to get him to eat his normal diet. Over time, he became depressed. Treatment had to focus not only on the original medical issue (the swallowing problem) but also on his depression and on counseling his family and others as to how to address his swallowing and eating issues.*

DIAGNOSIS

When we see an adolescent or adult with Down syndrome who is eating less or refusing to eat, our first step is to assess for underlying physical health problems. We do this even though the only symptom of a disorder may be a refusal to eat. If we were to assume that the eating refusal was completely behavioral in origin, we could miss a significant underlying health problem. If there were an underlying health problem and we failed to treat it, the result would generally be incomplete resolution of the eating problem and continuing, unnecessary discomfort for the person.

We consider the following medical conditions:

- gastroesophageal reflux and esophagitis (with and without esophageal stricture),
- peptic ulcer disease,
- dental problems,
- swallowing dysfunction,
- celiac disease,
- hypothyroidism,
- multiple other causes of nausea (e.g., kidney disease, diabetes, calcium abnormalities, pancreatitis, etc.),
- intracranial abnormalities (such as brain tumors or any cause for increased pressure within the brain),
- medication side effects,

◆ other possibilities that the history and physical might indicate such as sore throat, masses in the mouth or throat, and others.

We often find that stomach ulcers, inflammation in the esophagus, or other conditions in the gastrointestinal tract are the root cause of the problem. As part of the work-up for these problems, it is therefore often necessary to have the person undergo an upper endoscopy (esophagoduodenogastroscopy) to evaluate the gastrointestinal tract. This decision is not made without thorough discussion with the patient and family. An upper endoscopy involves placing an endoscope (a tube that can be looked through) into the mouth and advancing it through the esophagus down to the stomach and the first part of the small intestine. This is generally done under sedation, but many of our patients with Down syndrome require a greater degree of sedation and often require general anesthesia.

The decision regarding further testing is based on the findings of the history and physical. These include tests to assess for the problems noted above and others as guided by the findings.

TREATMENT

When there is an underlying medical problem, treating the problem sometimes results in a return to normal eating. No further treatment is needed. Other patients, however, continue to refuse to eat even after their physical problem is successfully treated. In these instances, we have found or suspected that the symptoms began due to a physical condition, but the medical condition served as a stressor and contributed to the development of compulsive behavior (i.e., the refusal to eat), depression, or other conditions. It is truly amazing how some people with Down syndrome in this situation seem to be able to ignore the body cue of hunger.

A frequently asked question is whether this problem is comparable to anorexia nervosa. Although there are some similarities, there are also differences between the presentation of anorexia nervosa in people without DS and the eating refusal we see in our patients. While our patients do avoid eating, we do not generally hear them express a concern that they are overweight or that they need to continue to lose weight— as is the case with patients who have anorexia nervosa. Instead, eating refusal appears most often as a response to a medical condition with subsequent development of the psychological issues of OCD or depression as outlined above.

If someone continues to refuse to eat once a medical problem is treated (or if we fail to find a physical problem underlying the eating refusal), treatment of eating refusal often involves treatment of an obsessive compulsive disorder or depression. These treatments can include:

1. counseling for the person with DS and for her family or caregivers,
2. swallowing therapy to promote eating trials,

3. support until the person is eating adequately, and/or
4. medications.

Support

Supportive therapy, reassurance, and redirection towards eating can all be helpful. When the physical problem has been treated, helping the person understand that the pain has resolved and eating will be pain-free can require ongoing support, "hand-holding," and encouragement. Often this needs to be done where the person lives (and eats). Therefore, her family and caregivers will also need to be part of the "team" that encourages and supports her. Other people who interact with her at school, work, and recreational settings will also have to be aware of the situation and be part of the solution.

The first goal is to make sure the person is eating enough to get the calories, vitamins, minerals, etc. she needs. As long as that is occurring, there is less pressure to push her to eat a "normal" diet. Therefore, if the person is refusing to eat solid foods, she may drink multiple cans of a supplemental drink (such as Ensure or Boost) and small amounts of food that add up to adequate calories, fluids, and other essential nutrients. Pressuring her to eat a "normal" diet may actually create anxiety and make it less likely she will consume the adequate amount she is presently. Support and gentle encouragement (and acceptance that this may be a slow process) are much more likely to be successful. They also give the adult with Down syndrome and the family time to work with the counselor, swallowing therapist, and/or medical practitioner to address additional treatments as outlined below.

Counseling

Coaching and counseling for the caregivers and families is usually necessary as well, since trying to encourage someone to eat can be very frustrating. The family and caregivers may need support to stay away from confrontational situations, "keep their cool," avoid taking the eating refusal personally, and reduce their frustrations. Confrontation often leads to the person with Down syndrome "digging in her heels" and can slow the healing process. A social worker, psychologist, or family therapist might provide beneficial counseling.

Swallowing Therapy

Swallowing therapy with a speech therapist can also be helpful. This therapy may be started as soon as the eating problem is recognized and while the underlying cause is being evaluated. Other times it is acceptable to wait until the underlying medical cause is found, because treatment of that problem may be all the treatment that is needed. The therapy consists of re-teaching the person to swallow and eat by progressively introducing foods. If some swallowing skills have been lost because the person has not swallowed appropriately in a long time, the therapy can help her regain these skills. Some adults with Down syndrome find swallowing therapy to be frightening or anxiety-provoking (just as eating may be). If so, anti-anxiety medications may be necessary before proceeding with the therapy.

MEDICATIONS

Medications are often part of the treatment for eating refusal. When depression or obsessive-compulsive disorder complicate the problem, antidepressant medications can be helpful. We have found paroxetine (Paxil) to be of particular benefit, because, like other antidepressants (SSRIs), it treats the depression or obsessive-compulsive disorder. In addition, many people with Down syndrome develop increased appetites and weight gain with paroxetine. In this situation, these side effects can be a real asset. Other antidepressants discussed in the chapters on depression and obsessive-compulsive disorder can also be helpful.

Sometimes, a thorough evaluation of the situation may lead to a diagnosis of a psychotic disorder (see Chapter 17). We have found all anti-psychotics to cause weight gain in some patients with Down syndrome. Olanzapine (Zyprexa) seems to be particularly associated with weight gain and can therefore be a good choice in this situation.

Medications to stimulate appetite can also be beneficial by increasing the person's motivation to eat. This, in turn, can help make her more receptive to other treatments. In our experience, megestrol (Megace) can be helpful in stimulating appetite in adults with DS who are refusing to eat. Blood sugar can become elevated on megestrol, however, so this needs to be monitored.

> Michael, 43, was brought to the Center because his sister was concerned that he was losing weight. His appetite had significantly declined and he had lost about 40 pounds, down to 110 pounds from 150 pounds. He had limited speech capabilities but could nod yes or no. He nodded that he didn't have any pain in his abdomen, although he appeared to have slight tenderness when his upper abdomen was examined. His hemoglobin (red blood cells) was a little low, indicating he was slightly anemic, which could have been due to inadequate intake of nutrients or because of blood loss.
>
> Michael was hospitalized to treat the dehydration that had occurred because of decreased fluid intake. While in the hospital, he underwent an endoscopy and was found to have a large stomach ulcer. He began treatment with a medication, omeprazole (Prilosec), to reduce the acid in his stomach. He was also treated with iron for his anemia. In addition, Michael was found to have and was treated for hyperthyroidism (overactive thyroid). Although hyperthyroidism can cause weight loss, it is often accompanied by an increased appetite (which was not the case with Michael).

Treatment for these conditions was only mildly successful in improving Michael's appetite and weight. He was diagnosed with depression based on his decreased appetite, his mood, his lack of interest in his usual activities, and increased sleepiness, and was started on paroxetine. His mood improved but he continued to struggle with eating. Megestrol was added and his appetite improved. As Michael gained weight and became more active, he regained strength and his overall demeanor markedly improved. Over the course of several months, he regained his 40 pounds. Megestrol and paroxetine were stopped, and he continued to eat well. Treatment to prevent further ulcers continued, as did his medication for hyperthyroidism.

Michael was a classic example of eating refusal. When he first stopped eating, he did not show symptoms of depression. These symptoms occurred later.

Paul, 33, required greater support. When we first saw him, he had lost 35 pounds, and was down to 105 pounds. Other than not eating, the only other problem his caregivers reported was a lifelong pattern of compulsive behavior. He tended to do most everything in a ritualistic, compulsive fashion. His physical exam was unremarkable except for his weight loss. Labs were all normal. Paul underwent an endoscopy, which showed just a little inflammation in his esophagus. Upon further questioning, there did seem to be a history of possible heartburn-type symptoms around the time he had begun eating less.

Paul was prescribed medications to reduce the acid in his stomach, but there was only minimal improvement in the amount he would eat. Despite counseling, paroxetine for presumed obsessive-compulsive disorder, and appetite stimulants, he continued to lose weight. Next he was fed through a nasogastric tube (a tube through his nose into his stomach). However, he continued to refuse to eat, and eventually a gastrostomy tube (a tube through his abdominal wall into his stomach) was surgically placed to feed him. Supportive nutrition was given through the gastrostomy tube while swallowing therapy, further counseling, and other medications were tried. Paul did get to a point where he would eat limited amounts "for pleasure," but he continues with a gastrostomy tube for nutritional support.

Paul's problem with eating demonstrates a fairly common finding. By the time the problem is evaluated, the original medical condition may be resolving. Alternatively, the medical condition may seem relatively minor. Paul, for example, was found to have minor inflammation in his esophagus. The problem, however, is that this relatively minor problem set off a progressively downhill course that resulted in an obsessive-compulsive disorder as well as behavioral changes. While it can't be stated for sure, it would seem that early intervention prior to the compounding of problems would improve the treatment of this condition.

> Another eating problem occurred for Jessica, 32. Jessica was placed on a strict, low-fat diet because of elevated cholesterol. Jessica was regularly reminded to avoid food that was higher in fat. Jessica had always been one who developed "grooves" (see Chapter 9) in her approach to her daily routine. She did this with her diet as well. Unfortunately, she developed such a groove that she became extremely selective in what she would eat. Her weight went down to her ideal body weight (120 pounds) and kept right on going, down to 101 pounds. Fortunately, we were able to redirect her and her family to support a healthy diet without going "overboard." Jessica was reassured that some fat was not only acceptable but good. Over time, her diet became more reasonable.

CONCLUSION

Eating refusal can be a very difficult problem that can pose a significant threat to health. In people with Down syndrome, there can be an interaction between both physical and mental health issues. A thorough evaluation for underlying physical health problems is an essential part of the diagnosis and treatment of the problem. Counseling, environmental evaluation and support, medications to treat associated psychological diagnoses, and medications to stimulate appetite may all be needed. Nutritional support may also be necessary. In adults with Down syndrome, significant weight loss is more the exception than the rule, so parents and other caregivers need to be vigilant about bringing changes in weight or appetite to the attention of healthcare professionals.

Chapter **19**

Challenging

· · · · · · · · ·

Behavior

· · · · · · · ·

Not all emotional and behavioral problems fit neatly into one of the diagnostic categories in the DSM-IV-TR. Yet, even though some behavior problems may not be formally labeled as disorders, they can still be challenging to deal with. In this chapter, we will use the term challenging behavior to refer to behavior that is maladaptive or disruptive to one's own or others' lives. Behavior problems may include:

- ◆ Verbal or physical aggression or damage to property;
- ◆ Oppositional, defiant, or disobedient behavior to authority figures;
- ◆ Antisocial or criminal behavior, including lying, stealing, or sexually inappropriate behavior, or behavior that is intentionally harmful to others;
- ◆ Behavior problems associated with impulsiveness, including behavior which is "discharged" without thinking or prior planning, such as blurting out inappropriate comments about others, darting into the street, grabbing food from others' plates, etc.

Behavior problems may also include behavior that is socially inappropriate or offensive but generally not harmful to others. This includes:

- ◆ Inappropriate behavior that is displayed in social or public places, including a lack of good hygiene, touching the genital area, expelling gas, nose-picking, etc.

Behavior problems occur less often for people with Down syndrome than for people who have other causes of mental retardation, but more often compared to the general population (Kahn, et al., 2002).

REASONS FOR CHALLENGING BEHAVIOR

Why do people with DS have behavior problems, and why do they have more problems than the general population? There are a number of possible reasons. Perhaps most importantly, adaptive and expressive language limitations may make it difficult to conceptualize and communicate the presence of problems or issues. Although this may be more obvious for people with limited verbal skills, it may also be the case for people who have better verbal skills. This is because adults with better verbal language may still not be able conceptualize and communicate thoughts or feelings around certain problems or issues. For example, one verbal young man turned a heavy dining room table over and threw many items in his room against the wall. He was also irritable and uncooperative with his family and his supervisor at work. This went on for a several weeks until his family brought him to the Adult Down Syndrome Center, where he was found to be suffering from a painful physical problem.

Another woman had similar incidents which were very uncharacteristic for her. Her family was at a loss to explain these changes until they learned that she had been recently dumped by her boyfriend and had also lost a close friend who moved to another town.

Any type of behavior problem, including aggressive, oppositional, or inappropriate social behavior, may communicate the presence of a problem. These behaviors may serve both to vent the person's frustration and to obtain attention from others. As a form of nonverbal communication, the message requires an interpretation by others (see Chapter 6). We have found that family members and other caregivers are usually able to help us interpret the message. Below are some of the most common causes of challenging behavior in adolescents and adults with Down syndrome.

UNDERLYING PHYSICAL CAUSES

It is particularly important to look for possible physical causes when evaluating a person with Down syndrome for difficulty with controlling behavior or aggressive behavior. Discomfort may lead to a reduced ability to control emotions or an exaggerated or aggressive response to another stimuli or event.

Malcolm, a 37-year-old man with Down syndrome who had obsessive-compulsive disorder, was being treated with Zoloft and redirection by the staff of his group home. The treatment was generally successful.

Periodically, however, he would become aggressive in response to the staff's attempts to redirect him. Malcolm had had mastoid (ear) surgery many years prior, and, periodically, the area would fill with debris and require suctioning. He was recurrently found to need this treatment during times of aggressiveness. He appeared to have discomfort associated with the physical problem but communicated this with his behavior, rather than words.

AD/HD. We also see individuals with behavior problems that are secondary to physiological or neurological conditions. People with these conditions may have more difficulty with controlling their impulses and behavior. Among the most common of these conditions is attention-deficit/hyperactivity disorder (AD/HD). AD/HD has impulsive behavior as one of the three core symptoms, along with attention problems and distractibility. Because of the impulsive behavior, the person with AD/HD may have more trouble waiting or difficulty keeping unflattering comments about others to himself. Some individuals may also have difficulty controlling their emotions and behaviors, and they may be likely to be aggressive when frustrated or stressed. Correctly identifying the physiological cause of the condition will help to ensure a more successful course of treatment. See below for more information about attention deficit disorders in adolescents and adults with Down syndrome.

Seizure Disorder. Occasionally we see adults at the Center who have aggressive or impulsive behaviors associated with simple or complex partial seizures. While relatively uncommon, these conditions need to be identified in order to provide the right pharmacological treatment. (See below and Chapter 14 for more on the use of anticonvulsant medications.)

Impulse Control Problems. We have also seen some individuals with DS who have impulsive behavior but show no evidence of either an attention deficit, a seizure disorder, or any other physical, emotional, or environmental precipitants. We continue to look for causes, but these people may simply have a greater disposition to impulsive behavior than others. As a result, like people with seizures and attention deficits, these individuals may have more difficulty controlling their impulses, and this may at times include antisocial or aggressive behavior.

ATTENTION DEFICIT DISORDERS

Attention deficit disorders are neurological disorders which have as core symptoms: problems with attention, impulsive behavior, and distractibility. The inattentive type (ADD-In) has only these core symptoms, while the hyperactive type (ADHD) has the above symptoms and the additional core symptom of hyperactivity. (Note that in the DSM-IV-TR, both types of attention deficit disorders fall under the umbrella category of attention-deficit/hyperactivity disorder, or AD/HD. To aid in making distinctions between the two subtypes, we will use the abbreviations ADD-In and ADHD, however.)

With studies showing prevalence rates at between 4 and 12 percent, AD/HD is one of the most common neurological condition diagnosed in children (Brown et al, 2001). Similar prevalence rates have been estimated among children with DS (Cohen and Patterson,1998; Myers and Pueschel 1991). AD/HD often has a disastrous impact on a child's academic and work performance as well as his social and emotional functioning and development. Attention problems and distractibility may make it very difficulty for people to focus and follow through in an organized fashion with essential tasks at home, school, or work. Additionally, because of impulsivity, relations with bosses and friends may suffer because the person may have trouble waiting or keeping his thoughtless or unflattering comments to himself. He may also have difficulty concentrating on conversations, which may make it appear as if he is disinterested in other people. Some individuals with this condition also have difficulty controlling their emotions and behaviors because of the impulsivity and may become aggressive when frustrated or stressed

Childhood AD/HD has been recognized for many years, but only recently has it been found to affect a significant number of adults. Adults may have the same problems with inattention, impulsivity, disorganization, and distractibility as children, and this may have the same effect on their social, emotional, academic, or occupational functioning as it does in children. Hyperactivity appears to be less common for adults with AD/HD, even in people who had hyperactivity as children. Apparently, people may grow out of the hyperactivity as they age into adulthood.

Although there is no available research on the rates of attention deficit disorders in teens and adults with DS, we have seen a significant number of individuals at the Adult Down Syndrome Center who have this condition. This includes many individuals with a history of attention deficit with hyperactivity who seemed to grow out of the hyperactivity in adulthood. Like adults in the general population, they often continue to have problems with attention and impulsivity and therefore often benefit from medication to help them better manage these issues. We have also seen some adults with DS who continue to have hyperactivity, even though ADHD with hyperactivity is less common in adulthood in the general population.

Symptoms of ADHD

What does ADHD (the hyperactive form of AD/HD) look like in adults with Down syndrome? To answer this question, it may be helpful to first describe typical symptoms in children. Although many children have high activity levels, children diagnosed with this disorder are so active that parents often describe them as "bouncing off the walls." Adults with DS who have ADHD will show some of the same overactive behavior which children show. Many have trouble sleeping, talk constantly and distractedly, and most cannot stay still or focus long enough to do sports activities, let alone essential school or work tasks. The level of activity in adults with DS may not be quite so intense as in children with ADHD (in either the general or DS population), but in comparison to other adults, their level of activity is quite extreme. Obviously, this type of behavior may be very trying for caregivers of adults as well as children. For example:

Marna, 21, was brought to the Center by her desperate and exhausted parents six months after she graduated from school. Marna was a friendly and good-natured young woman who was driving her parents and her boss crazy with her constant questions, distracted talk, and movement. At work, she could not stay in one place long enough to complete her job tasks. At home, she was only able to get ready for work or do other tasks if her parents were present to corral and prompt her at each step along the way. Marna was at her best when participating in sports, but even when engaged in these activities she had great difficulty staying focused. For example, Marna's coach described her as being "like a balloon with the air let out" when she was put into a game. She would fly around the field with great speed and intensity, but was not necessarily focused on the actual events in the game.

Marna's parents reported that she was hyperactive as a child and had been diagnosed with ADHD by a school psychologist and an experienced pediatrician. She was very active throughout her school years, but a stimulant medication, methylphenidate (Concerta), greatly helped to keep her hyperactivity, inattention, and impulsivity in check.

During the time after Marna graduated from school up until her appointment at the Center, her parents saw a marked increase in her ADHD, even though she was still on her medication. Marna's parents believed that the process of leaving school and starting her job may have been too stressful for her. Many of her friends were at the same worksite, but there was far more noise and distractions and less help available from staff than there had been at school.

At the Center, Marna showed no apparent health or sensory problems which could have aggravated her symptoms. ADSC staff confirmed the diagnosis of ADHD from her history and her current behavior and they began a course of treatment. Marna showed a positive response to bupropion (Welbutrin), an atypical antidepressant medication which is effective with adults who have ADD and ADHD in the general population. During this and subsequent meetings at the Center, Marna participated in counseling to discuss her feelings and expectations for herself. She was demoralized and her self-esteem was shaken, but she was encouraged to see herself in a more positive light, particularly as her hyperactive behavior and her inattention improved with the treatment.

For the first month, Marla continued to have some problems controlling her anger at work and settling down to sleep at night, but this improved with counseling and an increase in medication. During the second and third months, Marna's parents reported that her behavior was much improved at home and there were no negative reports from the workshop. At a six-month follow-up Marna was still doing well at home, but her parents reported receiving notice from her worksite that she could be suspended because of angry outbursts.

Shortly after this meeting, outreach staff from the Center arranged to visit the workshop to get a better understanding of the situation. What they found was enlightening. A number of participants in the worksite were aggravating Marna with taunting and teasing remarks. Apparently, these individuals had seen her overreact to situations before starting her medications and they seemed to want to goad her into making angry outbursts as she had in the past. Because Marna had a history of past outbursts (prior to starting the new medication) she was threatened with suspension from the program. After being informed that other participants were provoking Marna, workshop staff agreed to closely monitor the situation and to block the others from harassing Marna. After several weeks and several incident reports which named the other participants as provocateurs, the teasing and goading stopped.

It has been now three years since Marna's initial evaluation and she continues to be followed at the Center. She has had some minor problems and some medication adjustments, but overall she continues to do very well.

Is It ADHD or Something Else?

The good news about ADHD is that people get help because of the intensity of the symptoms and the stress and strain on caregivers. The symptoms simply cannot be ignored. Additionally, ADHD is one of the most researched and widely known conditions affecting children and adults. Because of this, teachers, pediatricians, and other practitioners are likely to diagnosis this condition when a child or adult with DS is brought in with hyperactivity. The bad news about the widespread knowledge of ADHD is that hyperactive behavior may be diagnosed as ADHD when in fact the hyperactivity is caused by something else.

In reviewing the referrals of people who have been previously diagnosed with ADHD who come to the ADSC, we have found that many have been misdiagnosed. Accurate diagnosis may be even more of a problem for people with DS who have a limited ability to verbally report problems or symptoms. For example, in our experience people with bipolar disorder may be misdiagnosed as ADHD because manic behavior may look like hyperactive behavior. However, manic behavior is only a part of the symptom picture, and viewing it this way may lead to treatments which may actually worsen the problem. For instance, stimulant medications may increase manic behavior or increase the intensity of mood fluctuations. Misdiagnosis as ADHD may be avoided if practitioners take a careful history, which may be more likely to show the mood fluctuations (between mania and depression) that are characteristic of this disorder.

Similarly, mania may also be misdiagnosed as ADHD. As with bipolar disorder, this may lead to the use of stimulants, which may worsen and intensify the mania. Taking a careful history may help to reduce this problem as well. Mania is often a condition that occurs cyclically and it often ebbs and flows, whereas ADHD is usually more consistent in presentation and intensity level.

We have also seen people with autism spectrum disorders who were misdiagnosed with ADHD. Although these individuals may have hyperactive-like behavior, particularly when anxious or over-stimulated, diagnosing them as having ADHD ignores such key aspects of the autism disorder as the lack of relatedness to others. Again, without a correct diagnosis individuals may not receive essential behavioral and medical treatment for the condition.

Anxiety may also be easily misdiagnosed as ADHD. This is particularly the case for people with DS who cannot verbalize their feelings but express anxiety through agitated and overactive behavior. How do you sort out anxiety from ADHD? We recommend being particularly sensitive to the history and longevity of the symptoms presented. ADHD is present in early childhood and occurs throughout the person's life. The intensity of the symptoms may change with age, but the disorder will still be present in some recognizable form in adulthood. On the other hand, if the person's "hyper" behavior seems to begin during a stressful time, then it is more likely that the behavior is actually anxiety in response to a stressor. Additionally, if the person's ADHD occurs in only certain environments, such as a school classroom, then this may simply mean that the environment is stressful. Often we find that the person is either over- or under-stimulated in the stressful environment.

Finally, and perhaps most importantly, symptoms of ADHD may simply be the person's preferred means of communicating behaviorally the presence of some type of stressor. Again, this is particularly likely for children and adults with DS who have limitations in verbalizing thoughts or feelings. Therefore, behavior that looks like ADHD may be communicating that there is a physical disorder, a sensory deficit (visual or auditory), a stressful change or loss, or an environmental stressor. As we have emphasized throughout this book, we can only get to the cause or source of a behavior if we, as practitioners and caregivers, become detectives and examine as many areas as possible (e.g., physical, sensory, environmental, life stage changes). This may be the only way to determine whether any other reasons or explanations for the person's behavior are possible.

SYMPTOMS OF ADD-IN

If ADHD is over-diagnosed, ADD-In (without hyperactivity) is under-diagnosed.

For children and adults with ADD-In who do not have hyperactivity, the good news for caregivers is that they are far less disruptive and difficult to manage. The bad news is that they may be far less likely to be diagnosed and treated for this condition. There is a growing body of evidence that a fairly large number of children and adults in the general population are not identified and treated for this condition because of the more subtle nature of the symptoms (especially when compared to people with hyperactivity) (Jensen and Cooper, 2002; Murphy and Barkley, 1996). We have found that diagnosis may be even more of a problem for people with DS than for other groups. Aside from the difficulty of identifying symptoms, ADD-In may not be considered because it may be too easily attributed to the Down syndrome, even when behaviors are not characteristic of DS (Reiss et al., 1982).

Children and adults with this condition may float along as if in a fog or dream-like state. They have great difficulty concentrating on school or work tasks. They may have trouble in social situations because they have difficulty listening to others or in reading social cues. The distracted, dream-like state may be even more of a problem for children with DS because they tend to have excellent visual memories which they may draw on to "space out" (see Chapter 5 for more on this).

Even if caregivers or teachers do not see the problem, these children may be teased by peers as being "space cadets" or "dreamers," but this is no laughing matter. ADD-In may have a profound negative effect on the individual's school, work, or social relations, and this in turn may have a disastrous impact on the person's self-esteem.

How, then, do we diagnose and treat ADD-In in people with DS, given the nature of the symptoms? We need to be very honest here with you, the reader. We have been treating adolescents and adults with DS for some time and yet we still have not identified many people with this condition. We simply need to do a better job with this. To this end, we have found that there are a number of clues which may help us as well as caregivers and parents identify ADD-In in this group. These clues relate to different symptom presentations in people with DS who have ADD-In compared to people with the disorder in the general population. There are also important differences between people with DS who do and do not have ADD-In which may be instructive.

First, regarding the presentation of symptoms, what is a key characteristic of people with ADD-In in the general population is that they are often chaotic and disorganized. They often have great difficulty setting up and following consistent routines, making it difficult to do daily tasks reliably and efficiently. The resulting lack of a predictable order is often very frustrating for themselves and for family members.

We have seen a similar pattern for some people with DS who have ADHD (AD/HD with hyperactivity), but not for people who have ADD-In (without hyperactivity). These individuals have a sense of order despite having attention deficit symptoms. They are often able to reliably complete daily living tasks, home chores, and work tasks, as long as these activities are part of their regular routine. Their routines and grooves then seem to carry them along despite their attention problems.

The key difficulty these individuals often seem to have is in dealing with free or unstructured time at home or work which is outside of their routine rather than an activity that is part of their routine. Although their routines usually carry them along, they have problems organizing activities when not doing their routines. This brings us to an important difference between people with Down syndrome who do and do not have ADD-In. In a nutshell, people with DS and ADD-In have great difficulty entertaining themselves. This is in contrast to the majority of people with DS, who are usually very good at entertaining and occupying themselves during free time activities.

Over thousands of interviews, we have heard time and again about adolescents and adults who have special activities they enjoy doing in their free time. Examples of these activities include drawing, copying words or letters, needlepoint, watching TV or movies, looking at family photographs, or even cleaning one's room. In fact, most people with DS are so good at entertaining themselves that parents and caregivers often complain that they may spend too much time doing these activities. Therefore, when someone cannot do this, it should be a red flag for caregivers and practitioners even if the person is otherwise able to follow daily routines. For example:

Alida, 23, was initially brought to the Center by her parents and case manager from her job because of several aggressive incidents that occurred at her job. Her parents and case manger were surprised and concerned because Alida had been a model employee for the two years she had been at her job. Her boss had been very pleased with her because she loved to do some of the most challenging jobs and her production rate was very high. Her parents and case manager also noted that she was very friendly and personable and was not prone to acts of aggression.

When questioned about possible changes in her job, the case manager reported that there had been an extended period of no work. This was the first time this had happened in the two years that Alida had worked at her job. She seemed to become more and more restless and bothersome to others during this period. She did not want to participate in some of the down-time activities, including doing arts and crafts or watching movies, which her case manager admitted were not very stimulating.

Alida's parents described a similar problem at home. Alida seemed to be fine when she could do things that were part of her regular routine. She enjoyed doing her daily chores, such as dusting the house and cleaning her room. However, when she had free time, she could not seem to settle down to do anything to entertain herself. Although her parents tried to give her things to do, such as watching a movie, drawing, or doing word search puzzles, she simply could not do these things for any length of time. Her parents stated that she had always had some problems with entertaining herself in the past, but she had three very active brothers who seemed to supply her with an endless number of interesting activities. Although her brothers complained at times that Alida was a "pain," they loved her and were very tolerant of her participation in their activities. Unfortunately, in the last year, two of her brothers had moved out of the family home, and the other was rarely around.

Alida's parents tried to keep her busy outside the house participating in social and recreation activities. She did fine in more active sports or recreation activities, but had a difficult time in more unstructured social gatherings. Unfortunately, her participation in outside activities did not seem to help her manage her free time at home.

Finally, Alida's school history was consistent with a diagnosis of ADD-In. Her family noted that she had had problems in grade school with staying on task. Her teachers had described her as having a short attention span. She also had some problems playing with others during recess activities, but they attributed this and her attention span to her Down syndrome. Alida had seemed to do better in high school, particularly in the last three years when she participated in an excellent vocational training problem involving experiences in a wide variety of jobs. She was very busy and challenged in this program, and this seemed to be the formula she needed. Indeed, she had found her job very challenging and satisfying until the sudden extended period of down time that had preceded her aggressive outbursts and her initial visit to the ADSC.

In order to verify ADD-In, we referred Alida to a psychologist who had expertise evaluating people with DS with attention deficit problems. She confirmed our suspicion that Alida had ADD-In. After a trial of several different stimulant medications, Alida showed a positive response to methylphenidate (Ritalin XR). On the medication, she was able to settle herself down and developed a healthy interest in a host of activities including needlepoint and word search puzzles. Equally important, she was far more able to tolerate down time at her workshop. We did, however, recommend to the workshop that they develop a more interesting program of free-time activities. Subsequently, a bank of computers was set up which Alida loved to use during her free time.

MEDICATIONS

Medications are an important part of the treatment for ADHD and ADD-In. The medications can help improve attention, reduce impulsivity, and reduce hyperactivity. The medications fall into two general categories: stimulant and nonstimulant.

Stimulant medications stimulate the central nervous system. Interestingly, this reduces the symptoms, including hyperactivity. The approved medications include: methylphenidate (Concerta, Metadate, and Ritalin), dextroamphetamine (Dexedrine), and dexmethylphenidate (Focalin). Amphetamine/dextroamphetamine (Adderall) is a non-FDA approved medication for ADHD and ADD-In that is also commonly used. Side effects of stimulant medications in adults include nervousness, difficulty sleeping, motor tics, palpitations, loss of appetite, and others. Finding the right medication may take some time. Even if someone doesn't respond well to one stimulant, he may respond to one of the other medications.

The other choice is a nonstimulant medication. At present, there is only one available choice, atomoxetine (Strattera). It inhibits the reuptake of the brain chemical norepinephrine, which is believed to play a role in regulating attention. It may cause side effects including: sleep problems, fatigue, increased sweating, fatigue, palpitations, and others. Some people benefit from using a combination of a stimulant medication and atomoxetine. Bupropion (Wellbutrin) is an antidepressant that has also been used for ADHD and ADD-In.

UNDERLYING MENTAL HEALTH DISORDERS OR STRESS

A behavior problem may signal the presence of a mental health problem. For example, at the ADSC, we have seen many people who become aggressive if prevented from doing their obsessive-compulsive behaviors and rituals. The presence of aggressive behavior often signals a marked increase in the severity of obsessive-compulsive symptoms. Caregivers who may be reluctant to seek treatment for obsessive-compulsive rituals may be more likely to seek help when symptoms are accompanied by physical aggression.

We have also seen similar patterns of behavior for some people with symptoms of depression (see Chapter 14.) This is particularly the case for individuals who withdraw and isolate themselves within the security of their bedroom or another private space. Although these individuals are not characteristically aggressive, they may display aggressive behavior when caregivers try, out of desperation, to get them to leave their rooms to resume normal social or work activities.

Challenging behaviors may also communicate the presence of more extreme environmental stress, such as due to intolerable living or work situations. One of the most common causes of environmental stress is conflicts or tensions with or between others.

Other causes of stress that may result in a behavior change include noxious or overwhelming sensory stimuli in the home, worksite, or the community. Loud cavernous worksites may be particularly to blame for this kind of stress, but other types of sensory input may be involved as well.

MORE SERIOUS BEHAVIOR PROBLEMS

The Diagnostic and Statistical Manual of Mental Disorders (DSM-IV-TR) has defined three major behavior disorders for the general population. Two of these, conduct disorder and antisocial personality disorder, are very similar except that the latter is diagnosed in adults and the former is usually diagnosed in children. The third is oppositional defiant disorder. We will define these disorders and discuss whether these behavior problems may be diagnosed for people with Down syndrome.

CONDUCT DISORDER/ANTISOCIAL PERSONALITY DISORDER

The diagnosis of conduct disorder is usually reserved for children under 18. This disorder is defined as a repetitive and persistent pattern of behavior in which the basic rights of others or major age-appropriate societal norms or rules are violated. The person exhibits aggression, criminal behavior, and wanton disregard for the feelings and well-being of others. The disorder may range from mild forms of antisocial behavior to more severe criminal behavior. The DSM-IV-TR has also defined antisocial personality disorder as the continuation of a conduct disorder into adulthood. As with conduct disorder, there is a lack of empathy and concern for others, as well as antisocial or criminal behavior. People with this disorder have been called "sociopaths" or "psychopaths" to describe their lack of feeling and remorse for their harmful behavior.

In our experience, it is rare for people with DS to have conduct or antisocial personality disorders. We have only seen a handful of people who have at least a moderate degree of conduct problems.

> *One individual, Hue, had a history of sexually inappropriate behavior throughout his childhood. We met him at the Center as a young adult when he was brought by a concerned older brother and staff from his group home and worksite. His brother and staff described a series of sexually inappropriate or sexually aggressive behaviors that had occurred in the bathroom at his worksite and at his group home residence. None of these had resulted in criminal prosecution, but Hue's brother believed that it was only a matter of time before this would happen. Hue's brother also revealed that Hue was the victim of sexual abuse by an uncle. This uncle was never prosecuted because the abuse was kept secret by the family. Unfortunately, like some victims of childhood abuse, Hue developed an insatiable desire for sexual gratification. He also seemed to have little concern for how his sexual behavior affected those he targeted to meet his needs.*
>
> *We developed a multimodal treatment approach to deal with Hue's difficult problem. It is important to understand that there is no definitive way to treat sexually deviant behavior except though strict monitoring and supervision. First, all his caregivers agreed to develop a highly structured environment for Hue. At no time would he be left alone with others without very close staff supervision. For example, he had his own bedroom and an alarm was rigged to go off if he left the room in the evening. As a second example, he was given a special changing room at the gymnasium where he exercised to keep him away from others in the locker room, especially children. Second, Hue was started on an antidepressant medication to reduce his sexual drive. (For Hue, the antidepressant effect of the medication was less important than the side effect of lowering sexual drive.) Because of the close supervision and the effectiveness of the medication, no further sexual incidents have been reported. Staff and family continue to meet at least every three months or more to ensure a continuation of the plan.*

A second example of a person with a conduct disorder can be seen in a 17-year-old teen with Down syndrome, Beatrice:

> *Beatrice had grown up in a household with a number of family members who had an extensive history of criminal behavior. She had spent much of her early school years in classrooms for students with behavior disorders because of her aggressive and oppositional behavior. She also had*

some of the same sexually inappropriate behavior as Hue, although not to the same degree, and a history of stealing money, food, and valuables from others. Her behavior continues to be difficult to manage in her current high school behavior disorders program and at home with her mother.

It is our belief, and that of her teachers, that Beatrice may continue to need a highly structured environment, similar to the program developed for Hue. However, Beatrice is much younger than Hue and her school and the appropriate state case-management agency are looking for a therapeutic facility for her. There is hope that in the right program she may have a chance to overcome her behavior problems. There is evidence that some children do grow out of conduct or other behavior disorders if they are given appropriate guidance and treatment before they reach adulthood.

Less Severe Sexual Conduct Problems

At the Adult Down Syndrome Center, we have seen a number of men and women with DS who have made inappropriate sexual comments or who have touched people inappropriately. These adults have generally responded to parent or staff attempts to stop or redirect their behavior. In a few instances, parents have had trouble stopping sexual behavior due to normal teenager-like resistance by the person with DS to parental control. In these cases we have collaborated successfully with parents to support their efforts to control the behavior through increased supervision. When we do encounter a problem of a sexual nature we have the adult with DS return for regular scheduled appointments (weekly or every other week) until we are satisfied that the problem is completely resolved or managed.

Behaviors Which May Look Like a Conduct Disorder

Stealing

Sometimes adults are brought to the Center by concerned parents or other caregivers because of incidents of stealing from others. Occasionally, there are concerns that this behavior may lead to other types of antisocial behavior. We generally find that this behavior has more to do with an intellectual or conceptual limitation in the person with DS than a problem of criminality. We often call this behavior "creative borrowing," rather than stealing, because the person may simply not understand the concept of stealing. Like many younger children in the general population, some people with DS have difficulty understanding that others have personal property, even when they are well aware of their own personal possessions.

For some people with Down syndrome, "stealing" may be related to a compulsion to save or hoard a special item (such as pens, paper, etc.). The person does not necessarily conceptualize this behavior as taking from others, but rather as simply adding to his collection (see Chapter 16 for more on hoarding).

In evaluating instances of "stealing" we look for the presence or absence of other forms of antisocial behavior to determine the severity of the behavior. Beatrice, discussed above, is a good example of a person with a conduct disorder. She stole from others and had many other serious behaviors such as a lack of sensitivity toward others' feelings, aggressive behavior, etc. For adults who just have instances of stealing, without other antisocial behavior, we work with caregivers to try to reinforce simple behavioral strategies to limit this behavior. For example, the person may earn a reward, such as buying a desired pen from a store, if he does not take the desired item from others. This allows him to acquire desired items without "borrowing" from others.

LYING

Parents and other caregivers sometimes have similar concerns about lying. This behavior, too, may involve a conceptual limitation. Some people with Down syndrome simply may not understand the concept of lying, just as many younger children do not. Another reason that people with DS may tell untruths or "lie" may be that they tend to be very sensitive to others. As a result, they may try to protect others from feeling bad by not telling them something that will hurt their feelings. They may also try to please the listener or even to protect themselves from the other's anger. The fact that they may not truly understand what it means to lie may make the "lie" less of a problem for them in certain situations, such as when protecting themselves or others from real or perceived harm.

Other times people with Down syndrome are thought to lie when in fact they are not lying. As discussed in Chapter 5, many people with DS have exceptional memories, but have difficulty understanding the concept of time. As a result, they may speak in the present tense about past events. If listeners are not aware of this lack of time orientation they may think the person is lying rather than describing a past event. A good example of this was a young man with DS who complained that he was abused by someone at his worksite. His mother was called to a meeting to discuss why he was lying about the abuse. Fortunately, she was able to explain that he was actually talking about a past event. However, it is easy to imagine that staff would interpret his statements as lies or false accusations if his mother was not present to explain the confusion. To avoid this type of problem, any comments need to be assessed as possibly having some basis in the past and not just the present.

Additionally, many people with Down syndrome may have difficulty with sorting out fact and fantasy, and may discuss imagined events or events viewed on TV or in the movies as if they are factual. What appears to be a lie may actually be the result of a very active and vivid imagination and memory. Special care should be taken to understand the confusion of fact and fantasy when assessing statements made by people with Down syndrome.

OPPOSITIONAL DEFIANT DISORDER

The DSM-IV-TR describes oppositional defiant disorder (ODD) as a recurrent pattern of negativistic, defiant, disobedient, and hostile behavior toward authority figures. Although this diagnosis is only used for children or teens in the general population, it may be applicable to adults with Down syndrome, because they often continue to have caregivers who are responsible for them.

We have seen a small number of people with DS who exhibit ODD behavior. Sometimes this seems to be something the person is born with (part of the person's temperament). Other times, the environment may play a role in the development of this problem. For example:

> Robin, 36, was raised by parents who were very strict and controlling of her behavior. After her parents died, she moved to a group home which she shared with three other women. The stated philosophy of the house was choice, independence, and a respect for the rights of others. This seemed to work for the other women but not for Robin. She seemed to experience the house as a place where she could dominate and control others like her parents had controlled her.

> Over time, Robin became more demanding and less cooperative with staff. When staff imposed some control over her, she rebelled and began to throw major tantrums and to harass and at times be aggressive to the other residents. After many unsuccessful attempts by staff to solve the problem, Robin was transferred to a therapeutic group home, which was set up to better manage people with behavioral issues. The house followed a structured behavior plan where people earned rights and freedoms for cooperating with the rules. After several intense months, Robin learned that cooperating with the rules allowed her to have some control over her own situation. Although she continued to struggle, she found that cooperating with the rules did not mean others controlled her. She also learned that if she respected others' rights, they would respect her rights too. After approximately three and a half years in the structured group home, she had shown enough maturity to move to a less structured house, and she has done very well ever since.

We have seen others like Robin who have problems with accepting caregiver authority. We should say, however, that we do not frequently diagnose them with ODD. As discussed earlier, we have found that the behavior may actually be an attempt to communicate the presence of a problem or an issue that people cannot easily verbalize. Again, this could be anything from a physical pain and discomfort to environmental stress. Therefore, whenever this type of behavior occurs, we recommend that the caregivers and professionals involved try to identify any message communicated through the person's behavior.

In addition, sometimes what caregivers call "oppositional behavior" is actually a message about inappropriate constraints being imposed on the person with Down syndrome. For example, we have had referrals from families who have difficulty with a son or daughter who is legitimately struggling for their own independence. In these situations, it is very important to diplomatically but emphatically support the person's legitimate need for independence. A good example of this type of situation may be seen in Andre's story in the family counseling section in Chapter 13.

Finally, another reason the diagnosis of ODD is not used as often as one might think is that oppositional behavior is often one symptom of a much larger problem or condition. For example, many people with bipolar disorder, a dual diagnosis of autism and Down syndrome, or even a conduct disorder may express some oppositional and defiant behavior toward caregivers as part of the condition, along with other behaviors and symptoms. The treatment for these conditions may be very different than for just ODD. For example, multimodal treatment approaches are often needed for bipolar disorder; autism may require very different behavioral strategies; and a more intensive behavior program may be required for someone with a conduct disorder, such as discussed for Hue above.

Disorders That May Be Misinterpreted as Behavior Problems

A number of disorders may be misinterpreted as behavior problems by professionals and caregivers. Most notably these may include obsessive-compulsive behaviors, tics associated with Tourette syndrome, and similar problems with stereotypic behaviors.

Obsessive-compulsive or groove-like behaviors may be misinterpreted as behavior problems. Uninformed or inexperienced authority figures may misinterpret the set routines and behaviors that people follow as oppositional behavior. For example, a teacher asked one of our teenaged students to stop what he was doing to do another task. Like many people with Down syndrome, this student continued doing the first task and did not move on to the new task. He was not trying to have a negative behavior or attitude but just to finish the first task out of a compulsive need.

If a teacher believed this kind of behavior was opposition or disobedience, he might intensify his efforts to force the student to stop. Force may work if the student is in fact oppositional, but if it is a compulsion, the teacher's behavior will usually only intensify the person's compulsive need to finish. See Chapters 9 and 16 for information on recognizing grooves and compulsions, as well as guidance on helpful responses to compulsive behavior.

Motor and vocal tics which occur as a result of the neurological condition Tourette syndrome may also be misinterpreted as a behavior problem. For example, verbal tics involving grunts, mouth noises, or the expression of certain words may be viewed by a teacher or employer as oppositional behavior, particularly when the person has difficulty stopping the behavior. An adult with stereotypical behavior (repetitive movements) such as hand flapping may also be erroneously labeled as oppositional, since attempts to block such behavior are often counterproductive. See Chapter 21 for information about appropriate ways of dealing with tics and repetitive movements.

TREATMENT

True oppositional behavior, aggression, difficulties with impulse control, and the other behaviors described in this chapter can be particularly problematic challenges. Whether it is an older person with Down syndrome who has begun to strike his elderly parents or a middle school student who is running out of the classroom and fleeing the school, these behaviors can be some of the most challenging. It is at least as important with these challenges as with any other behavior or mental health issue to assess for underlying physical causes, to assess the social context of the behavior, and to employ a multifaceted treatment approach with attention to psychological, social, and medicinal treatments.

The treatment of behavior problems can consist of:
1. behavioral treatment, and
2. medications.

BEHAVIORAL TREATMENT

Behavioral treatment can consist of reward systems, redirection attempts, and modeling of appropriate behavior and response to stressful situations. Families or other caregivers should look for a trained mental health counselor who specializes in behavioral therapy to assist them with behavioral treatment (see the Counseling section of Chapter 13 for more on this).

REWARD SYSTEMS

Reward systems can be used as part of the treatment plan for a variety of behavior issues in people with Down syndrome. This type of behavioral therapy is often directed only at responding to the occurrence (or absence) of an undesirable behavior. For example, if the person with Down syndrome has no aggressive episodes all week at work, he is allowed to purchase a soft drink on Friday afternoon. There are some additional features that should also be included in the behavioral approach.

First, make sure that the person is not being inadvertently rewarded for inappropriate behavior. If, in the example above, the person has repeated episodes of aggressive, oppositional, impulsive, or antisocial behavior throughout the week, he will not receive his soft drink at the end of the week. However, if he does not really care for the soft drink and what he is really looking for is increased attention from the staff, the attention he gets when he is aggressive may be much more rewarding than the soft drink. The behavioral program may actually be rewarding the behavior it seeks to extinguish.

The timing of rewards is another important aspect of the behavioral program. A reward that is three or four days away may have very little impact on some people with Down syndrome. Their attention span may be too short or the reward may be too distant in the future for them to link their behavior with the reward. Rewards that are given more frequently based on a shorter period of appropriate behavior are more likely to be meaningful to some adults with DS.

Preventing Problems

Another critical aspect of behavioral programs is usually the prevention aspect. This involves first analyzing the events that typically lead up to the problem behavior, and then figuring out what the person accomplishes with his behavior (does he receive attention? does he get out of doing something he does not want to do?). Afterwards, a variety of strategies can be tried to prevent the behavior from occurring. For example, if you learn that a behavior is apparently triggered by a certain event, you can try to prevent that event from occurring. Or, if you can anticipate the event that often provokes the behavior, you can redirect the person before he begins the behavior. Then again, if you learn that the behavior is related to difficulties the adult has in asking for a break, you can teach him a different way of communicating that message.

The systematic process of determining the function of a behavior by analyzing the antecedents (what happens before the behavior) and consequences (what happens after the behavior) is known as "functional behavior assessment" (FBA). It is beyond the scope of this chapter to go into detail about conducting an FBA. It is worth learning more about the process, however, if the adult with Down syndrome you care for has serious behavior problems. For an overview of the process, you may want to read the book *Functional Behavior Assessment for People with Autism* (Glasberg, 2006), or speak to a behavior analyst about conducting one. However, in the meantime, it may be very useful for you to try the redirection strategies described in the next section.

It is important to note that prevention may be more difficult where impulse control problems are involved. For impulse control problems, there is often no clear antecedent event that triggers the behavior. Therefore, preventing the problem may be difficult because it occurs "out of the blue." Sometimes, though, there are antecedent events that we are not recognizing. It is often worthwhile to observe the situation several times to see if something might be triggering the situation.

It may also be possible to reduce impulsive behavior if it is associated with a treatable physiological condition, such as AD/HD or a seizure disorder (see the section below on medication treatment).

Redirection

Rebecca, a young woman with Down syndrome, periodically would become so frustrated with some of her colleagues at work that she would turn over a table when she got home. Usually if she had had a frustrating day at work, she would pace back and forth in the doorway before entering her home. When they saw this behavior, the staff knew that if they interceded and guided Rebecca to her room to sit down and listen to music, they could usually help her relax and prevent an escalation of her behavior.

Rebecca's story shows how others can redirect a person with DS before they become aggressive. How and why does redirection work?

Redirection works when a person can successfully change a negative emotion or behavior to a positive emotion or behavior. A major principle of behavioral treatment is that people cannot have two contradictory emotions at the same time. If people feel calm and happy, they cannot experience the negative emotions of anger, sadness, etc., at the same time. Following from this, the goal of treatment is to identify the early stages of a negative emotion and behavior to help to redirect the person to a positive mood and behavior.

Keys to successful redirection:
- ◆ Redirection to positive emotions and behavior works best when started before the person is too far into a negative emotional state.
- ◆ In order to redirect someone before he becomes angry, try to identify early warning signs that he may display prior to expressing the anger. Rebecca's early warning sign was pacing in the doorway. Others may use a wide variety of different and idiosyncratic behaviors as early warning signs.
- ◆ Remember that warning signs may change, so continue to observe the person's behavior to identify new signs he may show before expressing anger.

Identifying positive alternatives:
- ◆ Regularly observe quiet time activities to identify activities the person enjoys and that are relaxing to him.
- ◆ Try to have a number of relaxing activities from which the person may choose. This gives him more of a say in the process.
- ◆ Giving someone a choice between relaxing activities is also a way to direct his attention to something positive without eliciting anger.

Attitude and behavior of caregivers:
- ◆ Be very careful in how you approach the person in these situations. If you are too forceful or confrontational, you run the risk of actually provoking anger rather than redirecting the person away from anger. For example, saying very calmly to someone who is getting angry, "Would you like to listen to music or draw?" is far more likely to succeed than to confront the person with, "You look like you are getting angry . . . You need to listen to music or draw something. Now!"
- ◆ A calm tone and attitude is particularly important for the parents of teens and young adults, who are far more likely to rebel against parental authority.

SELF-REDIRECTION
Sometimes adults with Down syndrome can be taught self-redirection. That is, the person may learn to identify his own early signs of anger and to redirect himself.

This is not an easy task for people with average intelligence and it may be even more difficult for people with Down syndrome. Nevertheless, we have found that with time and practice many people with DS can learn to redirect themselves. It may be possible to first teach the person with DS to respond to cues from others, particularly if a parent or caregiver cues him when early signs of anger are observed. Over time, he may be able to recognize his own patterns of behavior and to begin to cue himself when his mood and behavior changes.

It may also be possible to use self-talk to help someone redirect himself when he is feeling that he is about to act inappropriately. As described in the chapter on self-talk, people with Down syndrome will often say aloud what other adults would silently say to themselves. People can use their own self-talk to cue themselves to redirect an inappropriate behavior. Some will even speak to themselves in the third person when they are redirecting themselves. Annie, 37, periodically strikes out at other people. Many times others have witnessed her saying such phrases as, "Annie, don't hit Tommy" when she is agitated. People who hear this from Annie then take this as a cue that she needs to do an activity that is relaxing for her and assist her with this until she is relaxed.

For many other adults with DS, we have been able to take this self-talk redirection strategy a step further. Not only can some people learn to remind themselves not to express anger inappropriately, but they are also able to redirect themselves to do a positive or relaxing activity. For example:

> When Marvin began to feel himself getting angry and agitated, he would repeatedly say to himself "don't yell or throw things." Then he would tell himself to breathe deep. He would sit down and breathe in and out deeply for several minutes until he was calm and no longer agitated. At times Marvin had great difficulty practicing this strategy, especially if he was confronted too quickly or forcefully with a very stressful or frustrating situation. For example, once as he entered the dining room of his residence, he encountered a housemate who was having an angry, tantrum-like outburst. Marvin tried to start his redirection strategy, but he was too shaken by the other resident's anger. Fortunately, we had worked with staff to deal with just this type of situation. Several of them gave Marvin a prearranged sign (pointing their thumbs in the direction of the door). This was the signal for Marvin to leave the immediate situation. He then was able to go to the quiet living room to talk himself through his redirection and deep breathing exercise.
>
> Marvin has been very reliable with starting this strategy when he feels angry. In a few instances, he has needed another signal to remind him. This consists of staff members acting like they are taking a deep breath. This is usually enough for him to start his redirection and deep breathing exercise.

Steps to Take When Someone Is Already Expressing Anger

Sometimes, the person may already be angry and the opportunity to divert his anger to something positive is already past. In these situations the following guidelines for moderate or more severe angry behavior may help to deal with the problem.

More Moderate Degree of Anger. Assess the degree of anger. If the person is out of control and there is a risk that he could hurt himself or someone else, then follow the recommendations in the section below on "More Extreme Anger and Aggression." Otherwise, the following steps may be helpful for managing the anger:

1. Remain calm and in control of your own anger, if any. Caregiver's anger will only serve to further anger or agitate the person with DS.
2. If possible, give the person room to express his anger. It is particularly important to get children or others who may not understand the danger out of the way. Remember, too, that in a fit of passion any behavior is possible. Therefore, clear away anything that can be thrown or used as a weapon.
3. Once the worst of the storm has blown over, approach the person in a unthreatening way.
4. In a calm voice, gently coax him to sit down to be in a more relaxed physical state. Once he is seated, repeat calming statements.
5. Family members may also gently hug or hold the person with DS to help him relax if he is comfortable with this.
6. Once he is calm, try to engage him in an enjoyable activity, such as listening to music, looking at pictures, etc.
7. When the situation is stable, examine the sequence of events that led to the anger. This may help you identify and resolve whatever problems led to the outburst. It may also help to identify behavioral precursors to the anger that can cue you to redirect the anger.

More Extreme Anger and Aggression

Dealing with the Immediate Crisis. Assess the aggressive behavior. If the person is out of control and there is a risk that he could hurt himself or someone else, he may require an immediate intervention. If he lives in a larger group home, there may be set procedures for dealing with more extreme aggressive behavior. Usually these procedures involve some form of physical restraint which is maintained until the person calms down. For example, one larger residential agency has approximately eight staff members who are specially trained by a psychologist. When there is an incident, at least four of these staff are paged to respond immediately to the situation. Following planned procedures, these individuals then carefully but firmly hold the person down so that he cannot hurt himself or others.

If the person lives at home, in a small residence, or anywhere where there is no procedure for managing aggressive behavior, then outside help may be needed. Sometimes experienced staff or family members are able to calm the person down when others cannot. For example, one staff person was called at home when Georgia had an outburst because she had a particularly good rapport with Georgia. She responded immediately by coming to the group home and Georgia responded very positively to her presence. In another situation, an angry adult with DS calmed down after talking on the phone to his mother.

Sometimes the police may be called when interventions tried by family or staff have not been effective. The presence of police officers may help to calm down some people who have aggressive behavior. This is usually the case when the person does not have an extensive prior history of aggressive behavior. However, caregivers may need to be very active any time the police are called. Most police officers have very little experience or training in dealing with people with Down syndrome or other disabilities. They will often look to the caregiver for guidance. Caregivers may use the police presence to help stabilize the situation but not necessarily to make decisions about treatment options (discussed below). However, the police may be enlisted to transport the person to a treatment facility if needed (discussed below). Otherwise, if the person is calm, the staff or family members may be able to safely transport the person to an appropriate facility, if deemed necessary.

Seeking Treatment. Once the adult is calm and the crisis is over, there are two primary courses of action involving outpatient or inpatient treatment. Many times staff will bring people with more extreme aggression to the attention of mental health professionals. This usually involves a consultation with a behaviorist and/or mental health professional in a medical or mental health outpatient setting. At the ADSC, we have been asked on an emergency basis to assess and treat many people who display more extreme forms of aggression. In our experience there are many different causes, explanations, and possible treatments for these behaviors, which we have discussed in detail throughout this chapter and throughout the book.

Sometimes when adults with Down syndrome have extreme behavior, they are taken by staff, police, or their families to a hospital emergency room to be assessed for possible hospitalization in a mental health ward. In larger cities, there may be hospitals with wards specifically for people with intellectual disabilities. However, in most cases, the only option is a general psychiatric ward.

We have found that hospitalizations are not always as beneficial as people would hope. Ideally, hospital staff attempt to identify and treat mental health and health conditions and to work with family and staff to identify sources of stress. Too often, though, staff do not have enough experience or comfort with diagnosing and treating people with DS for mental health or behavioral problems. They often neglect to do other medical testing to identify health problems. Hospital staff may also not make an effort to contact the family or staff to help identify and resolve environmental conflicts or stress. As a result, the hospitalization may become little more than an extremely expensive respite, which buys time, and gives family and staff a break, but solves none of the problems or issues that may have caused the problem to begin with.

Sometimes hospitalization actually worsens the problem. This is because caregivers may rely heavily on hospitalizations for crisis management, but this does not necessarily help to resolve the problems leading to the behavioral outbursts. Additionally, some people with DS actually like the experience of being hospitalized. They may be doted over by staff and there may be little pressure on them to do anything constructive. Some adults with DS experience this as a type of vacation. Unfortunately, this is an extremely expensive "vacation," and again, not necessarily productive if there is no attempt to identify the underlying problem or to teach the person how to better manage his behavior.

We have also found that many hospitals will not admit people with intellectual disabilities to the psychiatric ward even if they are seen in their emergency rooms. Sometimes hospital staff do not feeling comfortable treating a population for whom they have little experience. Often the person who is taken to the ER will eventually calm down, even if he is still agitated upon arrival. Some may lose their anger and hostility when they see others in the ER who have more serious physical or emotional conditions. Waiting to be seen for hours in an ER may also deaden any anger that remains. Failing to be hospitalized is not necessarily a bad thing. This is especially the case if the hospitalization is not geared to identify and resolve the problems causing the behavior, as discussed immediately above.

Additionally, many times people who are turned away from the ER will then look for resources in the community. Once the immediate crisis is over, they may have more time to locate an outpatient facility with more experience serving people with disabilities. These facilities will have professionals who may have more success with resolving the causes of the behavior problem.

Evaluation of the Causes of an Extreme Behavior. Once the crisis of an extreme aggressive incident is over, a thorough evaluation of the possible causes of the problem needs to commence. Efforts to treat without this evaluation may lead to failure if the real reasons behind the angry outbursts are not identified and resolved. Often, once the cause of the problems is dealt with, the behavior will become more manageable. Once this occurs the guidelines discussed above for more moderate forms of anger may be used to help manage any remaining aggressive outbursts that occur.

Some of the most common causes of extreme behavior:

- The behavior may be due to extreme environmental stress. Consider this possibility particularly if there is no history of prior behavioral outbursts. For example, Bret had simply had it with being victimized by a bully in his residence. His behavior was a "wake up call" to staff to move or to better manage the behavior of the bully, who had been abusing a number of people in his residence. Once this problem was solved, there were no more outbursts from Bret or any of the other residents in the household.
- As mentioned previously, health problems may create extreme pain and discomfort and may contribute to or cause extreme behavior

changes. A thorough physical exam should be conducted whenever there are changes in behavior, especially more extreme changes.

◆ Extreme behavior may also be related to a mental health problem. As mentioned throughout this book, many people with DS have limited ability to communicate problems and issues verbally. A mental health problem may surface as an extreme change in behavior. Therefore, if the person's aggressive behavior problem is not explainable by environmental stress, by a medical condition, or by any other type of behavior disorder (conduct disorder, oppositional defiant disorder, etc.), then a consultation with a mental health professional may be advisable. For example, people with previously undiagnosed bipolar disorders have been brought to our office with a recent history of aggressive outbursts.

MEDICATIONS

As discussed previously, behavior problems, and especially impulsive behavior, may be caused or aggravated by physiological or neurological conditions such as AD/HD, seizure disorders, Tourette syndrome, and tic disorders. The behavior problems which result may be far more manageable with the use of medications to treat these conditions. For example, people with attention deficit disorders may greatly benefit from a stimulant medication, while those with seizure disorders may respond positively to an anticonvulsant medication, and those with Tourette syndrome/tic disorders may respond to anti-psychotic medications. Similarly, we have found that some individuals with more severe impulsive behavior may respond to anticonvulsant medications even when there is no apparent physiological cause. This may be due to the fact that seizures are difficult to detect because they occur intermittently.

Certainly, a host of other medical conditions may also cause or aggravate behavior problems, as discussed previously. This may include thyroid disorder, B12 deficiency, and other disorders discussed in detail in Chapter 2. As discussed previously, appropriately treating physical problems that are contributing to behavioral problems is necessary to optimally reduce the abnormal behavior.

Additionally, medications may be helpful when mental health symptoms coexist with behavior problems. One of the most common of these symptoms is anxiety, which is often manifested as agitation and body tension. We also find mood disorders to be fairly common with behavior problems. A mood disorder may include the more severe fluctuations in mood and behavior associated with bipolar disorder (see Chapter 14), but far more often it includes less severe symptoms of moodiness and irritability.

The anticonvulsant (anti-seizure) medications are an effective treatment approach for behavior problems with mental health symptoms. Valproic acid (Depakote, Depakene) and carbamazepine (Tegretol) are good choices. People on these medications need to have periodic blood tests to check medication levels, as well as tests such as CBC, liver function tests, and electrolytes to check for side effects. We have also had some success with gabapentin (Neurontin), which is not as widely recognized as a choice and is probably not as effective as the others. The advantage of gabapentin is that there is less need to monitor blood work, and therefore it is more tolerable for our patients who dislike blood drawing. We have also recently started to use lamotrigine (Lamictal) with some success. Blood test monitoring is indicated when using this medication as well. None of these medications are FDA approved for these behavior issues.

Antipsychotic medications can also be quite beneficial in treating these types of behavior problems with mental health symptoms. Risperdone (Risperdal), olanzapine (Zyprexa), queitapine (Seroquel), ziprasidone (Geodon), and aripiprazole (Abilify) have all been effective in some of our patients with Down syndrome. As indicated in Chapter 17, however, monitoring for sedation, weight gain, and elevated blood sugar is necessary.

Antidepressants are not generally beneficial when used on their own to treat these types of behavior problems, but may be helpful in combination with other medications (such as the anti-seizure medications). The antidepressant trazodone (Desyrel) can be particularly helpful as an adjunct medication in treating behavior and mental health problems. It is especially helpful as a sleep aid. Therefore, it may be a good addition for patients who have sleep disturbance as part of their symptoms. Similarly, use of melatonin (a hormone used for sleep disturbance and jet lag) or other sleep aids such as zolpidem (Ambien), eszopidone (Lunesta), or zaleplon (Sonata) may play a role in treating these conditions.

Finally, if the challenging behavior is associated with an obsessive-compulsive disorder or with major depression, then an antidepressant medication that treats these conditions may help to reduce the behavior problems associated with these disorders.

CONCLUSION

When an adolescent or adult with Down syndrome is aggressive, impulsive, extremely oppositional, or is engaging in other challenging behaviors that interfere with daily life, it is extremely important to try to determine what is triggering this behavior. A careful assessment for underlying medical issues, as well as for possible environmental triggers, is essential. As with the treatment of other mental health problems, addressing psychological, social, and biological aspects increases the likelihood that treatment will be successful.

Chapter 20

Self-Injurious

Behavior

On the surface, self-injurious behavior may seem one of the most difficult-to-comprehend mental health problems. Most of us do not expect people "in their right minds" to willingly hurt themselves. Actually, however, self-injurious behavior is not always a symptom of mental illness. When it occurs, though, it always requires diagnosis and treatment, which is why it is included in the Mental Illness section of this book.

Self-injurious behavior can be a means to express discomfort, displeasure, or even pleasure. It can be seen in a variety of mental health problems. In addition, it may be a means of communicating physical pain.

WHAT IS SELF-INJURIOUS BEHAVIOR?

By self-injurious behavior, we mean behavior that causes injury to oneself. This may include striking oneself, biting oneself, falling, running into walls, and other activities that cause injury.

Self-injurious behavior is not common in adults with Down syndrome, but does seem to occur more often than in people who do not have developmental disabilities. One reason is that self-injurious behavior often appears to be a form of communication. Often the person who does self-injurious behavior has limited communication skills. This makes it that much more difficult to develop an understanding of the problem and to treat it.

CAUSES

In people with DS, self-injury may occur for a variety of reasons, including:
1. The person finds self-injurious behavior pleasurable or rewarding.
2. The person has autism in addition to Down syndrome.
3. Self-injury helps relieve anxiety or stress.
4. Self-injury is an effective means of communication.
5. Self-injury is related to pain or a medical condition.

Finding Self-injury Pleasurable: Difficult as it may be to believe, self-injury seems to be rewarding for many people who engage in it. They don't seem to experience this injurious behavior as painful and it may actually be pleasurable. Difficulties in understanding how this injurious behavior is pleasurable or rewarding to the person can make it difficult to understand and to develop an effective behavior program. However, endorphins may play a role. Endorphins are a natural substance produced by the body in response to pain (and certain other causes) that stimulate the opiate receptors, reduce pain, and can cause euphoric or positive feelings.

Self-injury in Autism: Self-injurious behavior may be one of the symptoms seen in autism spectrum disorders. There are a number of theories as to why this behavior is seen in autism. It may be part of self-stimulation, may release endorphins and cause pleasure, may be a way to get attention, or it may be a symptom of a sub-clinical seizure. Autism is discussed in Chapter 22.

Relieving Anxiety: If someone is feeling anxiety or stress, self-injury might reduce that sensation. It may also distract her from the anxiety. For example, if you are worrying about something and accidentally cut your finger or drop something on your foot, you immediately start thinking about your finger or your foot instead of your worry. In addition, if the person is overwhelmed by the anxiety, she may respond irrationally when the anxiety "boils over." That is, she may respond to the sense of loss of control caused by the anxiety by striking or otherwise injuring herself. Some people with an intellectual disability have less ability to control their actions or to understand what an appropriate response is.

Self-injury Related to Medical Problems: Self-injurious behavior can be a symptom of a variety of physical health problems. Its purpose may be to inform others of the discomfort or perhaps to eliminate the pain. For example, we had a patient who was depressed and had a chronic sinus infection. Whenever discomfort from the sinus infection occurred, he would repeatedly strike his head. Once the infection was diagnosed and treated, he stopped striking his forehead.

Often the person will strike a location on her body that is different from the location of the discomfort. This appears to be a general display of pain or frustration or a generalized call for help. We have seen a number of people who bit their hands, struck their chests, or hit their head against objects when uncomfortable.

Self-Injury as Communication: Self-injurious behavior can be a wonderfully effective communication device—particularly if the goal of the behavior is to gain attention. When someone observes a person who is performing self-injurious behavior, a very natural reaction is to attempt to stop him or her. This effort rewards the person with attention.

Self-injury can also be a very effective way to demonstrate displeasure with something that is going on in the environment.

> Samir would slap himself in the face whenever he was displeased with what someone else was doing. His roommate, Oscar, had a tendency to quietly tease Samir in such a way that the staff members of their group home were unaware that it was happening. However, whenever Samir would slap his face in response to Oscar's teasing, the staff would intervene and tell Oscar to stop bothering Samir.
>
> Telling Oscar to stop teasing Samir whenever Samir slapped his face did stop the slapping immediately. However, it also encouraged Samir to continue to slap his face to get Oscar to stop his teasing. After assessing the situation, the staff observed Oscar more closely for teasing behavior. They worked on intervening before Samir started hurting himself. In addition, they watched for early signs that Samir was beginning to get agitated (if they had missed Oscar's teasing). When they saw these signs, they praised Samir for not injuring himself and redirected Oscar away from his teasing.
>
> Samir learned that he did not need to strike himself to cause a change in his environment. Over time, the staff taught him to use a picture communication book that included a picture that indicated he was unhappy with something. He and the staff were able to learn a new way for him to communicate and he no longer felt the need to communicate by striking himself.

When assessing self-injurious behavior, it is important to ascertain if it is a form of communication. Some steps to assess the behavior as communication include:

- ◆ Analyze what the person "gets" as a result of the injury. (Does he get attention, removal from a situation he finds troubling, or something he wanted?)
- ◆ Consider whether the behavior may be linked to a health issue (or is there some other indication that he may be in pain or have an illness)?

As discussed in the chapter on depression (Chapter 14), suicide seems to be uncommon in people with DS. This generally does not seem to be the motivation for self-injurious behavior.

TREATMENT

Treatment depends on the underlying reason for the self-injury. If it's a form of communication, as described above, the solution is often to teach the person a different way of communicating the problem. A speech-language pathologist may need to be involved, especially if the person is not very verbal and may need an alternative communication system.

REDIRECTION

When there is no apparent "cause" for the behavior or no apparent communicative intent for the behavior, just redirecting the person away from the behavior is sometimes the most effective intervention. For example:

> Louise, a nonverbal woman aged 43, had a tendency to strike herself in the head. We found no evidence that she was trying to communicate something, that she was in pain, or that there was an underlying physical problem. Whenever she would begin to strike herself or look like she would strike herself, the staff would initiate a clapping game with her. Eventually, she was able to initiate the clapping game on her own.

Keys to redirecting someone away from self-injury include:
- Choose a substitute behavior that is incompatible with the self-injury. In Louise's case, she struck herself with her hands so a clapping game occupied her hands (as well as her attention) and reduced the self-injurious behavior.
- Watch for warning signs that the behavior is about to occur and intervene before the behavior starts.
- If the person is using something readily accessible (such as a sharp corner of a piece of furniture) to cause injury, safety-proof the house.

Helping someone learn to redirect herself is a very effective way to reduce self-injurious behavior. One way is to have the person tell herself out loud not to hit herself. Start by asking her to repeat the phrase after she hits herself. Next, work with her to say it during an episode of hitting. Finally, watch for warning signs and work with her to say the phrase before she hits herself. Interestingly, many of our patients who use this technique address themselves in the third person when they do it. For example, when David redirects himself, he says, "David, don't hit."

COUNSELING

Counseling may also be effective for some adults with Down syndrome. Particularly if a stressful situation tends to trigger the self-injurious behavior, counseling may help the individual discover the event or events that lead to the behavior. Counseling may be done with the individual alone or with the family or caregiver participating in the session. It depends on the individual. However, it is often fruitful to give the person with DS an opportunity to participate in individual therapy with the counselor. If she is nonverbal, alternative means of communicating may be tried such as drawing pictures, communication boards, etc.

Through counseling, adults with DS can be taught other ways to deal with stress. Use of devices to promote "self-redirection" may be effective. For example:

> Sandy had a tendency to strike herself when she became anxious or agitated. Sandy was able to communicate this concern, which allowed the counselor to help her see the connection. They were also able to develop a system together to allow her to redirect herself. Sandy agreed that when she was feeling anxious, she would pull her "worry stone" out of her pocket and rub it instead of striking herself.

Similarly, other people have been able to learn to go to their rooms, sit down, listen to music, and relax when they are feeling anxious.

MEDICATION

In addition to behavior techniques and counseling, medication can be beneficial for people with self-injurious behavior. There may be an underlying psychological problem that causes or contributes to self-injurious behavior. An assessment for an underlying psychological problem will help guide the medication selection. Further information on the medications discussed below can be found in Chapter 13.

HELPFUL MEDICATIONS WHEN ANXIETY AND DEPRESSION ARE INVOLVED

When anxiety is associated with self-injurious behavior, anti-anxiety medications can be helpful in reducing self-injury as well as anxiety (see Chapter 15). We have had limited success with buspirone (Buspar), but it often takes several weeks to see the benefits. The benzodiazepine medications (e.g., alprazolam, lorazepam, etc.) can be used while waiting for the effects of buspirone to be felt. In addition, the benzodiazepines can be used as the primary treatment. The longer-acting choices, in particular, can be used on a regular basis. However, the potential for developing tolerance, addiction, and withdrawal symptoms (when the medication is discontinued) may limit their benefits.

Several of the antidepressants are also beneficial in treating anxiety. Venlafaxine (Effexor) as well as the SSRIs, paroxetine (Paxil), escitalopram (Lexapro), and sertraline (Zoloft), have been approved by the FDA for treating social and or generalized anxiety. The other SSRI medications as well as bupropion (Wellbutrin) have been beneficial for some patients. These medications can all contribute to reduce self-injurious behavior when anxiety is a contributing factor.

When self-injurious behavior is a manifestation of depression, antidepressants can again be quite beneficial. As indicated above for anxiety, the selective serotonin reuptake inhibitors are very effective for depression. In addition, we have found venlafaxine (Effexor) and bupropion (Wellbutrin) to be effective.

Helpful Medications When Sleep Disorders Are Involved

As discussed in Chapter 2, sleep disturbance is more common in people with Down syndrome. When sleep disturbance is chronic, it can lead to agitation. Self-injurious behavior may be the expression of the agitation. Restoring a more normal sleep pattern can be a very effective way to reduce agitation and any self-injurious behavior associated with it.

Sleep apnea is more common in people with Down syndrome and can cause agitation. If an adult with DS has sleep apnea, it should be brought under control as much as possible through CPAP or BIPAP, supplemental oxygen, position change, or surgery such as tonsillectomy (see Chapter 2). Otherwise, long-term damage to the lungs or heart can result.

Sleep disturbances due to other causes, or unknown causes, might be treated with supplements or medications. We have found melatonin (a hormone used for sleep and to treat jet lag) to be beneficial in reducing self-injury associated with poor sleep. The antidepressant trazodone (Desyrel) is also an effective treatment for self-injurious behavior, particularly when there is sleep disturbance. In our experience, trazodone seems to work better as a sleep aid than as an antidepressant in people with Down syndrome. We have also prescribed short courses of other sleep aids such as zolpidem (Ambien), eszopiclone (Lunesta), or zaleplon (Sonata).

Once the person gets back on a regular sleep pattern with the help of the drugs, she may continue to sleep well (at least for awhile) without the sleep aid. However, it is important to watch for recurrence of sleep disturbance and self-injury and to prescribe the drug again, if necessary. Some individuals require long-term use of a sleep aid to optimize their sleep (and behavior).

Other Medications

Anti-seizure Medications: Anti-seizure medications (anticonvulsants) can also be an adjunct to behavior techniques in treating people who have self-injurious behavior. For example, valproic acid (Depakote) has FDA approval for mania and has been found to be beneficial for agitated behavior, impulse control disorder, and self-injurious behavior. Carbamezepine (Tegretol) and oxcarbazepine (Trileptal) have also been used for these problems.

Gabapentin (Neurontin), another anti-seizure medication, is less well known as a treatment for self-injurious behavior, but limited research data supports its use in mania. Although we knew there was neither FDA approval for this medication for self-injurious behavior nor a history of recognized benefit, we first tried it in several patients with self-injurious behavior who would not allow us to draw blood. (Drawing blood to monitor for possible side effects is usually recommended for other anti-seizure medications such as valproic acid and carbamezepine.) We found that gabapentin is an effective treatment for some individuals for self-injurious behavior, aggressive behavior, and impulse control disorder. It can be used with less concern about the need for blood test monitoring (although not no concern.)

Atypical Anti-Psychotics: The atypical anti-psychotics are quite beneficial in treating self-injurious behavior in people with Down syndrome. We have successfully reduced self-injurious behavior with risperdone (Risperdal), olanzapine (Zyprexa), ziprasidone (Geodon), quetiapine (Seroquel), and aripiprazole (Abilify). Unfortunately, we have seen tremendous weight gain in some of our patients on these medications. We have also seen significant elevations of blood sugars (necessitating discontinuing the medication) in some individuals.

It is important to note that the people with Down syndrome and self-injurious behavior we have seen generally do not have clear psychotic symptoms. We are not using the medication to treat psychosis in this situation, nor using it as a sedative. In fact, if sedation occurs as a side effect, we usually reduce the dose or change the medication.

Naltrexone (ReVia). As mentioned above, some people may find self-injury pleasurable because pain can cause the body to release natural substances called endorphins. Endorphins stimulate the opiate receptors in the nervous system and this may cause the person to perceive the sensation as enjoyable. For this reason, medications developed to block the effect of opiates (narcotics) on the opiate receptors can be helpful in treating self-injurious behavior. Apparently, by blocking the opiate receptors from working as usual, any pleasurable effects of self-injury can be blocked as well. The opiod antagonist (blocker) we have had some success with is naltrexone. Since it can be difficult to tell whether someone with Down syndrome "gets pleasure" from self-injurious behavior, naltrexone may be tried even in individuals who don't seem to find the self-injurious behavior pleasurable.

EATING FECES

Another problem that appears to be similar to self-injurious behavior is eating feces. This behavior has significant potential to hurt the individual.

In people with Down syndrome, eating feces often seems to occur in association with one of a couple of issues. First, we have seen a few people whose vision was declining and may not have recognized that what was on their hands was not food. In these cases, treating the vision problem often helps reduce the eating of feces.

Second, some people with Down syndrome seem to find eating feces pleasurable. As with self-injurious behavior, it is difficult to understand how this can be so. Generally, we have found that our patients who eat feces are more severely cognitively challenged and have limited or no verbal skills. Some also have autism or pica (eating inedible substances). Counseling is often of little benefit in these situations.

Redirecting and closely monitoring the person may improve the situation. Giving her something else to eat, especially food that is a similar consistency and texture, may be helpful. Sometimes giving the person something else to hold in her hands helps, but some people might eat that instead.

Tailoring clothing to make it harder for the individual to reach stool may be helpful. Long-legged pants or one-piece garments that open in the back where the person can't reach have been successfully used. We generally only recommend this strategy for people who are not able to use the toilet independently because this clothing would prevent independent toileting.

Medications are usually the mainstay of treatment. The medications discussed above may also be helpful to reduce eating feces.

Clearly, it is also important to monitor and treat the person for illnesses such as diarrhea or upset stomach resulting from eating feces.

CONCLUSION

Self-injury can be quite harmful to the person who is doing the behavior. It is usually quite disturbing to those around the person as well. Careful assessment is needed while keeping in mind that the adult with Down syndrome may be using self-injury to communicate that she is in pain. Counseling, redirection, behavior programs, and medications may all be part of the treatment for individuals with this problem.

Chapter 21

Tics and

· · · · · · · · · · · · · · ·

Movement

· · · · · · · · ·

Disorders

· · · · · · · · · · · · · · · ·

Many people with Down syndrome repeatedly make movements or sounds that others may consider odd or annoying.
For example, they may grind their teeth, hum to themselves, wring their hands, or
rock back and forth when listening to music or watching television.

Sometimes these movements and sounds are what are called stereotypic or self-
stimulatory behavior. Stereotypic behavior is defined as a motor behavior that is repetitive, often seemingly driven, and nonfunctional (DSM-IV-TR). Stereotypic behavior includes repetitive motor behaviors and the repetitive movement of objects. These
motor behaviors may at times interfere with normal activities and may result in self-
inflicted bodily injury.

Sometimes repetitive movements may be related to other things such as compulsions, although compulsions are usually more complex than stereotypic behaviors.
Stereotypic behaviors involve the repetition of more simple behaviors, such as hand
flapping, whereas compulsions often entail a more complex series of steps such as
arranging personal items so that they are "just so." Repetitive movements may also
be manifestations of stress, agitation, anxiety, or excitement rather than stereotypic
behaviors. In addition, some types of motor movements are side effects of neurolep-

tic medications (see Chapter 13). Some movements may also be related to medical conditions such as seizures or to a seizure-like condition in Alzheimer disease, or to less common health conditions such as Huntington's disease or strokes. There are also repetitive movements which are actually tics, or involuntary sounds or actions that are due to biochemical differences in the brain. Tics may at times be difficult to differentiate from stereotypic behavior, but the main difference is that stereotypic behavior seems to be under more voluntary control than tics.

Because repetitive movements and sounds are so common among people with Down syndrome, it is important to understand the different underlying reasons for them, as well as what, if anything, should be done to reduce their occurrence. With tic disorders, for instance, medical treatment may be extremely beneficial, but with stereotyped movements, medical treatment may not help and may sometimes actually do more harm than good.

STEREOTYPIC BEHAVIOR

* * * * * * * * * * * * * * * * * * * *

> Denise's whole body gets involved when she is excited about something.
> For example, at home, when watching a favorite DVD, she frequently wrings
> her hands when she knows a "good part" is coming, or she may shoot
> her arms straight out in front of her and scrunch up her face in a happy
> grimace, her eyes wide with pleasure. She may wring her hands, stretch
> her fingers out, and grimace dozens of times in the course of a movie. If
> someone asks her what she is doing, however, she usually stops right away.
> And at school or in other settings where she is less relaxed and more aware
> of others' reactions, she rarely, if ever, wrings her hands or grimaces.

Like Denise, many people with Down syndrome have some seemingly odd, purposeless actions that they do over and over again. These stereotypic behaviors are presumed to occur more frequently in people with developmental disabilities. At the Adult Center, we have found that many types of stereotypic behaviors are fairly common and occur regardless of the person's level of skill or functioning. Common stereotypic behaviors include:

- ◆ hand flapping or hand wringing,
- ◆ rocking back and forth or side to side,
- ◆ humming or making other types of mouth noises, and
- ◆ manipulating objects in some repetitious way (rubbing, twirling, etc.).

Of course, people have their own idiosyncratic versions of these behaviors based on the types of objects they manipulate or the unique movements or sounds they may make.

FREQUENCY OF OCCURRENCE CONTINUUM

Among people with DS, there is a continuum from a very high rate of stereotypic behaviors to a very low rate of occurrence, with the vast majority of people with DS falling somewhere in the middle. At the low end, there are a relatively small number of people who rarely display these behaviors and at the higher end, a small number who have a high rate of behaviors.

PEOPLE WITH A HIGH RATE OF STEREOTYPIC BEHAVIORS

Many of the people at the high end of the continuum spend a considerable amount of their waking hours engaged in stereotypic behavior. These individuals tend to have more severe impairments in intellectual and adaptive functioning. This may also include people with autism spectrum disorders, and especially those with significant social and expressive language limitations.

These individuals often have the same types of stereotypic behaviors as those in the more moderate group (discussed below), but the frequency and duration of these behaviors greatly inhibit functioning in other important life spheres. Many of these individuals also display self-injurious behavior and a sizable number display more severe forms of this behavior. Examples of self-injurious behavior include rubbing, biting, or chewing on hands, knuckles, or other body parts, as well as picking at skin and at sores. Often there is also a history of hitting or slapping themselves in the face or body, head banging, or other forms of self-injury.

Some people in this group may have more odd types of behaviors. For example, they manipulate objects in unusual ways, such as dangling or shaking action figures, or manipulate unusual objects such as strings, paper items, pieces of clothing (socks, underwear, etc.), or shiny metal objects.

Some stereotypic behaviors may pose a significant challenge to caregivers. For example, some people may have more onerous behaviors, such as licking or smelling objects or people, anal digging, fecal smearing, masturbation, or grabbing at genitals, etc. The treatment for these severe problems is an intensive and often lifelong process of diverting the person's attention to more productive social and adaptive behavior. (For more on the treatment of these behaviors, see Chapter 20.)

PEOPLE WITH MORE MODERATE FREQUENCY OF STEREOTYPIC BEHAVIORS

As mentioned above, the vast majority of people with Down syndrome do have a measurable amount of stereotypic behaviors. These may include such behaviors as hand flapping or wringing, rocking or swaying, mouth noises, and manipulating certain objects. Some of these individuals may also have self-injurious stereotypic behaviors, particularly when anxious or stressed.

For people with more moderate displays of stereotypic behaviors, we have found that there are ways to predict when these behaviors are more or less likely to occur. These behaviors are less likely to occur when people are engaged in work, social, or recreation activities which require more of their attention and physical engagement. Stereotypic behavior is more likely to occur when people have down time, such as when they are idle at work or when relaxing at home in the evening listening to music or watching TV. Often stereotypic behavior also occurs at a greater frequency and intensity when the person is having some type of emotional experience, such as the pleasure and excitement which Denise felt in the above example. On the other hand, stereotypic behavior may also increase when the person experiences negative emotions, such as stress or anxiety.

WHAT CAUSES STEREOTYPIC BEHAVIORS?

There are theories but no definitive answers for what causes stereotypic behavior or why it occurs more frequently in persons with developmental disabilities. Understandably, much of the research has focused on people with more severe impairments who have a higher frequency of stereotypic behavior. Still, these theories may help those with more moderate frequency and intensity of these behaviors as well. Some researchers believe stereotypic behavior may be caused by a deficiency in the central nervous system resulting in a need or craving for intense stimulation. This could help explain the increase in stereotypic behaviors when someone is relaxing and is mildly under-stimulated. Other theorists believe the opposite, that people are over-stimulated and use stereotypic behavior to try to block input from their environment. Still others believe that stereotypic behaviors may be self-soothing.

Each of these theories may have validity for some people. On the other hand, in many situations (such as in the example of Denise, above), stereotypic behavior may simply indicate the presence of something that is stimulating and not necessarily something that is under- or over-stimulating. Then again, it may be possible that stereotypic behaviors may simply be a complement to whatever else people do to relax, such as play music, watch TV, etc.

Understanding stereotypic behavior which results in self-injurious behavior may be more difficult. As discussed previously, we have seen a relatively small number of individuals who do more serious self-harm. What causes this? Ironically, this behavior may actually be self-soothing for some individuals. Researchers have found evidence that more severe self-injurious behavior may release pleasurable endorphins in the brain.

Although the release of endorphins may help to explain the contradictory behavior of people who seem to find pleasure in hitting or harming themselves, it may not help to explain the more moderate forms of self-injury we encounter more frequently in our clinical work. Examples include picking at skin or sores, scratching, and chewing or biting at fingers and knuckles. In our experience, these more moderate self-injuries seem to occur when people experience, or are over-stimulated by, some degree of stress in their lives.

WHEN TO SEEK HELP FOR STEREOTYPIC BEHAVIOR

Families are often concerned as to whether these behaviors are pathological or an indication of an autism spectrum disorder. The key question here is whether the behavior interferes with normal life activities or is harmful to self or others. If it does neither of these, then we recommend that caregivers try to ignore the behavior, particularly if done in a private space.

There are some situations, however, when the behavior itself is not the problem but rather when and where it is displayed. For example, hand flapping or rocking back and forth may be a problem if done in a shopping center, community job, or in some other public setting. If this behavior occurs in public, it may draw attention and lead to possible ridicule from others. If so, the person may need to learn to limit this behavior to a private space. For instance, a capable young woman who worked in a bank was approached by her parents and her supervisor because her hand flapping was drawing attention from others. After talking out possible solutions, she decided on her own to curb this behavior. As she explained to her teacher and parents, she wanted to "fit in." In other situations, the solution may be for others to change, rather than the person with Down syndrome. For example, in the case of a 15-year-old boy in high school, enlightened school staff used sensitivity training to educate other teens as to the normalcy of this behavior, and the teasing stopped.

Of course, there may be other important considerations such as the type of behavior, the attitude of caregivers who are present, and when the behavior is displayed. For example, many people with DS (like Denise above) briefly display hand flapping, a rocking behavior, and facial grimacing when they are happy or excited. These behaviors may be expressed and then over with fairly quickly. Many family members simply tell others that this is the way the person shows excitement and enthusiasm.

Although some people briefly display rocking when excited, more pronounced rocking may be a problem in public. The bad news about rocking is that compared to hand gestures or other forms of stereotypic behavior, rocking is a bigger and bolder behavior and often more obvious to others. More importantly, others are more likely to associate this behavior with people with intellectual disabilities. As such, it may serve to mark the person as disabled like a big neon sign and thus may make it more difficult for him to go about his normal business in public. Obviously, this may be even more of a problem at school, where the teen with DS may be subject to ridicule from peers.

The good news about rocking behavior is that it is also more obvious to caregivers, and if they are present, they are often able to remind the person with DS to stop the behavior fairly quickly. Try to find less obvious ways of reminding the person that he is rocking, such as by touching his shoulder. You might also develop private signals to alert him when this is going on. It may also be possible to predict when this behavior is more likely to occur and help him find alternative ways of expressing himself in these situations.

When Stereotypic Behavior May Need to Be Changed

In some situations, the stereotypic behavior itself is harmful or it interferes more prominently in the person's life and therefore requires more of an intervention to correct or change it. Following from the research, it may be helpful to regard more problematic stereotypic behaviors as possible indications that the person is under- or over-stimulated.

In our experience, one of the major causes of unproductive stereotypic behavior, including self-injurious behavior, is under-stimulation in the workplace. This is particularly the case for people with DS who are conscientious about their work. Being idle or having "down time" at work can be deadly for them. Too often, supervisors respond with activities that fill this time but are not interesting or stimulating. For example, many worksites show movies or TV or fill the time with what one gentleman called the "same old tired busy work" (unpaid assembly tasks such as sorting different sizes of nuts or bolts solely to pass time).

Worst of all, some agencies do absolutely nothing. Employees are simply left to their own devices. We have heard from many families that they try to find ways to help their sons and daughters deal with down time. They often send them in with their favorite free-time activities, such as paper or books to write or draw on, magazines, needlepoint, CD players, etc. These activities can occupy people for some time, but asking them to entertain themselves all day is ludicrous. Naturally, this kind of down time results in an increase in stress and anxiety and an increase in unproductive stereotypic behaviors.

During down time at work, we strongly recommend providing activities that are physically and mentally stimulating. This may include:

1. Beneficial recreation programs such as dancing, aerobics, or walking clubs;
2. Higher caliber arts and craft programs which challenge and incite people to produce high quality work;
3. Outings into the community to more mundane places such as shopping centers, but also to more interesting places such as museums and cultural events;
4. Interesting volunteer work in the community (for example, one worksite has a very popular outing where people work doing a variety of clerical and janitorial tasks at local churches).

On the other hand, people with excessive stereotypic behavior may also be communicating the presence of a stress or condition which is overwhelming or over-stimulating to them. We recommend the following to resolve these problems:

1. First, try to identify and reduce the cause or source of the stress. For example, people with DS are often very sensitive to the feelings, emotions, and conflicts of others and especially to significant others (see Chapter 13). Some people may be victimized by others (see Chapter 5). Life changes or losses may also be especially stressful for people with DS, who crave consistency in their lives (see Chapter 9). People may also be exposed to situations that overload their senses such as loud group homes or worksites.
2. After reducing stress, try to keep people busy with interesting activities. This helps to distract them from their preoccupations and stress.

3. Finally, when the stereotypic behavior itself is a problem, remember that it is easier to divert the behavior to something more appropriate than to try to stop the behavior altogether. For example, an adult who picks at his skin may need activities that occupy his hands. Some people may find rubbing worry stones (small, smooth stones) helpful. These stones may be rubbed while in the person's pocket or they may be small enough to not be noticed by others. Keeping a pad and pencil handy to write on may help some people keep from scratching or some other behavior. Still others may find that chewing on a toothpick, gum, etc. may help to keep them from biting nails or fingers.

TIC DISORDERS

People who have tic disorders, like people with stereotyped behavior, also make seemingly odd or purposeless movements or sounds. The major difference, however, is that stereotypic behaviors are voluntary, whereas tics may be suppressed for short periods of time but are otherwise not under the person's voluntary control.

The DSM-IV-TR describes several types of tic disorders. Some of these involve just motor (movement) or vocal tics, persisting for varying lengths of time. In our experience, people with DS are not more likely to have these types of tic disorders than other people are. However, they do seem to be at increased risk of having a more complicated type of tic disorder; namely, Tourette syndrome.

TOURETTE SYNDROME

Tourette syndrome (TS) is a hereditary, chronic neuromuscular condition consisting of motor and vocal tics. Tics are sudden, involuntary, brief, repetitive, stereotypic motor movements and vocalizations.

Examples of motor tics include: jerking movement of the head, sudden movement of the extremities, facial twitches, and others. Examples of vocal tics include: guttural sounds, yelling out, repeating a word or phrase, and others.

Symptoms begin in childhood and can change in location, number, frequency, and complexity over time. For a diagnosis of Tourette syndrome to be made, the tics need to begin before age 18, be present for at least one year, and not be due to a stimulant medication or a medical condition. In addition, people with classic TS always have at least two motor tics as well as one vocal tic, but not necessarily concurrently. Attention deficit disorders and/or obsessive-compulsive disorders often occur with Tourette syndrome (DSM-IV-TR).

We have seen a number of adults or adolescents with Down syndrome with a To-urette-like presentation. We label this as Tourette-like (or atypical Tourette syndrome) because the full complement of criteria are usually not present. (Most commonly there is an absence of the vocal tics.)

SYMPTOMS

Most of the people we have seen with both Down syndrome and Tourette syndrome have obsessive-compulsive symptoms which began in adolescence or adulthood. These patients have usually been diagnosed with attention deficit disorder in childhood. Further questioning will lead to the discovery of the tics.

Motor Tics: Motor tics may include repetitious and at times sudden mouth, tongue, face, head, trunk, or limb movements. Tics appear fairly odd or bizarre—for instance, facial contortions, twirling, squatting, eyes deviated up or to the side, sniffing at objects.

Vocal Tics: The people with DS plus TS that we see often do not have vocal tics in combination with motor tics. They sometimes have motor tics without vocal tics. However, we have seen a number of individuals with vocal tics that may include the expression of words as well as such sounds as clicks, grunts, sniffs, hoots, snorts, coughs, throat clearing, and other types of mouth noises.

In the general population, people with Tourette syndrome occasionally have coprolalia, or the involuntary expression of obscenities or other inappropriate expressions. We have not seen coprolalia in our patients. However, we have seen several people with DS who have vocal tics that include negative comments along with other vocalizations. These comments often resemble expressions of self-talk (see Chapter 8), but they have a different look and feel. They appear to be more sudden and spontaneous compared to regular self-talk and it appears that these comments are not under the person's conscious control.

Waxing and Waning of Tics: In Tourette syndrome, tics change over time. A tic may persist for several months, and then be replaced by a different tic. The intensity and frequency of tics change over time, too. Sometimes, a tic may only occur several times an hour; at other times, it may occur dozens or even hundreds of times an hour. Often stress seems to increase the type, intensity, and frequency of tics. For example:

> We have followed Reggie, 33, for many years at the ADSC. Like many people with Tourette syndrome, he has an attention problem, as well as obsessive-compulsive disorder, and both motor and vocal tics. Additionally, he is overweight and has an associated sleep apnea problem. He has lived in a number of residential living situations which have been extremely stressful for him—due primarily to the staff's mismanagement of other residents' behavior problems.

Reggie's Tourette's symptoms have been greatly affected by the stress of his health and environmental difficulties. Under stress, his obsessive-compulsive behaviors are more incapacitating. He often gets "stuck" and refuses to move at transition points in his day. At these times, his motor and vocal tics also increase markedly. His motor tics include repetitious head and trunk movements. His vocal tics include frequent outbursts and expressions that often sound like self-criticism, as well as nonsensical comments. (Although these comments often resemble self-talk, they appear suddenly and are seemingly out of Reggie's control.)

When his Tourette's symptoms increase, he moves less. As a result, his weight and sleeping problems also worsen. This in turn makes him more tired and sluggish in the daytime.

DIAGNOSIS

We have found that misdiagnosing the symptoms of Tourette syndrome may delay the effective treatment of the disorder in people with Down syndrome. This often happens when motor and vocal tics are misdiagnosed as behavior problems. For example:

Dawn, 16, was referred to the Center by her school. Dawn attended a public school for children with disabilities who have behavioral and learning challenges because she had been diagnosed with an attention problem at a younger age.

The school had dealt with the attention problem through a structured curriculum, but they had recently noted a significant increase in compulsive behavior. Dawn had become more rigid in her routines and less capable of adapting to changes. Her teacher and family also noted an increase in "odd" ritualistic behaviors such as bending her knees every five feet when she walked and other repetitious movements of her arms and head. Most problematic to the school, she frequently uttered nonsensical words and other sounds that were becoming louder and more disturbing to her teacher and the other students.

At the Adult Center, we diagnosed Dawn with Tourette syndrome because of the presence of attention issues, obsessive-compulsive behaviors, and the tics. For the school, it was most helpful to hear our opinion that not only were her "odd" ritualistic behaviors tics, but that her expressions of words and other mouth sounds were tics as well. With this knowledge, school staff and her parents began to see that these behaviors were not under Dawn's willful control. Consequently, the school began to reduce their insistence that she control her mouth noises. Interestingly, once teachers stopped pressuring Dawn to stop these sounds, the intensity and frequency of her vocalizations markedly decreased. The literature on Tourette syndrome has reported similar results when caregivers understand the nature of tics as involuntary behaviors (Rosen, 2002).

The school followed up with an effective behavior plan to deal with Dawn's vocalizations when they became too disruptive. This included plenty of activities to divert her attention from the tics. Additionally, when her vocalizations became a little too loud, she would be asked very quietly and diplomatically if she would prefer to leave the class to express herself more freely in a vacant room next door. Rarely, Dawn took advantage of this invitation, but in general this was not necessary. She was also treated with an antidepressant to reduce the intensity of her compulsive behavior, which helped her to be more flexible with her daily schedule.

If you suspect that an adolescent or adult with Down syndrome may also have Tourette syndrome, the first step in diagnosis is to get an assessment of his history. Looking back to the person's childhood is important. As discussed above, a previous diagnosis or symptoms of AD/HD are commonly present in people with DS and TS. Compulsive symptoms are also often seen, often beginning later than the AD/HD symptoms (often starting in adolescence). Often the tics are the unrecognized symptom. They may have been overlooked or thought to be side effects of medications. (Tics can increase with the stimulants frequently used for AD/HD.) The person's family doctor may be able to make the diagnosis and provide appropriate treatment, or a referral to a neurologist or psychiatrist may be necessary.

TREATMENT

Our treatment for Reggie, described above, has been multifaceted to meet his needs. He has responded positively to an anti-psychotic medication that has helped to reduce his tics and the "stuck-ness" of his compulsive behaviors (see more on medication below). This, in turn, has helped him better manage his weight and to sleep better in the evening. We have also targeted his environmental stresses by advocating for him to move from several different problematic residences. These interventions have helped to get his symptoms under control and allowed him to get on with his life.

In general, the treatment for people with Down syndrome who have TS is the same as for people in the general population who have TS. In our experience, people with a dual diagnosis of Down syndrome and Tourette syndrome respond best to a multifaceted approach to treatment, involving both behavioral interventions and medications.

BEHAVIORAL STRATEGIES AND INTERVENTIONS FOR TOURETTE SYNDROME

A number of chapters in the book deal with the obsessive-compulsive symptoms and the attention problems which often coexist with tics in people who have TS. This section will emphasize behavioral strategies for dealing with tics because they have not been discussed elsewhere.

In many respects, the behavioral strategies for dealing with tics and stereotypic behaviors are similar. For example:

1. Stress may increase the occurrence of both conditions. Therefore reducing the source of the stress may be helpful. (See above.)
2. Additionally, both conditions occur less often when people are engaged in more active pursuits such as sports or recreation activities.
3. We have also found it helpful to keep the body part that is most often engaged in the motor movement busy. For example, if the tic or stereotypic behavior involves the hands, it may help to engage the person in favorite hand activities, such as needlepoint, writing, drawing, video or computer games, etc. As an added benefit these activities are often stimulating yet relaxing and therefore they may also help reduce stress.
4. Certain items may be used to keep hands busy when tics result in such self-injurious behavior as picking at skin or sores. These items may include the worry stones described above, or items with a sensory texture. These items may be chosen by the person himself. For example, we have seen small rubber hoses, paper bags, and small stuffed animals used. By helping to reduce the incidence of self-injury, these items may also help to reduce anxiety created by the response of others to the self-injury.
5. Finally boredom and under-stimulation may increase the occurrence of tics. As suggested above in the section on stereotypic behaviors, it may be very important to find work that is interesting and mentally challenging. People who are productive and busy are generally happier and less stressed, and, as a result, may be less likely to display tics and stereotypic behaviors. At home, mental activities that are interesting such as educational computer games, word search puzzles, reading, or even video games may help.

There is a major difference between tics and stereotypic behaviors which may result in very different treatment and behavioral strategies. The primary difference is that stereotypic behaviors are under the person's voluntary control, while tics are not. People may be able to repress tics for short periods of time, but not control them. For example, students may keep their tics suppressed or less obvious when in class, but then may need to let loose with a barrage of tics after class. This difference needs to be appreciated by family members and other caregivers.

Caregivers may have one of three strategies for dealing with tics based on how well-informed and experienced they are regarding tics and Tourette disorder.

1. Those with less understanding may try to block or stop the person from engaging in the tic. This may work for a short period but will in-

evitably fail because of the involuntary nature of the tic. Not surprisingly, the anxiety this creates in the person with DS will often result in more tics.

2. Those with more understanding may have some success by trying to redirect the tic, particularly if redirecting to something that is of great interest to the person with DS. However, this may also backfire, particularly if the person with DS experiences this as just another attempt to block the tic.

3. Those with the most understanding and experience often back off and let the tic run its course. This strategy often reduces stress on the person, which then helps reduce the incidence of the tics.

MANAGING THE EFFECT OF TICS AND TS ON OTHERS

Families may need to develop strategies for dealing with tics when they affect the relationships between people in the home and other key settings. This may occur when tics are annoying or disruptive to others, adversely affect the demands and expectations of the person with DS, or are misinterpreted by others as behavioral or attitude problems. Finally, we will discuss when to seek professional help for tics that interfere with daily life or become harmful.

DEALING WITH DISRUPTIVE OR ANNOYING TICS

One issue that families need to sort out is how to deal with tics that are disruptive or annoying to family members. Families who do a better job with this educate their other children to be tolerant of the tics. They are also aware of the effect of tics on the other family members, however, and try to plan effective strategies to reduce the possibility of conflicts and tensions. For example:

> John, 22, who has tics and DS, had a job he loved. Still, he came home from work very stressed sometimes. As a result, he would have vocal tics which were loud and disruptive to his two young sisters who were trying to do their homework, read, or watch TV. His sisters responded to his tics by yelling at him to stop or complaining to their mother to make him stop. This only seemed to make the tics worse because John felt upset and persecuted by the complaints.
>
> To deal with this problem, John's parents had a family meeting and proposed the following solutions. John's sisters would not yell at him or complain to his parents. Instead they would ask him politely to go to his room, where he could relax and unwind by listening to his favorite music. This suited him fine. Additionally, John's father agreed to help John to better insulate his room. This would allow him to tic as loud as he needed without disturbing others. In time, John was even able to remind himself to go to his room when he had a stressful day.

Not surprisingly, we have run across similar issues in residential settings. We often recommend similar meetings between residents of group homes to sort out how to deal with tics that become annoying to others. In many cases, a resolution can be found which reduces annoyance to others and stress experienced by the person with the tics.

DEMANDS AND EXPECTATIONS

In our experience, families and others caregivers have to be careful not to let the person's tics affect the demands and expectations for him to behave normally in every other respect. For example, if a parent of a teen who tics asks him to do his homework or to pick up his room, the presence of tics should not prevent this from happening. If it does then, this may actually reinforce the expression of more tics or tic-like behavior. The teen may learn that expressing tics may "let him off the hook" for homework or other jobs he is expected to do. It may be a simple task to fake a tic "when needed." Excusing the teen from obligations may also create tension with siblings, who may feel the teen is given special treatment. There may be other repercussions as well. For example, the teen may experience anxiety at the school if his homework is not completed.

In order to prevent tics from altering demands or expectations, we recommend the following:

1. Discuss with the person with DS and TS that he has the same responsibility to do chores or obligations as everyone else in the family, regardless of tics. Couch this in positive terms; for example, by stating that the tics should not affect his ability to develop his talents, skills, and independence.
2. It may help to explain that if a tic is disruptive, a task may be delayed, but only temporarily, until the tic is no longer an interference.
3. Be very careful to follow through with this expectation. If a tic is allowed to stop and not just delay the completion of a task, this will reinforce maladaptive patterns of responding to tics.
4. If a tic is not disruptive to the person or the task, then the person should be encouraged to complete a task whenever possible.
5. Being mindful that stress may increase the expression of tics, assess situations in which demands are made on the person with DS and TS. If the task is challenging but still in line with the person's ability, then you should encourage him to do the task, even if it results in a tic.
6. Provide assistance with a task only because it is too difficult and not because of the presence of a tic. As a test of this, ask yourself if you would be helping if the person did not have tics.

Similar problems with decreased demands or expectations may result in settings other than the family home. Schools, worksites, and residential settings may also give the person with Down syndrome and Tourette syndrome special treatment or "let him off the hook" because of the tics. As in family households, this may result in resentment from others. It may also result in an underestimate and the possible underdevelopment of the person's skills and abilities based on a misperception or misunderstanding of tics and TS.

MISINTERPRETATION OR MISUNDERSTANDING OF TICS AND TOURETTE SYNDROME

Sometimes families have to deal with a lack of understanding by people in different settings who may not be familiar with Tourette syndrome or tics. This can be very challenging, particularly if family members encounter service providers who assume the person's tics are actually the result of an attitude or an oppositional behavior problem. You can avoid or decrease this problem by educating caregivers on the nature of tics, as shown in the previous example of Dawn (above).

In order to avoid this type of situation, we recommend the following:

1. Meet regularly with any staff or authority figures in your child's educational, work, or residential settings to educate them about the presence and nature of tics.
2. When needed, enlist the help of knowledgeable professionals to help educate staff who work with or serve as caregivers for your son or daughter.
3. Even if meetings are held with providers, problems may recur if there are changes in staff. Monitor these changes to avoid problems developing over an extended period of time.
4. If staff cannot or do not want to understand the nature of tics, then some changes should be made to avoid undo hardship and trauma for your child. When Tourette syndrome is accurately diagnosed, it must be viewed like any other handicapping condition or disability. If caregivers do not accept this diagnosis and this has a negative effect on the person with DS, then the family has a right, and an obligation, to change either the offending person or the agency.

WHEN TO SEEK PROFESSIONAL HELP

Even the most experienced and effective of families seek professional help for their sons and daughters when the tics and other symptoms result in physical harm or interfere in normal life activities. When this happens, the family may try to reduce stress, keep the person occupied with interesting activities, and try to patiently wait for the tics to subside. Sometimes this may still not be enough to reduce a problem with tics. In these situations, medications may reduce the intensity and frequency of the tics to better allow the behavioral strategies to work.

MEDICATIONS

Our behavioral interventions worked successfully for Dawn for close to one year. However, by the middle of her second school year, her tics were once again very disruptive in school and her compulsive behavior more and more debilitating. She was brought to the Center after she responded with physical aggression to her teacher's attempts to encourage her to remove herself from the classroom. We discovered a new health problem that was treated successfully. When her vocal tics and her behavior continued to be a problem, a small dose of an anti-psychotic medication was added, and this helped to turn the corner on the problem.

At this point, Dawn is back in school. She still has some disruptive vocal tics and some inflexibility with her rituals and routines, but to a much lesser degree. We continue to follow her progress very closely to insure that this positive progress is maintained.

We have found that the reason why some of our patients did not respond well to medications for AD/HD or OCD was that they actually have Tourette syndrome (or atypical Tourette syndrome). The usual treatment medications for the symptoms of AD/HD and OCD do not seem to work as well when those symptoms are part of TS.

Generally, when these patients were treated as children with the usual medications for attention deficit disorders, their response was less than optimal. For example, Dawn responded to her structured school curriculum, but did not show a positive response to stimulant medication. Her attention did not improve significantly and her family also noted the presence of "odd" behaviors (most likely tics) with the use of the medication. Other parents have also reported that tics were first observed when their child took medications for attention deficit disorder. And in fact, among people with Tourette syndrome who don't have Down syndrome, tics often seem to be triggered by stimulant medications used in the treatment of AD/HD. Other caregivers have reported that tics were not observed until adolescence or adulthood, although it is quite possible that tic activity occurred at a younger age but was not observed and diagnosed as a tic.

We have found too that for many of the people we have seen with Tourette syndrome—including both Dawn and Reggie—obsessive-compulsive symptoms generally became more noticeable or problematic in adolescence or adulthood. Attempts to treat the obsessive-compulsive disorder has had mixed results for these individuals. Treatment with the usual antidepressant medications is generally less than optimally successful. For example, an antidepressant medication temporarily helped to reduce the intensity of some of Dawn's compulsive behaviors, but it was not helpful for her tics and seemed to be less effective for her compulsions after approximately one year. Reggie also had a trial of an antidepressant medication for his compulsive behaviors, but it had no effect in reducing the problem symptoms.

We have had the best success in treating Tourette syndrome in people with Down syndrome with anti-psychotic medications. These medications are especially helpful in reducing the intensity of tics and of the more debilitating compulsive behaviors. We have used pimozide (Orap), risperdone (Risperdal), olanzapine (Zyprexa), quetiapine (Seroquel), and aripiprazole (Abilify) generally with good results. Only pimozide, however, is FDA approved for treating TS. Side effects can be a limiting factor.

Weight gain and sedation are particular problems, and elevated blood sugar and type 2 diabetes mellitus can also occur. Since people with Down syndrome are at greater risk for type 2 diabetes mellitus any way, we recommend monitoring blood sugar on a periodic basis while taking these medications.

THE NEED FOR LONG-TERM FOLLOW-UP

In people without DS, if the tics abate before adulthood, they generally do not recur. However, if they continue into adulthood, they tend to be persistent and recurrent. In our experience with adults with Down syndrome (albeit limited to up to 14 years of follow-up), symptoms tend to be persistent and recurrent. Often, some of the tics resolve, but they are generally replaced with others. We recommend regular monitoring of the symptoms. Most of our patients have required ongoing treatment with medications.

Chapter 22

Autism

. . . .

Autism is a disorder that primarily causes problems in three domains:

1. Significant difficulties in communication skills;
2. Significant difficulties in social skills;
3. Repetitive and ritualistic behaviors and interests (that is, seemingly odd or purposeless behaviors combined with an intense interest in relatively few topics or activities).

Autism is not a mental illness. It does, however, usually contribute to emotional and behavioral problems that complicate life at home, school, and in the community, and these problems will not get better without appropriate treatment. For this reason, we have chosen to include autism in this volume.

Until recently, many professionals believed that autism could not coexist with Down syndrome (Ghaziuddin, Tsai, and Ghaziuddin, 1992). It was assumed that these individuals had a more severe form of cognitive impairment rather than autism. As discussed below, there have also been questions about the diagnosis related to age at onset.

There is now greater recognition that some people with Down syndrome also have autism. This is due in good part to the efforts of a number of parents, advocates, and expert professionals who have worked tirelessly to educate others on the coexistence of this disorder for some persons with Down syndrome. Perhaps most notable is a volume of the *Disability Solutions* newsletter (volume 3, issue 5 & 6), edited by Joan Medlen, a dietitian and the mother of a son with Down syndrome and autism. This volume included key articles by a number of experts in the field, including Drs. George Capone, Bill Cohen, and Bonnie Patterson.

Because the recognition that Down syndrome and autism can coexist has only occurred in the last few years (and because some professionals still doubt that the dual diagnosis is possible), we have seen some adults with Down syndrome who have autism but were never diagnosed as children. The diagnosis of autism is often extremely important even for adolescents and adults. For families, the diagnosis gives a name and an explanation for why their family member is different, and why she may have had a dramatic loss of function since childhood. There are other major benefits as well. State agencies often allocate additional funding for individuals with this diagnosis to receive special programs and services because of their greater needs. For example, funding may be available for behavior management, as well as communication and social skills training, which may greatly reduce the more debilitating and isolating symptoms of autism.

WHAT IS AUTISM?

Autism is a disorder that is displayed in a spectrum that ranges from mild to severe. Consequently, the term "Autistic (or Autism) Spectrum Disorder" (ASD) is now often used to describe the range of findings and behaviors in people with autism. People on the milder end of the spectrum may have fewer symptoms or symptoms that are less disabling, while people on the more severe end of the spectrum will often have more symptoms that are more debilitating.

UNIQUE CHARACTERISTICS OF PEOPLE WITH DOWN SYNDROME AND ASD

Clinical researchers have found that people with DS and ASD show somewhat less impairment in social relatedness compared to people with only ASD (Lord et al., 2000). Still, most people with DS and ASD have major deficits in social skills, particularly in the areas of empathy and sensitivity to others. In this respect, they are more like others with ASD and less like people with Down syndrome, who are generally quite sensitive to others (see Chapter 4). Ironically, there may be some negative consequences from the greater social relatedness. Some parents believe this may confuse clinicians and made them slow or reluctant to diagnose ASD in people with Down syndrome.

We have found too that people with Down syndrome and ASD tend to have more significant deficits in intellectual functioning and expressive language compared to others with just ASD. For example, most children with DS and ASD have mental retardation, which is not the case for all children with just ASD. Additionally, most children with DS and ASD have speech articulation problems in addition to the other communication problems, which again is not necessarily the case for individuals with just ASD.

In addition to differences in social relatedness, intellectual functioning, and speech skills, children with DS and ASD tend to be diagnosed later than children with just ASD. According to the DSM-IV-TR, symptoms of autism must be present before the age of three for the diagnosis to be made. Parents of children with Down syndrome, however, often report observing symptoms of autism for the first time at around five or six and even as late as seven or eight years of age. Because of the comparatively late onset of autistic symptoms in children with the dual diagnosis, there has been discussion as to whether this is autism or childhood disintegrative disorder (CDD), which has the same cluster of symptom as ASD but is diagnosed later than three years of age.

Does this mean that the children with Down syndrome do not have "classic" autism? Do they have childhood disintegrative disorder instead? There are no definitive answers to these questions. However, one thing to consider is that DSM-IV-TR criteria are not always 100 percent applicable to people with Down syndrome. For example, we have had to adapt DSM-IV-TR criteria to diagnose depression, anxiety, and psychotic disorders in people with Down syndrome. Perhaps we may need to adapt the criteria for ASD to a later age for persons with DS to better fit their pattern of symptoms. As George Capone has noted in the *Disability Solutions* article on DS and ASD, "If it looks like a duck, quacks like a duck …. Guess what?"

Practically speaking, as clinicians treating teens and adults, we are less concerned with age of onset and more concerned with how to help people to get the treatment and services they need. To this end, the diagnosis of autism spectrum disorder is understood by far more people than is childhood disintegrative disorder and is thus more likely to lead to appropriate services and treatments. For all of the above reasons, then, at our Center we diagnose adolescents and adults who show symptoms of autism as having autism spectrum disorder.

The next section will explain how symptoms of autism may manifest themselves in people with Down syndrome.

SYMPTOMS

As mentioned above, people with autism spectrum disorders have particular difficulty in three areas: 1) communication skills, 2) social skills, and 3) repetitive and ritualistic interests and behavior. Since people with Down syndrome who do not have autism also may have trouble in these areas, it is important to understand what is and is not normal for someone with Down syndrome.

IMPAIRED COMMUNICATION AND SOCIAL SKILLS

People with autism spectrum disorders have impairments in both expressive and receptive language. That is, they have problems in expressing themselves to others and in understanding what others are saying. People with DS and ASD also have these types of impairments, but tend to have more problems with speech articulation, which make it more difficult for them to be understood when they *are* able to communicate. People with DS who do not have ASD often have similar problems with speech articulation, but they do not have the same problems with receptive language and are generally quite good at picking up social cues.

People who have autism spectrum disorders usually have difficulty understanding other people's thoughts and perspectives. This can be particularly noticeable in a person with Down syndrome because many people with Down syndrome have an innate ability to sense the feelings of others. Even nonverbal people with DS and more significant intellectual impairments seem to have a sensitivity to others that is missing or at least deficient to some degree in people with Down syndrome and ASD. In other words, in people who have a dual diagnosis, we find debilitating symptoms in the area of social skills that they do not share with others with just Down syndrome, regardless of the person's level of skill and functioning.

Often people with autism spectrum disorders have deficits in basic social skills. They may have difficulty maintaining eye contact. Many do not like to be touched or to be in close proximity to others. They may feel unsure and even afraid in social situations. They may also have a sensitivity to sensory stimuli (see below for more). For example, they may have difficulty tolerating the level of sound that occurs when people get together to talk in groups.

People with Down syndrome and ASD may have limited abilities to respond to parents or siblings in a caring and affectionate way. They may also have great difficulty interacting with peers and even greater difficulty establishing and maintaining friendships. In short, social exchanges are fraught with stress and difficulty for many people with autism spectrum disorders.

RESTRICTED AND REPETITIVE INTERESTS/BEHAVIOR

Typically, people with DS and ASD have repetitive motor behaviors. For example, many flap their hands or make similar body movements that are commonly seen in people with autism. They may also repeat unusual vocalizations such as humming or "raspberry-like" sounds. In addition, many are preoccupied with certain inanimate objects such as shoelaces, paper bags, and other items people do not normally play with. They may also play with toys in very restricted and compulsive ways such as by placing toy cars or soldiers in perfect lines. Many people with DS and ASD watch movies over and over or do certain tasks repetitively, such as putting their desk in order or opening and closing the doors in the house, or arranging furniture in nonsensical ways. Many also save items, including unusual items such as lint or specific paper products.

It is important to note that people with Down syndrome who don't have ASD may also have these kinds of repetitive movements or compulsive behaviors. However, they usually do not have these behaviors to the same degree or intensity as people with DS and ASD. More importantly, they do not also have the significant problems with communication skills and social skills that individuals with a dual diagnosis of DS and ASD have.

OTHER SYMPTOMS

Sensory Issues: The ability to take in and organize sensory input may be impaired in people with Down syndrome and ASD. Of particular importance may be:

1) the ability to understand where the body is in relation to the environment; 2) balance control; and 3) tactile input through the skin. The person may be sensitive to the environment in ways that are difficult to understand. For example, while a gentle touch from someone may be reassuring to most people, it may be frightening to someone with an autism spectrum disorder. Spinning, staring at lights, sensitivity to sounds, or other unusual sensory responsiveness may be present.

Behavioral Issues: People with a dual diagnosis of autism and Down syndrome may have self-injurious behavior, as discussed in Chapter 20. There may also be increased anxiety, irritability, hyperactivity, attention problems, significant sleep disturbances not related to sleep apnea or another medical problem, compulsive behaviors and rituals, and difficulty with transitions.

DIAGNOSING AUTISM IN AN ADULT WITH DOWN SYNDROME

◆ ◆ ◆ ◆ ◆ ◆ ◆ ◆ ◆ ◆ ◆ ◆ ◆ ◆ ◆ ◆ ◆ ◆

If autism is suspected in an adolescent or adult with Down syndrome, the diagnostic process is similar to diagnosis of any disorder. A complete and thorough evaluation requires that all other explanations of the person's behavior be looked at and ruled out. For example, a complete physical exam should be conducted to rule out any health problems that may cause behavior change. Extreme stress in the person's environment may also cause behavior that is characteristic of autism. There may be other less obvious explanations as well, such as those related to the person's culture and language. For example, an English-speaking psychologist or physician may attribute social and communication problems to autism when the problem is simply a lack of facility with English (Geisinger and Carlson, 1992).

Having ruled out other possible explanations, the next step is for a trained and experienced professional or team of professionals to assess the presence of the three primary deficits of autism spectrum disorders, which are described above. Optimally, families should try to locate a center whose staff has experience with people with autism, and, preferably, the dual diagnosis of autism and Down syndrome. If you have a family member who displays the behaviors described in this chapter, you should seek help from experienced professionals in your community. Local parent organizations serving people with ASD and DS may be able to provide names of local centers or practitioners who diagnose and treat autism.

The challenge in diagnosis is to obtain a history regarding the childhood of the adult with Down syndrome who is suspected of having autism. If you, the parent, are bringing your adult child for an evaluation, your observations and experience with your child is essential to any diagnosis. Additionally, any records or observations documented by teachers and other caregivers over the years may be very helpful. The same is true of tests or evaluations by medical or psychological practitioners.

These records often help to show a pattern of behavior which is very helpful in diagnosing the disorder.

In addition, some families may want to bring in videotapes or family films showing the person's behavior. This may be particularly helpful if the person displays behavior at specific times and locations, or if the behavior occurs intermittently or in response to certain stimuli such as those at a shopping center, social gathering, etc. Films/videos may be very helpful too if the person with DS tends to be "perfect" (act normal) in certain situations, such as when the parent wants her to display some of the problem behavior for the doctor.

TREATMENT

Many volumes have been written on strategies for managing behavior and assisting learning in individuals with autism spectrum disorders. We can only begin to touch on some of the methods that, in our experience, can be helpful for adolescents and adults with a dual diagnosis of autism and Down syndrome.

BEHAVIORAL APPROACHES

HELPING THE ADULT DEAL WITH SENSORY ISSUES

As mentioned above, people with autism may have unusual reactions to sights, sounds, smells, and other sensations in the environment. Appreciating this difference can be very important to understanding and helping the individual. A sensory integration assessment by a qualified occupational therapist (OT) can be very helpful in understanding the person's needs and in developing useful strategies for dealing with these issues. For example, many individuals with sensory integration issues may benefit from a "sensory diet," which is a list of sensory-related tasks (such as the use of a weighted blanket, brushes for the skin, etc.).

Recommended strategies and activities may go a long way to make someone comfortable, increasing her willingness to cooperate with daily living and learning tasks in the home, work, or school environments. It may also be useful to consult with an OT about ways to adapt the environment to make it more palatable to the person with autism—for instance, getting rid of lights that make a humming sound or figuring out what sounds are calming to her.

PROVIDING STRUCTURE AND CONSISTENCY

Adults with Down syndrome and autism typically benefit from a structured environment. Routine is important. The structure helps them manage their day. They often respond better to pictures or visual cues than to spoken or written words. Picture calendars and schedules help them understand and appreciate what will be happening in their day. Without this understanding, the person may become more frustrated and irritable. Even after she has learned the task, the person may still need visual and picture schedules for support. You may find the book *Activity Schedules for Children with Autism* by Patricia Krantz and Lynn McClannahan useful in learning ways that picture schedules can help individuals with autism (Woodbine House, 1999).

Consistency in the way tasks are done and explained is also beneficial and comforting. For example, it may be helpful for caregivers to teach tasks the same way every time. If different family member or staff in a residence are teaching a given task, it may be helpful to give each teacher a written task list to ensure consistency and necessary structure for learning tasks. It is also helpful to allow the person adequate time to process requests and to figure out what it will take to perform a task. Limiting other stimuli also encourages the person to focus on the task.

Sharing information with all people who regularly interact with the person is very important. This increases the likelihood that the environment will be responsive in a consistent manner. For example:

> Adam's parents have written a short book on Adam. They have recorded a list of typical behaviors, what he is usually trying to communicate with the behavior, and how the family usually responds. The staff at his day program regularly reviews this information, and new staff members are instructed on the use of the book. The use of this book is very beneficial for Adam, as he is happier and less frustrated when staff members are consistent. In addition, less staff time is spent dealing with challenging behaviors and more time is spent helping Adam and other people in the day program to learn and participate in the activities.

HANDLING TRANSITIONS

Due to a strong reliance on compulsive, ritualized, and repetitive patterns of behavior, transitions from one event to another can be very challenging for most people with autism spectrum disorders. It is very important for others to appreciate and respect this characteristic. Providing "warnings" (especially visual warnings) that it is going to be time soon to switch to a new activity helps with transitions. Then, explaining the transition to the person (with pictures, if necessary) as it occurs may make it less likely she will resist the transition.

TEACHING ABOUT SOCIAL SITUATIONS

As mentioned above, people with autism usually have great difficulty putting themselves in another's shoes. We recommend helping the person with autism improve her understanding of others' feelings by discussing how these feelings relate to her experiences.

Basic instruction on what to do and say in social situations is also beneficial. Many autism experts recommend using "Social Stories" (Gray, 1993) to help individuals with autism learn new social skills. Social stories are custom made to help someone learn to handle a situation that is problematic for her. A parent, teacher, or other service provider writes a simple story describing the situation and how the individual with autism appropriately deals with it. The story might then be illustrated with photos or drawings of the person engaged in the situation. The story is read to the person with autism before she encounters the situation and at other times when she can learn from the story.

PREVENTING INFORMATION OVERLOAD

Slow processing is another feature of autism spectrum disorder (and of Down syndrome). People who just have autism may have problems understanding others because of receptive language limitations, problems with picking up social cues, etc. People with DS and ASD have these difficulties too but also have a slower processing speed related to their Down syndrome. Therefore, it is important to give the person an opportunity to process what has been said or asked before giving her additional instruction or input. Presenting the material in a concrete form (especially in picture form) is beneficial. Waiting for an answer or giving the person a chance to answer at a later time helps prevent information overload. In addition, limiting the input to one voice or one person helps reduce overload.

TEACHING TO HER STRENGTHS

Learning new information is often difficult for a person with autism. If the information is presented in a way that enables her to use her strengths, the learning process is much more likely to be successful. Use of abstract thinking, imagination, social intuition, interpretation, and rapid responding are not typically learning strengths of people with autism spectrum disorders. Learning will more likely be easier and more complete if:

1. New information is presented **visually** (such as showing a person how to brush her teeth).
2. The information is presented in as **concrete** a form as possible. For example, it is best to simply show the steps for brushing teeth and not to discuss the benefits of oral hygiene.
3. **Hands-on** learning is best. Information may be easier to absorb if the person can first observe and then do the task herself.
4. The information is broken down into **sequential steps** that are easier to master. For example, learning how to brush one's teeth could include such steps as grasping the toothbrush, putting on toothpaste, turning on the water, moving the toothbrush up and down, etc.
5. Even if there are multiple teachers, the **order of the sequence of steps** is not altered in the learning process. This is why it is useful to use pictures showing the sequence of steps.
6. **Rote learning** or repeating the task numerous times helps to ensure that the task is learned.

These methods of learning may be particularly strong in a person with an autism spectrum disorder; even beyond what might ordinarily be expected based on the person's other abilities.

MEDICATIONS

Individuals with autism spectrum disorders may have challenging behaviors, including aggressive or self-injurious behavior. If the behavioral approaches discussed above are not sufficient, medications may be necessary. The atypical anti-psychotics can be beneficial in reducing aggression. Those we tend to use most include risperdone (Risperdal), quetiapine (Seroquel), olanzapine (Zyprexa), ziprasidone (Geodon), and aripiprazole (Abilify). Please see Chapter 17 (Psychotic Disorders) and Addendum 1 for information on side effects and other aspects of these medications.

In addition, anti-seizure medications may help with the behavior challenges. They can be particularly helpful with aggressive behavior. They are further discussed in Chapters 19 and 20, as well as in Addendum 1. Clonidine (Catapres) may also reduce agitation and aggression.

When there is an accompanying mood disorder, antidepressants may be helpful. Their use is described in Chapter 14. Anti-anxiety medications are also sometimes beneficial when anxiety symptoms complicate autism (see Chapter 15).

IN-HOME BEHAVIOR SUPPORT

Because life with a child or adult with ASD and Down syndrome can be extremely challenging, family and other caregivers have a critical need for support. For example, the most successful group homes and work sites for adults with DS and ASD have a high ratio of staff to residents. Equally important, staff in these settings have training in positive behavior management techniques and other useful strategies for supporting the adaptive functioning of people with ASD.

Without at least some outside assistance, families may be overwhelmed with the challenges of having a person with ASD in their household. We have written a number of letters to state funding sources to secure in-home behavior support for families. We recommend that parents who have an adolescent or adult with a diagnosis of DS and autism find a professional in their community who is willing to do the same for them. This may include the physician, psychologist, or other professionals who were involved in the diagnosis of your son or daughter, or similar professionals with whom you are in contact. The following is an example of one such letter we wrote for Tony, a 14-year-old boy with ASD and DS:

> "Tony's behavior challenges are so severe that, if left unsupported, his family would be severely taxed and possibly at risk for adverse effects to their own health and well-being. At home, Tony is extremely demanding of his parents' time and attention. This is limiting to them but also detrimental to his three siblings who are 9, 11, and 15 years of age. At home, he is frequently not cooperative with activities, which then diverts attention away from the others. Perhaps more frustrating to his siblings is that he will also not cooperate with normal and typical family activities outside the home, such

as outings to a sibling's sports event, church, evenings out to a restaurant, etc. He often reacts to these outings by dropping on the ground and refusing to move. If his parents attempt to force him to move, he may escalate his behavior, which then compounds the problem.

Of importance, Tony is usually more cooperative with teachers and experienced respite staff than with his own parents. In this way, he is no different than any other teenager. Unfortunately, unlike most teenagers who revel in their freedom, Tony is extremely resistant to leaving his own house. Thus, at a time when most children become less demanding of parental time and attention, he is even more demanding, while still possessing the uncooperative attitude of a teenager.

In-home behavior support would have a number of critically important benefits for Tony and his family. A trained in-home behavior analyst would help to build on Tony's compulsive tendencies to help establish a functional routine for the completion of daily living tasks. Additionally, important skills such as safety training could be reinforced in the home environment. This would free his parents from having to micromanage his behavior, while giving him independence and a sense of pride. Equally important, in-home behavior support would allow his family to return to a more normal pattern of family life. For example, if Tony refused to go out to a community function with his family, he could stay with his trainer. The trainer would also be able to accompany Tony when they do go on outings. It would also be extremely beneficial to Tony's parents and siblings to have more quality time with Tony, especially if they are not responsible for his care 24 hours per day.

States may have funding available for in-home behavior support, although the amount of support varies. In Illinois, families are allowed 15 hours per week of in-home support. Most families will state that they can use more than 15 hours but that this amount is often sufficient to their needs. They also report that anything less than 15 may be inadequate, given that people with ASD crave sameness and consistency in their daily lives. If less than 15 hours of in-home care are allotted, the person barely has enough time to get familiar with the staff person before he or she is gone. This may actually create more stress on the family if they have to deal with the aftereffects of too much change and upheaval in the person's life

Given enough time and contact, in-home behavior support staff are able to successfully implement picture schedules and behavior management programs and to assist with general care-giving tasks. These in-home behavior support staff are usually trained by agencies and centers to serve the needs of individuals with autism. Usually a psychologist or behavioral analyst will develop behavioral management and picture schedules, which are then implemented by the in-home support staff. This professional may also provide ongoing consultation to support staff to help to better tailor the programs to meet the person's needs.

FINDING SUPPORT FOR YOUR FAMILY

Support groups for families who have children with autism spectrum disorders and other challenging disorders may be helpful to you. No one quite knows and understands the challenges of living with a child or adult with autism like another family who is facing the same challenges.

In Chicago, the National Association for Down Syndrome (NADS), the parent group that is the driving force behind our Center, has had a number of innovative programs to support families of children and adults who have Down syndrome and ASD and other challenging problems. For example, since 1998 they have run a weekend retreat for ten individuals with severe challenging behavior and their families. The retreat is held at a hotel and the parents and children/adolescents are separated into two groups. The children stay with a small army of trained staff and volunteers, who manage their care for the entire weekend. Interestingly, the staff who do this often come back every year because they enjoy what they do. The parents and family members attend classes taught by experts on such topics as positive behavior support, medication, and sensory integration strategies. Perhaps more importantly, they receive support from the other families who know what it is like. Many people exchange creative ideas and solutions to common problems encountered in the care of their family member with ASD. It is easy to see why this event is so highly regarded by families.

Participants to the NADS retreat are referred by one of several clinics serving children with Down syndrome and also from the Adult Down Syndrome Center. For families who live outside of Chicago, the retreat may serve as an excellent model of what could be. It may be possible to run such a retreat through your local Down syndrome support group or even through an autism support group in your community.

CONCLUSION

Autism spectrum disorders begin in childhood. However, there are many benefits to assessing and treating adults with Down syndrome who have not been previously diagnosed with autism. Understanding the unique issues that autism spectrum disorder presents can significantly affect the care of someone who has both Down syndrome and ASD. Behavioral approaches, medications, and other therapies should be considered.

If at all possible, we recommend at least one visit to a doctor or clinic with expertise in treating people with Down syndrome and autism. At present, Down syndrome clinics that have staff knowledgeable about these issues include those at the Kennedy Krieger Institute in Baltimore, Maryland; The Thomas Center for Down Syndrome at the Cincinnati Children's Hospital; and The Family Clinic at the Institute on Disability and Human Development at the University of Illinois at Chicago, which also specializes in evaluating people who are bilingual in Spanish and English. Additionally, there are major medical centers around the country which specialize in evaluating autism, and they would most likely be able to diagnose autism for a person with Down syndrome.

Chapter 23

Alzheimer Disease

· · · · · · · · · · · · · · · · · · · ·

and Decline

· · · · · · · · · · · · · · · ·

in Skills

· · · · · · · · ·

Alzheimer disease is one of the most commonly diagnosed and misdiagnosed mental disorders in adults with Down syndrome. On the one hand, the condition is often blamed for a decline in skills when the real culprit is depression, a treatable medical condition such as thyroid disease, a change in hearing or vision, or any of a number of less serious causes. On the other hand, Alzheimer disease can appear at an earlier age in people with Down syndrome. In addition, while the incidence of Alzheimer disease in people with Down syndrome is not clearly defined, some data suggest that it is more common and some suggest that the incidence is similar to that in the general population, but beginning at a younger age. Since the condition can greatly complicate the care of any adult, including one with Down syndrome, accurate diagnosis is very important.

WHAT IS ALZHEIMER DISEASE?

· ·

Alzheimer disease (AD) is a progressively degenerative neurological condition that affects the brain. Alzheimer disease is a form of dementia. There is progressive destruction of brain cells, especially in certain parts of the brain. People with Alzheimer disease experience progressive impairment of memory, cognitive skills, and daily living skills, as well as psychological changes. There is presently no cure for Alzheimer disease, but there are treatments that can, at least temporarily, reduce its effects.

Alzheimer disease is characterized by plaques and tangles in the brain. The plaques are the build-up of amyloid protein between neurons (nerve cells). In AD, the protein builds up to form hard plaques. The tangles are the remnants of collapsed microtubules. The microtubules are a normal part of the nerve cell whose function is to transport nutrients and other substances in the cell. In AD, a protein (tau protein) that is an important part of the structure of the tubule is abnormal, leading to the collapse of the microtubules into tangles. There is no clear way to detect these changes without examining a piece of brain tissue (generally only done after a person's death) under a microscope. However, as the disease progresses, Computerized Tomography (CT) or Magnetic Resonance Imaging (MRI) scans of the brain can depict the destruction of many cells because the brain begins to atrophy or shrink.

The cause of Alzheimer disease remains unclear. In a few cases, however, there seems to be a familial link associated with a gene on chromosome 21.

How Common Is Alzheimer Disease?

In the general population, the incidence of Alzheimer disease is increasing as the population ages. The incidence of AD in the general population is listed as 10 percent for people in their 60s, 20 percent for those in their 70s, 40 percent for those in their 80s, and 50 percent or more after age 85.

The incidence among people with Down syndrome is not known, although a great deal has been written about Alzheimer disease in Down syndrome. A number of years ago, when researchers did autopsies on people with Down syndrome who had died from a variety of reasons, they found changes in the brains of all those over age 35 that were similar to those found in the brains of adults with Alzheimer disease. Much discussion and investigation has taken place since then. Some believe that because of these changes in the brain, all people with Down syndrome will get Alzheimer disease if they live long enough. Others believe that not all people with Down syndrome get clinical Alzheimer disease (decline in cognitive skills and other symptoms outlined later in the chapter).

Our experience suggests that not all people with Down syndrome develop the symptoms of Alzheimer disease. We suspect that the incidence of clinical Alzheimer disease might be similar to that in the general population but that it occurs, on average, 20 years earlier than in adults without Down syndrome. The youngest person with DS we have seen with symptoms of AD was in his late 30s. Whether the incidence is the same or higher in people with DS, AD does not seem to be universal when one considers the development of symptoms. There are other causes for a decline in cognitive skills (as discussed later in the chapter), and, therefore, it is important to remember that people with DS deserve an evaluation for these other causes rather than an assumption that any decline is secondary to Alzheimer disease.

We have treated many older adults with Down syndrome who showed no evidence of mental decline. One was a woman believed to be the oldest, well-documented person with Down syndrome. She died in 1994 at the age of 83, with no evidence of decline (Chicoine & McGuire, 1997). In one study published in 1996, researchers showed a small decline in function with age in adults with Down syndrome (Devenny et al., 1996). This decline was comparable to that seen in healthy adults who do not have mental retardation. Other researchers showed a similar lack of decline in function except for those with Alzheimer disease (Burt et al., 1995). So, despite the universal finding of changes in the brain, we do not see the decline in function that would be expected if all adults with Down syndrome were getting clinical Alzheimer disease.

DIAGNOSING THE CAUSE OF DECLINING SKILLS

What if we assumed the diagnosis of Alzheimer disease in all adults with Down syndrome over the age of 40 whose cognitive skills were declining? Because studies suggest that all people with DS over the age of 35 have microscopic changes in the brain consistent with Alzheimer disease, this conclusion is sometimes made. When we evaluated our patients, however, that is not what we found. In fact, if we had assumed that all of our patients over the age of 40 with declines in function had Alzheimer disease, we would have been wrong 75 percent of the time. Only 25 percent had Alzheimer disease. The other 75 percent are being treated successfully for other conditions. There is no cure for Alzheimer disease at this time, so detection of treatable conditions is a vital element of patient care.

Since many other health problems can cause dementia, it is imperative to evaluate for these other conditions before making the diagnosis of Alzheimer disease. Unfortunately, this is not always done for people with Down syndrome. One of the concerns expressed by the parents who asked that we start a clinic for adults with Down syndrome was that their sons or daughters were not being given an appropriate work-up when a decline in skills was noted.

There is no specific test that definitely diagnoses AD. Finding a pattern of decline in neurological and psychological function makes the diagnosis. The medical and behavioral health team must also rule out other illnesses and conditions that cause symptoms that are similar to those seen in AD. This diagnostic process is similar for adults with and without Down syndrome.

When a patient comes to us because of a decline in abilities, we provide a thorough medical and psychological evaluation. In our evaluation, we assess for a variety of conditions, particularly those that are more common for adults with Down syndrome (see Chapter 2).

CONDITIONS TO RULE OUT

To rule out causes of decline other than Alzheimer disease, we consider:

- Depression and other psychological concerns
- Sleep apnea
- Thyroid disease
- Vitamin B12 deficiency
- Metabolic diseases such as kidney disease, diabetes, or calcium abnormalities
- Celiac disease
- Loss of hearing or vision
- Atlanto-axial instability or other cervical (neck) problems
- Heart disease
- Seizure disorder
- Normal pressure hydrocephalus
- Medication side effects
- Additional possible causes that we have not seen in our patients:
  - Syphilis
  - Acquired Immune Deficiency Syndrome (AIDS)

Another consideration is chronic, undiagnosed pain. Adults with Down syndrome sometimes have a global decline in function in response to pain and illnesses that do not directly cause a loss of function. This appears to be an emotional or psychological response to the trauma of pain or illness.

In addition, as discussed in Chapter 10, people with Down syndrome seem to age more rapidly than others, so that when they are 55, we consider them to be more like someone without Down syndrome at 75. It is important to remember that there may be aging changes at a younger age in a person with Down syndrome. We have seen a number of patients who were slowing down because of age and age-associated health issues. Often these factors were not being considered or addressed and the changes were attributed to behavioral challenges. Addressing them from an aging perspective put the changes in a whole new light.

TESTS FOR DECLINE IN FUNCTION

The tests we recommend for all our adult patients who are experiencing a decline in function include:

- CBC (complete blood count)
- Electrolyte panel including serum calcium
- Thyroid blood tests
- Serum Vitamin B12 level
- Vision and hearing testing

Additional tests that may be indicated based on the findings on the history, physical, and lab tests include:

- Lateral cervical spine x-ray in flexion, extension, and neutral positions
- Liver function tests
- RPR (for syphilis)
- HIV testing (for AIDS)
- CT scan or MRI of the brain
- Blood testing for celiac disease (anti-tissue transglutaminase antibody or anti-endomysial Ig A and anti-gliadin IgG and IgA).
- EEG
- Sleep study

Neuropsychological testing is part of the evaluation for Alzheimer disease for people who do not have an intellectual disability. However, this testing is more difficult in people with Down syndrome and other intellectual disabilities. The underlying intellectual disability makes it difficult for people with DS to perform most of the tests and, therefore, the tests are less accurate. There are, however, a few tests (see below) that, when done sequentially over time, are thought to be more effective. Usually, however, we find that by the time a cognitive decline is evident on the testing, the decline and diagnosis are clear from the person's behavior. In our experience, referring our patients for these tests is not beneficial. We are able to get similar information by asking parents and other caregivers to update us on symptoms, particularly over time.

There are also three tests specifically designed to measure symptoms of Alzheimer disease in people with Down syndrome. These include the *Dementia Scale for Down's Syndrome* (Huxley et al., 2000); *The Dementia Scale for Down Syndrome* (Gedye, 2000); and the *Dementia Questionnaire for Mentally Retarded Persons* (Evenhuis et al., 1990). These tests may be an aid to diagnosis for trained mental health or medical professionals, as they help point out key areas that need to be considered when ruling out other causes. However, these tests should not stand alone as the diagnosis of Alzheimer disease. There is still no definitive test to make the diagnosis. The diagnosis is still based on a process of excluding every other possible cause of the person's skill loss. The three tests mentioned here should only be part of a total assessment involving a thorough physical exam, and extensive information gathered from caregivers regarding skill and memory loss, environmental and developmental stressors, etc.

SYMPTOMS OF ALZHEIMER DISEASE IN ADULTS WITH DOWN SYNDROME

The symptoms of Alzheimer disease we see in our patients with Down syndrome are:

- Memory impairment (in early Alzheimer disease, short-term memory loss is primarily affected, while memory of events and people from the distant past are preserved. In late AD, however, both short- and long-term memory is lost.)

- Decline in skills (this may include cognitive skills such as reading and math and ability to do activities of daily living such as teeth brushing, hygiene, etc.) The first sign of decline is often the need for more prompts. Early on, the person may still have the ability but needs more guidance or direction.
- Incontinence of urine and/or stool
- Gait disturbance (gait apraxia) (we often seen poor balance, leaning to one side—later this occurs even when sitting—and falling).
- Personality or psychological changes
  - depressed mood
  - aggressiveness
  - paranoia
  - compulsiveness
  - loss of interest in activities
- Seizures
- Swallowing dysfunction (this may be seen as a fear of eating, apparently due to a sense that swallowing abilities are changing. It generally progresses to an inability to swallow without choking, gagging, and often aspiration of saliva or food into the lungs)
- Sleep changes (day-night reversal, daytime fatigue)
- Altered appetite and thirst (most commonly, a decrease in eating and drinking).

Most of these symptoms are similar to those seen in people with AD who don't have Down syndrome, with the exception of seizures, gait problems, and swallowing difficulties. Seizures tend to occur much more frequently and at an earlier stage in Alzheimer disease in people with Down syndrome. Recurrent, uncontrolled seizures can lead to a more rapid decline. People with DS are also more likely to lose the ability to walk earlier on and to have earlier difficulty with swallowing and with aspiration. The aspiration becomes especially problematic if it is associated with recurrent pneumonia or decreased eating or drinking.

Particularly earlier in the disease, the functioning level of a person with Alzheimer disease often fluctuates. These fluctuations may occur over several days or weeks, from day to day, and even within minutes or moments. A skill may come and go over these periods of time. As the disease progresses, the person's skill level will decline and her periods of better functioning will be shorter and not as functional as before.

TREATMENT OF ALZHEIMER DISEASE

There is no treatment presently available to cure Alzheimer disease. Various medications and other treatments, however, may be prescribed in an attempt to slow down the progression of the disease, or to treat medical problems associated with it.

MEDICATIONS TO DELAY DECLINE

Some data suggest that anti-inflammatory agents (such as ibuprofen), vitamin E, and selegiline (Eldepryl) may prevent, delay, or slow down the decline associated with Alzheimer disease. However, ongoing studies are needed to further evaluate these treatments.

Researchers have proven that medications that slow down the breakdown of choline can improve the function of people with Alzheimer disease. Nerve cells communicate with each other via neurotransmitters (chemicals) that pass from cell to cell. One of these transmitters, choline, is the chemical used for communication by many of the cells that are destroyed in Alzheimer disease. Medications that slow down the rate of breakdown of choline prolong the ability of the choline to transmit the message to the next cell. Blocking cholinesterase, the chemical that breaks down choline, does this. This improves the function of the cells, and thus the function of the person with Alzheimer disease. Unfortunately, this improvement is temporary and the effectiveness of the medications decrease as more cells are destroyed and fewer cells are sending and receiving signals via choline. The medications presently available include: donepezil (Aricept), galantamine (Razadyne), rivastigmine (Exelon), and tacrine (Cognex).

Tacrine (Cognex) is rarely used now because of liver toxicity side effects and the need for frequent monitoring of blood tests. The others—donepezil (Aricept), galantamine (Reminyl), and rivastigmine (Exelon)—seem similar in their benefits and side effects. One side effect to watch for is gastrointestinal upset and/or anorexia (decreased appetite). Many people with Alzheimer disease require assistance and encouragement to consume enough calories and appropriate nutrition any way. If they develop these side effects, it may be even more difficult to maintain good nutrition. In addition, seizures, although not common, can be a side effect as well. If the person is taking one of the medications and develops seizures, the question arises whether the seizures are secondary to the medication or the Alzheimer disease. Unfortunately, there is no way to determine which is the cause. A decision must then be made as to whether the benefit of the medication exceeds the downside that it could be causing seizures.

A newer medication is memantine (Namenda). It may slow calcium influx into cells and nerve damage. In our experience, the medication is effective in temporarily stabilizing or even improving function, and it is generally well tolerated. It is indicated for moderate to severe Alzheimer disease and we usually add it to one of the cholinesterase inhibitors. Unfortunately, as with the medications that block the breakdown of choline, memantine does not stop the destructive process of Alzheimer disease. Eventually, too many cells are damaged and the effect of the medication diminishes.

TREATMENT OF ASSOCIATED SEIZURES

The seizures seen in Alzheimer disease may be tonic-clonic (grand mal) or other types. In addition, myoclonic jerks are often seen. Phenytoin (Dilantin), carbamazepine (Tegretol), valproic acid (Depakote), gabapentin (Neurontin), and other anti-seizure medications can be effective, depending on the type of seizure. The seizure medications can cause drowsiness and increased confusion. We have found this to be particularly true of phenytoin (Dilantin).

We wait until seizures develop before starting anti-seizure medications, in light of the potential side effects and the fact that not all people develop seizures. It is important, however, to bring the seizures under control as soon as possible. Uncontrolled seizures seem to contribute to a more rapid rate of decline.

TREATMENT OF PSYCHOLOGICAL, PERSONALITY, AND BEHAVIORAL CHANGES

Psychological, personality, and behavioral changes are common in Alzheimer disease. Changes may include sleep problems, depression, anxiety, agitation, compulsiveness, paranoia, hallucinations, and others. These symptoms can often be reduced through behavioral management. Sometimes medications are also beneficial. Further information regarding specific medications for specific symptoms is addressed below.

One key issue for treating people with Alzheimer disease is to limit the negative impact of the medication. People with AD are often more susceptible to side effects of medications such as sedation, increased confusion, and further loss of skills such as walking or swallowing. Therefore, careful monitoring of the medications and the benefits and negative effects is important. In addition, smaller doses, less frequent dosing, and shorter duration of use may be effective while at the same time limiting side effects.

OBSESSIVE-COMPULSIVE DISORDER

Some degree of compulsiveness is common in people with Down syndrome. However, the development of AD may increase this behavior. Some of our patients developed obsessive-compulsive disorder that was, in retrospect, the earliest sign of Alzheimer disease. Chapter 9 covers how to assist people with compulsive tendencies, but in short, helping someone use these tendencies in a positive manner is likely to be more effective than trying to use behavioral techniques to eliminate this tendency. If the problem is not responding to behavioral approaches and is affecting the person's ability to participate in daily life, we generally recommend the use of medications. We have found the selective serotonin reuptake inhibitors to work well. Medications for obsessive-compulsive disorder are discussed in Chapter 16.

DEPRESSION

Depression is common in people with Alzheimer disease. Depression can be seen independent of Alzheimer disease, it can mimic Alzheimer disease (which is why checking for depression is part of the diagnostic process), and it can be part of the symptoms of Alzheimer disease. Supportive treatment is essential for a person with depression, whether Alzheimer disease is part of the depression or not. Offering reassurances, listening to concerns, and encouraging participation in activities are some of the many ways to support a person with depression.

Medications are also necessary sometimes. We have found the newer antidepressants, sertraline (Zoloft), paroxetine (Paxil), citalopram (Celexa), escitalopram (Lexapro), and venlafaxine (Effexor), to be particularly effective. Although any of the antidepressants may cause some agitation, fluoxetine (Prozac) seems to cause it more often in people with DS. Typically, the agitation does not begin immediately but is delayed until the person has taken the medication for several weeks. Paroxetine (Paxil) causes agitation less frequently than fluoxetine (Prozac), but when it does cause agitation, it tends to occur sooner, within several days to a few weeks after starting the medication.

Another choice is bupropion (Wellbutrin), but it has a greater theoretical risk of seizures (which are already a concern in Alzheimer disease). The older antidepressants such as amitriptyline (Elavil), desipramine (Norpramin), and others are probably effective as well. However, we tend not to use these medications because of their greater incidence of anti-cholinergic side effects. People with Down syndrome seem to be more sensitive to these side effects even when they do not have Alzheimer disease. There is also the concern that blocking the effect of choline will result in a greater decline in skills. As indicated previously, medications that promote choline activity may reduce the symptoms of Alzheimer disease.

SLEEP DISTURBANCE

Many people with Alzheimer disease have sleep disturbances. Often they are confused with regards to typical day-night sleep cycles. The person sleeps during the day and is awake at night. This may not be harmful if the person can get adequate sleep, just at a different time. If the environment can allow for this pattern, then it is reasonable not to intervene.

There are several reasons to consider intervention, however. Safety is often the most important reason. If care providers sleep at night, the person with Alzheimer disease is not as well supervised at night. In addition, often stimulating activity is only available during the day. Therefore, even if safety could be maintained at night, the person would have no activity to participate in during his wake time, which can lead to further decline, as discussed previously. In addition, the person who is up at night may be very disruptive to others who sleep at night. Continued sleep deprivation can be very stressful for caregivers.

Interventions for sleep changes can include both nonmedicinal and medicinal treatments. We have outlined our nonmedicinal recommendations in the "Sleep Hygiene" section in Chapter 2. When these recommendations are unsuccessful, additional measures are available. We have had some success with the natural product melatonin. We generally recommend starting with 2 mg and increasing to 4 mg in a few weeks if 2 mg is not adequate. There are several other over-the-counter agents, but many of them contain diphenhydramine (Benadryl), which has anti-cholinergic side effects. As noted above, anti-cholinergic side effects can, particularly in someone with Alzheimer disease, include confusion. Therefore, we tend to stay away from these products. Prescription medications such as zaleplon (Sonata), eszopiclone (Lunesta), or zolpidem (Ambien) are effective in many patients. A short-acting benzodiazepine such as oxazepam (Serax) may also be effective. We have also found trazodone (Desyrel) to be helpful.

ANXIETY

Anxiety can be part of the psychological decline in Alzheimer disease. Some anxiety may stem from a direct neurological impairment. We suspect that some of it may result from the person's fear of the inability to understand what is happening to him as he declines. Often, anxiety seems to occur during earlier stages, which would seem to go along with the latter idea. It can be very disconcerting to sense that you are losing skills but not have the ability to understand why. Ways to reduce anxiety include:

- Providing reassurances (gentle verbal reassurance, encouraging and helping the person do the task that he is having difficulty with, etc.)
- Helping the person find tasks at which he can be successful
- Providing written or picture cues that help the person find his way or do things (we find pictures to work best)
- Removing reminders of things that he can no longer do (e.g., if it frustrates him that he can't cook his own meals any more, removing the microwave may reduce anxiety)
- Not arguing with him when he is recalling something incorrectly (unless there is a safety issue involved)

Medications can also be used. The newer antidepressants, as discussed above, can help with anxiety. A shorter-acting benzodiazepine can also be helpful. We have used alprazolam (Xanax) and lorazepam (Ativan) with good success. We generally use very small doses and use them less frequently than would generally be recommended. Real care must be used when using these medications in a person with Alzheimer disease. Sedation, unsteady gait, depressed mood, and increased confusion are common side effects.

We have generally found that there is a relatively short period of time (weeks to a few months) that the anxiety requires medications, although some of our patients had anxiety for a longer period. We recommend careful observation for side effects and discontinuing the medications if side effects occur. In addition, wean the medication as soon as possible, as anxiety symptoms decrease.

Agitated Behavior

Agitated behavior is another problem that can occur in people with Alzheimer disease. When it occurs, careful assessment is important. An evaluation for medical problems and physical sources of pain may find a cause that is not directly related to Alzheimer disease. Because of the person's reduced ability to understand or inform others of his discomfort, he may be using behavioral changes to communicate. In addition, depression, increasing obsessive tendencies or compulsivity, anxiety, and sleep disturbance may cause agitated behavior. Treatment for the appropriate condition may reduce or eliminate the agitated behavior. Sometimes, however, no other underlying cause is found.

Sometimes agitated behavior can endanger the person with AD or others. In addition, it may be associated with hallucinatory behavior or paranoia. If this is disturbing to the person or is a safety issue, medications can be beneficial. We have found the newer anti-psychotics helpful. Risperidone (Risperdal), olanzapine (Zyprexa), ziprasidone (Geodon), aripiprazole (Abilify), and quetiapine (Seroquel) have all reduced symptoms. But we have also seen increased sedation, increased confusion, unsteadiness, and increased incontinence in patients taking these medications. However, we start with very tiny doses—e.g., risperidone (Risperdal) 0.25 mg at bedtime—and this has reduced the incidence of side effects.

Some recent findings in people without DS who have AD suggest that there may be an increased incidence of stroke when they take these medications. Vascular disease seems to be less common in general in people with Down syndrome, so this would theoretically appear to be less of a concern in people with DS. However, studies have not been done to assess this risk in people with DS, so be sure to discuss these concerns with the doctor if these medications are prescribed for an adult with DS and AD under your care.

Hallucinatory behavior and paranoia can also occur without agitated behavior. If this is a significant problem for the person, treatment as described above can be beneficial.

Keeping Activities at the Right Level

Another aspect of caring for a person who has developed Alzheimer disease is maximizing his level of function. We recommend encouraging him to participate in activities that are of the appropriate cognitive level. Engaging him in activities that are not too easy and not too difficult will help maintain a higher level of function for a longer period of time. Tasks that are too difficult will be frustrating and can lead to a more rapid loss of skills, as well as emotional changes, stress-related behaviors, and unhappiness. Similarly, tasks that are too easy will not allow the person to use the skills that he has and will lead to greater erosion of skills.

Assessing the appropriate skill level of tasks can be difficult, particularly if the person's skill level fluctuates. What was appropriate yesterday may not be appropriate today but may again be appropriate tomorrow. This can be a challenge for a caregiver both from an assessment standpoint and from an emotional standpoint. Caregivers can begin to "take it personally" when the person with Alzheimer disease can't do a task that he could do just recently. They may feel that the person with AD is not trying, is being lazy, or is not doing it to spite them. Although the caregiver may have previously helped the person with Down syndrome develop new skills and greater independence, this emphasis on improving skills must be reassessed when AD is diagnosed. The focus must shift to maintaining skills or limiting the decline in skills.

THE RIGHT ENVIRONMENT

In our experience, it is usually best for the person with AD to remain in a familiar environment. A change in environment can be confusing, require learning new skills, and be emotionally upsetting. Compare a change in environment to changing the furniture in the house of a person with severe vision impairment. It requires new learning in order to function in the environment. With the declining intellect of a person with Alzheimer disease, this can be difficult. However, the environment will need to be adjusted as the person's skills decline (adjust the environment to meet the needs of the person, not the person to meet the needs of the environment).

The flexibility of the environment is crucial to optimizing the care of the person with AD. When skills first begin to decline, someone may do well in the same environment. As the person's skills further decline, however, his adaptability does too. Often he will be most comfortable (or perhaps only comfortable) in his home. Going to work may become too stressful, especially as Alzheimer disease progresses. If the person lives somewhere where leaving the building and going to work is a required part of the schedule, this may become a significant problem. Flexibility in the schedule is helpful to the person with Alzheimer disease who is declining. There may be days when it is apparent that he would best be served by staying home. The environment must allow for the assessment of the person's level of function and the benefit of work versus the stress of work. In addition, an alternative program at home should be available on days that the person would be best served by remaining at home.

Safety issues may also develop. Loss of judgment related to appliances, hot water, and other potential household hazards can lead to potentially serious accidents. In addition, as the person's walking skills decline, stairs and other obstacles can become safety hazards. Wandering is another potential safety issue that may need to be addressed with alarms on doors, the person's bed, and other sites. Assessing the safety of the environment is critical. A "Home Safety Inspection" by an occupational therapist can be of significant benefit.

Besides assessing how the environment affects the person with Alzheimer disease, it is necessary to assess how the person with Alzheimer disease affects the environment. For example, how does he affect the other people who are living with him? For a person of "normal" intelligence, the stress of caring for, or just living with, a person with Alzheimer disease can be substantial. While we have seen people with Down syndrome and other intellectual disabilities "rise to the occasion" when someone they live with develops Alzheimer disease, we have also seen it become an overwhelming stress. One group of three women who lived with a woman with Down syndrome who developed Alzheimer disease initially "blossomed" with regards to their own caregiver skills. However, later they found the situation too much to handle and a different living situation was arranged.

Whenever possible, we encourage letting roommates or housemates with intellectual disabilities try to provide care for the person with AD. Many people with Down syndrome or other intellectual disabilities get "done for" their whole lives with little opportunity to "do for." Assisting someone with Alzheimer disease can provide a real boost to self-esteem for the care provider.

However, sometimes the stress of something that seems relatively minor can create problematic tension in the house. This might occur, for example, when the person with Alzheimer disease is no longer expected to participate in life skills classes, go to work, or follow the daily schedule. The sense of "injustice" can create emotional or behavioral problems for the others. At other times, people with Alzheimer disease may recurrently yell or talk loudly, have irregular sleep patterns that disturb others' sleep, or need changes in the environment that are stressful for the others. Sometimes the changes in the person with AD just become too great a stress. All these issues may create a situation where reassessing the environment becomes necessary.

A Change in Environment

If an environment does not allow for the adult with AD to stay home during the day when he needs to, this can result in significant stress for him. The continuous expectation to do tasks that are too difficult or too stressful can lead to emotional, behavioral, and cognitive changes. If he feels overwhelmed by expectations, the person might give up and seem to have fewer skills than he actually has. Moving to an environment that allows for the necessary flexibility can be of significant benefit. This benefit often outweighs the negative impact a move to a new residence can have.

Moving may also be advisable if safety issues cannot be resolved. The presence of stairs or potentially dangerous household appliances or the inability to assure that the person does not wander away can all be significant safety issues that may not be correctable in the present living situation. In these instances, a move to a safer residence can be a real benefit.

Finally, it is often best for the person with AD to move to another residence if his caregivers or the people he lives with are overwhelmed with the situation and appropriate in-home assistance is not available. This can be necessary both when the person lives at home with his family or when he lives in a residential facility.

We have participated in a number of successful, appropriate moves to different residences for our patients with Down syndrome and Alzheimer disease. Nursing homes, particularly if they offer specialized care for people with AD, can be appropriate. Some agencies have residences for "seniors" that are able to provide appropriate care. Moving back home with family (if the person is living in a residential facility) has also worked for some. Generally, however, this requires some additional in-home assistance.

DURATION OF ALZHEIMER DISEASE

The duration of Alzheimer disease in adults with Down syndrome is not clear. In the general population, the course of the disease is thought to be approximately ten to twelve years. Particularly in people with Down syndrome who have a higher degree of functioning before the onset of Alzheimer disease, an overall course of ten or so years might be expected. However, our experience suggests that the duration is shorter for many, particularly in those who have a lower level of functioning prior to the onset of Alzheimer disease. In a sense, the further the person has to fall cognitively, the longer it generally takes. We have seen people live one year from the time of diagnosis to the time of death. On average, though, the time from the development of symptoms to death is usually in the three- to six-year range.

Again, the development of seizures (particularly if they are difficult to control) seems to accelerate the decline in some people. Losing the ability to walk and swallow and the complications seen when these skills are lost also seems to increase the rate of decline.

FUTURE CONSIDERATIONS

At present, a great deal of research is addressing the issue of Alzheimer disease, not only for people with Down syndrome, but for those without. People with DS receive particular attention when it comes to AD because studies suggest that they all develop the neuropathologic changes that are seen in Alzheimer disease. Since these changes appear to be universal, researchers wonder why all people with DS do not appear to get the symptoms of AD. Is there something else that is coded on the twenty-first chromosome that may be protective for some people with Down syndrome against Alzheimer disease? This question has not yet been answered. It should be noted, however, that people with Down syndrome rarely develop heart attacks and coronary artery disease, so there may be something about Down syndrome that protects against some diseases.

The findings in people with Down syndrome may be important keys in unlocking the mysteries of Alzheimer disease. In addition, there is a great deal of interest in discovering whether what helps AD may help people with DS when they are younger (before AD is apparent). For example, donepezil (Aricept) is being studied for its potential benefit to younger people with Down syndrome. In addition, there is a great deal of interest and study around the potential benefit of vitamins and other medications and how they might benefit or prevent Alzheimer disease in people with Down syndrome. Similar research is being conducted as to whether vitamins, supplements, and other treatments may also benefit the cognitive, speech, and other skills of people with DS. There appears to be much to learn that may benefit people with Down syndrome, people with Alzheimer disease, and people with both.

SUMMARY

◆ ◆ ◆ ◆ ◆ ◆ ◆ ◆ ◆ ◆ ◆ ◆ ◆ ◆ ◆ ◆ ◆

Decline in function does not appear to be inevitable in older adults with Down syndrome. When a decline in function is noted, a thorough evaluation is indicated to look for potentially reversible causes. While there is currently no cure if the diagnosis is Alzheimer disease, there are many ways to temporarily improve a person's level of function and make him more comfortable.

Addenda

1. Medications by Class (PAGES 402-413)

The addendum on pages 402-413 is a selection of medications that are used to treat mental health conditions in people with Down syndrome. The medications are presented by class of medication. We have used most of the classes of the medications for our patients when they have a condition that necessitates the use of medications. We have included some others that we don't use but that might be used by other practitioners. In the "Notes" column we have briefly shared some of our experiences with that class of medications. Further information can be found in the chapter on that condition. A list of the definition of terms used in the table is provided on page 413.

2. Psychotropic Consent Form (PAGE 414)

The addendum on page 414 is an example of a consent form that can be used before starting a psychotropic medication. Consent and assent are discussed on pages 248-249.

Addendum 1: Medications by Class

Class	Drugs	Chemistry	Uses	Side Effects/Chronic Use	Notes
Acetylcholine receptor inhibitor	benztropine (Cogentin)	Antagonizes acetylcholine and histamine receptors	Treat extrapyramidal side effects of other medications	Psychosis Rapid heart rate Dry mouth Constipation Urinary retention Sedation Confusion	
Alpha adrenergic anti-hypertensive	clonidine (Catapres) guanfacine (Tenex)	Stimulates central nervous system alpha adrenergic receptors	Anxiety* Attention-Deficit/Hyperactivity Disorder*	Lower blood pressure Dry mouth Dizziness Constipation Sedation Weakness Decreased appetite Nausea	We have had only limited success with these medications.
Anti-anxiety (non-benzodiazepine)	1. buspirone (Buspar) 2. chloral hydrate	Mechanism unknown	Anxiety (1) Insomnia (2) Sedation for procedures* (2)	Dizziness Drowsiness Nausea Headache Fatigue Agitation Depression Dependency (2)	We have not often found these to be beneficial in people with anxiety. Buspirone has been helpful in some people with anxiety and agitated behavior when used in combination with other medications. Chloral hydrate has limited benefit in use as a sedative for procedures.

An asterisk (*) indicates a use that is not approved by the FDA (Federal Drug Agency).

Anti-anxiety, Benzodiazepines, Short acting	1. alprazolam (Xanax) 2. oxazepam (Serax)	Binds to benzodiazepine receptors and enhances GABA effects	Anxiety Insomnia (short-term)	Respiratory depression Withdrawal, dependency (usually with longer-term use) Sedation Nausea Unsteady gait Depression Sleep and sleep cycle disturbance Agitation	Useful medications particularly on short term before effects of other medications are realized. Short acting are best for use as mild sedatives if needed for blood drawing, x-rays, etc. Alprazolam also available in a sustained-release form that can be given once a day.
Anti-anxiety, Benzodiazepines, Mid-Acting	1. lorazepam (Ativan) 2. temazepam (Restoril)	Binds to benzodiazepine receptors and enhances GABA effects	Anxiety (1) Insomnia (short-term) (1,2)	Respiratory depression Withdrawal, Dependency (usually with longer-term use) Sedation Nausea Unsteady gait Depression Sleep and sleep cycle disturbance Agitation	Useful medications, particularly on short term before effects of other medications are realized.
Anti-anxiety, Benzodiazepines, Long Acting	1. diazepam (Valium) 2. clonazepam (Klonopin) 3. librium	Binds to benzodiazepine receptors and enhances GABA effects	Anxiety Insomnia (short-term) *Above indications are not FDA approved for clonazepam; it is FDA approved as an anti-seizure medication.	Respiratory depression Withdrawal, Dependency (usually with longer-term use) Sedation Nausea Unsteady gait Depression Sleep and sleep cycle disturbance Agitation	Useful medications, particularly on short term before effects of other medications are realized.

Class	Drugs	Chemistry	Uses	Side Effects/Chronic Use	Notes
Antidepressant, not specified	1. bupropion (Wellbutrin) 2. trazodone (Desyrel) 3. venlafaxine (Effexor) 4. mirtazapine (Remeron) 5. duloxetine (Cymbalta)	Inhibits uptake of norepinephrine, serotonin, and dopamine (1) Inhibits serotonin reuptake (2) Inhibits norephinephrine, serotonin, and dopamine reuptake (3) Antagonizes serotonin and norephinephrine reuptake (4,5)	Depression Insomnia* (2) Aggressive behavior* (2)	Seizures Heart block (rhythm disturbance) Agitation Dry mouth Fast heart rate Sleep disturbance Nausea and vomiting Prolonged erection Tremor Constipation Sedation Weight loss or gain	Bupropion sometimes contributes to weight loss, which can be a benefit when increased appetite and weight gain are a part of the depressive symptoms. We have not found trazodone to be a very effective anti-depressant. It often causes sedation, however, and we have found it to be an effective sleep aid. It is also sometimes beneficial with agitated or aggressive behavior. Particularly at higher doses, the norepinephrine reuptake blocking effect of venlafaxine is seen and can provide some degree of stimulation for those for whom decreased activity is part of the depression.

Antidepressants, Selective Serotonin Reuptake Inhibitors (SSRIs)	1. citalopram (Celexa) 2. escitalopram (Lexapro) 3. fluvoxamine (Luvox) 4. paroxetine (Paxil) 5. fluoxetine (Prozac) 6. sertraline (Zoloft)	Selectively inhibits serotonin reuptake	Depression (1,2,4,5,6) Obsessive-Compulsive Disorder (3,4,5,6) Anxiety (2,4) Panic disorder (4,5,6) Social anxiety disorder (4,6) Post-traumatic stress disorder (4,6) Premenstrual Dysphoric Disorder (6)	Weight gain Sedation Dry mouth Agitation Tremor Decreased sexual drive Gastrointestinal upset Diarrhea Headache	Paroxetine has caused the greatest weight gain. Fluoxetine most likely to cause agitation but it is often delayed several weeks. Therefore, we do not generally use fluoxetine. Paroxetine second most likely to cause agitation and most often occurs in the first 2 to 4 weeks after starting the medication or increasing the dose. Higher doses often needed with Obsessive-Compulsive disorder. All except Fluvoxamine available as liquids, which can be useful for patients who can't swallow pills or need doses adjusted minutely.
Anti-depressants, tricyclic	1. clomipramine (Anafranil) 2. amitriptyline (Elavil) 3. doxepin (Sinequan) 4. nortriptyline (Pamelor) 5. imipramine (Tofranil)	Inhibits reuptake of serotonin and norepinephrine	Obsessive-Compulsive Disorder (1) Depression Chronic pain (2)	Seizures Dry mouth Tremor Headache Drowsiness Constipation Sleep changes Difficulty urinating	We have found this class to generally have more side effects than the selective serotonin reuptake inhibitors (SSRIs). Doxepin sometimes beneficial as sleep aid but tends to cause more side effects than other available choices.

Class	Drugs	Chemistry	Uses	Side Effects/Chronic Use	Notes
Antihistamines	1. hydroxyzine (Atarax) 2. diphenhydramine (Benadryl)	Blocks histamine receptors	Anxiety* Sedation* Insomnia*	Dry mouth Sedation Confusion Dizziness Unsteady gait Agitation Slurred speech Headache	Anti-cholinergic effects can be particularly problematic for people with Down syndrome, especially those with Alzheimer disease. We have generally found the antihistamines to not be effective for psychological use or as a sleep aid.
Anti-psychotic, atypical and other	1. ziprasidone (Geodon) 2. risperdone (Risperdal) 3. quetiapine (Seroquel) 4. olanzapine (Zyprexa) 5. aripiprazole (Abilify)	Antagonizes dopamine and serotonin receptors	Psychoses/ Schizophrenia (1,2,3,4,5) Agitation (1,4) Bipolar disorder (1,2,3,4,5)	Neuroleptic malignant syndrome Tardive dyskinesia Extrapyramidal side effects Elevated blood sugar Heart rhythm disturbance Drowsiness Headache Nausea Constipation Decreased enthusiasm/ "energy" Elevated prolactin level Menstrual irregularities Weight change	Weight gain can be a particular problem with these medications. (Olanzapine appears to be particularly a problem for people with DS.) Drowsiness can be a significant side effect. This can be an advantage when sleep disturbance is part of the illness. Olanzapine appears to have the greatest potential for sedation.

Anti-psychotic, typical	1. haloperidol (Haldol) 2. thioridazine (Mellaril) 3. thiothixene (Navane) 4. pimozide (Orap) 5. trifluoperazine (Stelazine) 6. chlorpromazine (Thorazine)	Antagonizes dopamine receptors	Psychosis (1,2,3,5,6) Tourette syndrome (1,4) Acute agitation (1) Anxiety (5)	Neuroleptic malignant syndrome Tardive dyskinesia Extrapyramidal side effects Low blood pressure Heart rhythm disturbance (particularly life-threatening with Mellaril) Drowsiness Headache Nausea Constipation Decreased enthusiasm/"energy" Elevated prolactin level Menstrual irregularities Agitation Sleep disturbance Breast enlargement	Particular caution with thioridazine in light of the potential for severe heart rhythm disturbance.
Anti-seizure	1. valproic acid (Depakote, Depakene) 2. gabapentin (Neurontin) 3. carbamezepine (Tegretol) 4. oxcarbazepine (Trileptal) 5. lamotrigine (Lamictal)	Unknown	Mania (1) Bipolar illness (3,5) Aggressive behavior* Impulse control disorder*	Liver disease (1,3,4,5) Low blood sodium level (1,3,4) Bone marrow suppression (decreased platelets, decreased white blood cells &/or decreased red blood cells) (only white blood cells for Neurontin) Nausea Sedation Tremor (1,3,4) Weight changes Nervousness	Although gabapentin is less well recognized as being beneficial in these conditions, we have had some success with it. It has been particularly helpful when a patient has difficulty complying with blood drawing because less monitoring of blood work is necessary. Lamotrigine indicated for bipolar maintenance.

Class	Drugs	Chemistry	Uses	Side Effects/Chronic Use	Notes
Appetite stimulant	megestrol (Megace)	Inhibits pituitary gonadotropin release	Appetite stimulant*	Adrenal suppression Diabetes mellitus Blood clots Congestive heart failure Hypertension Sleep disturbance Urinary frequency Abdominal pain Hot flashes Hair loss	We have found this to be beneficial when eating refusal or severe anorexia is part of the symptomotology.
Attention-deficit/hyperactivity disorder (see also stimulants)	atomoxetine (Strattera)	Exact mechanism unknown; selectively inhibits norephinephrine reuptake	Attention deficit disorder	Tachycardia (fast heart rate) Hypertension (elevated blood pressure) Low blood pressure Dry mouth Decreased appetite Urinary difficulty (hesitancy) Fatigue Dysmenorrhea (painful periods) Sleep disturbance Abnormal dreams	An effective, non-stimulant treatment for AD/HD.
Beta Blockers	1. atenolol (Tenormin) 2. propranolol (Inderal)	Blocks beta receptors	Anxiety* Impulse control disorder* Aggressive behavior*	Congestive heart failure Brochospasm (asthma) Fatigue Weakness Constipation Diarrhea Low blood pressure	Is sometimes used for these uses but we have not had much success with these medications.

Contraceptives, Birth Control Pills	Many brands e.g., Alesse Tri-Noriny Tri-Levlen Ortho-Novum	Inhibits ovulation by suppressing LH and FSH (hormones in the brain)	Contraception Dysmenorrhea* (painful periods) May benefit some women with premenstrual syndrome*	Blood clots Myocardial infarction (heart attack) Stroke Hypertension (high blood pressure) Gall bladder disease Abnormal uterine bleeding Headaches Swelling Weight changes	We have used it as an additional therapy in some women who have painful periods that contribute to behavioral changes. Can also be useful in premenstrual syndrome.
Contraceptives, other	medroxyprogesterone (Depo-Provera)	Inhibits ovulation by suppressing LH and FSH (hormones in the brain)	Contraception Dysmenorrhea (painful periods)*	Blood clots Menstrual irregularities Absence of menses Weight gain Headache Depression Hair growth Hot flashes Fluid retention Decreased libido	Often causes absence of periods (while medication being taken) which can be a benefit when uncomfortable periods are a problem or when managing periods is a significant problem for the woman. Given as injection every 3 months. Periods may be significantly irregular for first year or so.

Class	Drugs	Chemistry	Uses	Side Effects/Chronic Use	Notes
Cholinesterase inhibitors	1. donepezil (Aricept) 2. tacrine (Cognex) 3. galantamine (Razadyne) 4. rivastigmine (Exelon)	Inhibits cholinesterase (reduces destruction of acetylcholine)	Alzheimer Dementia	Seizures Nausea Weight loss Headache Sleep disturbance Depression Urinary frequency and incontinence Liver toxicity (2)	Temporarily improves cognitive function and benefits behavior and emotional changes associated with Alzheimer Dementia Some early data suggest it may help language in people with DS who don't have AD. Tacrine generally not used because of liver toxicity and the need to regularly monitor blood tests.
Lithium		Alters sodium transport in nerve cells	Mania/Bipolar	Seizures Heart rhythm disturbance Tremor Urinary frequency Vomiting Drowsiness Blurred vision Dry mouth Diarrhea Muscle weakness Fatigue	We have not used this a great deal because of concern regarding toxicity.

Melatonin		May affect serotonin	Insomnia*		Can be a beneficial treatment to help people with DS fall asleep when sleep disturbance is a primary problem or part of a mental illness such as depression.
NMDA Receptor antagonist	memantine (Namenda)	Binds N-methyl-D-aspartase receptors	Alzheimer disease	Dizziness Confusion Headache Constipation High blood pressure Cough Somnolence Vomiting Fatigue Hallucinations	We have found memantine to be beneficial in temporarily improving cognitive function in adults with DS who have Alzheimer disease.
Nonsteroidal anti-inflammatory agents, (Non-selective inhibitors)	1. naproxen (Anaprox) 2. ibuprofen (Motrin) 3. naproxen (Naprosyn)	Inhibits prostaglandin synthesis	Arthritis (1,2,3) Pain (1,2,3) Dysmenorrhea (painful periods) (1,2,3) Gout (1,3) Fever (2)	Gastrointestinal bleeding Kidney failure Reduced blood clotting Upset stomach Abdominal pain Fluid retention Ringing in the ear	If discomfort with a woman's periods is noted, we often recommend one of these be started 3 to 5 days prior to the anticipated onset of the period. May also decrease the amount of menstrual flow.
Opioid antagonist	naltrexone (ReVia)	Antagonizes opiate receptors	Self-injurious behavior*	Suicide ideation (thoughts) Opiate withdrawal symptoms Insomnia Nausea Vomiting Anxiety Headache Decreased appetite Abdominal pain	Helpful in some people to reduce self-injurious behavior.

Class	Drugs	Chemistry	Uses	Side Effects/Chronic Use	Notes
Sleep agents	1. zolpidem (Ambien) 2. zaleplon (Sonata) 3. eszopiclone (Lunesta)	Interacts with GABA-benzodiazepine receptor complexes	Insomnia (short-term)	Gait disturbance Hallucinations Headache Drowsiness Muscle aches Dizziness Nausea Constipation Depression	We generally use melatonin first. Trazodone also useful (see antidepressant, not specified).
Stimulants	1. amphetamine-dextroamphetamine (Adderall) 2. dextroamphetamine (Dexedrine) 3. methylphenidate (Concerta) 4. methylphenidate (Ritalin)	Stimulates Central Nervous System	1. Attention-Deficit/Hyperactivity Disorder (2,3,4) 2. Narcolepsy (1,2,4)	Psychosis Dependency Loss of appetite Sleep disturbance Nausea Diarrhea Seizures Irritability Tics	We have had particular success with methylphenidate (Concerta and Ritalin). Amphetamine-dextroamphetamine in particular seems to agitate some people with DS.
Thyroid supplement	1. Dessicated Thyroid (Armour Thyroid) 2. levothyroxine (Synthroid)	Thyroid hormone	Hypothyroidism	Heart rhythm disturbances High blood pressure Nervousness Fast heart rate Tremor Intolerance of heat	Side effects minimal if blood tests are followed and dose adjusted accordingly. When starting the medication, some people tolerate it better if started at a lower dose and work up gradually to appropriate dose.

*Non-FDA approved use

DEFINITION OF TERMS USED IN ADDENDUM 1

Antagonize: Prevent the function of. For example, acetylcholine receptor antagonists prevent the effect of acetylcholine on the acetylcholine receptors.

Anti-cholinergic: The effect of blocking cholinergic receptors. This results in side effects such as dry mouth, constipation, urinary hesitancy, and visual changes.

Dependency: The need to use increasing doses over time to achieve the same effect. Usually used in reference to medications that are potentially addictive such as benzodiazepines or narcotics.

Extrapyramidal: Involuntary muscle contractions, rigidity, or restlessness. Parkinsonism (symptoms like Parkinson disease) can occur.

Neuroleptic malignant syndrome: Potentially fatal side-effect that includes muscle rigidity, tremor, high fever, sweating, fluctuating blood pressure, impaired thought processes, and dysfunction of the autonomic nervous system.

Respiratory depression: Reduction in the normal, automatic drive to breathe. This results in a reduction in oxygen in the blood and an increase in carbon dioxide.

Sleep cycle: The normal flow of sleep, including the proper order of the different stages of sleep.

Suicide ideation: Thinking of committing suicide.

Tics: Habitual and repeated contractions of certain muscles. These result in stereotypical movements or actions. They can only be voluntarily suppressed for brief periods of time.

Unsteady gait: Imbalance with walking with a tendency toward frequent falling.

Urinary retention: Inability to completely empty the urinary bladder.

Withdrawal: Symptoms that occur when a medication is reduced or discontinued. Usually used in reference to a medication for which a dependency occurs over time, such as a benzodiazepine or narcotic.

Name _____   Date _____

Psychotropic Consent Form

A psychotropic medication has been prescribed for the above named patient.

Name of medication: _____

Diagnosis: _____

Range of Medication: _____

Reduction Plan: _____

_____

_____

Information is provided/attached about the medication and its potential side effects.

I recommend the above medication and have completed the above information.

Physician signature:_____ Date _____

I have reviewed the above information, have had an opportunity to have my questions answered, and I consent to the use of this medication.

Patient signature: _____ Date _____

Explain if patient unable to sign: _____

_____

_____

Guardian/Family Consent: _____ Relationship? _____

Date _____

References

Anderson, L.M., Shinn, C., Fullilove, M.T., et al. (2003). The effectiveness of early childhood development programs: A systematic review. *American Journal of Preventative Medicine 24* (3 suppl.): 32.

Breiter, H. C., Rauch, S. L., Kwong, K. K., et al. (1996). Functional magnetic resonance imaging of symptom provocation in obsessive-compulsive disorder. *Archives of General Psychiatry 53* (7): 595-606.

Brown, R.T., Freeman, W.S., Perrin, J.M., Stein, M.T., Amler, R.W., Feldman, H.M., Pierce, K., and Wolraich, M. L. (2001). Prevalence and assessment of Attention-Deficit/Hyperactivity Disorder in primary care settings. *Pediatrics 107* (3): e43

Buckley, S., and Le Prevost, P. (2002). Speech and language therapy for Down syndrome children: Guidelines for best practice based on current research. *Down Syndrome News and Update 2* (2): 70-76.

Carey, W. B., and McDevitt, S, C. (1995). *Coping with children's temperament: a guide for professionals.* New York: Basic Books.

Chen, H. Down syndrome. www.emedicine.com/ped/topics615.htm.

Chicoine, B., and McGuire, D. (1997). Longevity of a woman with Down syndrome: A case study. *Mental Retardation 35,* 477-79

Chicoine, B., McGuire, D., Hebein, S., and Gilly, D. (1994). Development of a clinic for adults with Down syndrome. *Mental Retardation, 32* (2): 100-106.

Cohen, W. I. and Patterson, B. J. (1998). Neurodevelopmental disorders in Down syndrome. In *Down syndrome: A promising future, together,* T. Hassold and D. Patterson (eds.). New York: Wiley-Liss.

Cohen, W., ed. (1991). Health care guidelines for individuals with Down syndrome. *Down Syndrome Quarterly 4* (3). (Available online at www.denison.edu/collaborations/dsq/health99.html)

de Vinck, C. (1990). *The power of the powerless.* New York: Doubleday.

Diagnostic and Statistical Manual of Mental Disorders, Fourth Edition, Text Revision. (2000). Washington, DC: American Psychiatric Association.

Diaz, R., and Berk, L. (1991). *Private speech: From social interaction to self-regulation.* Mahwah, NJ: Lawrence Erlbaum Associates.
    (Private speech is the term used for self-talk in literature on child development. This volume includes a wide range of references on the uses of private speech.)

Down Syndrome & Autism Spectrum Disorder (September/October 1999). *Disability Solutions 3, 5 & 6:* 1-40.

Dowrick, P.W. (1991). *Practical guide to using video in the behavioral sciences.* New York: New York: Wiley.

Eddy, M. F., and Walbroehl, G.S. (1998). Recognition and treatment of obsessive-compulsive disorder. *American Family Physician 57* (7), 1623-28.

Evenhuis, H. M., Kengen, M. M. F., and Eurling, H. A. L. (1990). *Dementia questionnaire for mentally retarded persons.* Zwammerdam, Netherlands: Hooge Burch.

Frank, E., Kupfer, D.J., Derel, J.M., Cornes, C., Mallinger, A.G. Thase, M.E., McEachran, A.B., and Grochoncinski, V.J. (1990). Three year outcomes for maintenance therapies in recurrent depression. *Archives of General Psychology 47:* 1093-99

Gamage, K. L., Hardy, J., and Hall, C. R. (2001). A description of self talk in exercise. *Psychology of Sport & Exercise, 2* (4): 233-47.

Gedye, A. (1995). *Manual for the Dementia Scale for Down syndrome.* Vancouver, BC: Gedye Research and Consulting.

Geisinger, K. F., and Carlson, J. F. (1992). Assessing language-minority students. *Practical Assessment, Research & Evaluation, 3* (2).

Ghaziuddin, M., Tsai, L., and Ghaziuddin, N. (1992). Autism in Down syndrome: Presentation and diagnosis. *Journal of Intellectual Disability Research 36:* 449-56.

Glasberg, B. (2006). *Functional behavior analysis for people with autism: Making sense of seemingly senseless behavior.* Bethesda, MD: Woodbine House.

Gray, C. (1993). *The Original Social Story Book.* Arlington, TX: Future Horizons.

Greenspan, S., and Granfield, J. M. (1992). Reconsidering the construct of mental retardation: Implications of a model of social competence. *American Journal on Mental Retardation, 96* (4), 442-53.

Greenspan, S., and Shoultz, J. (1981). Why mentally retarded adults lose their jobs: Social competence as a factor in work adjustment. *Applied Research in Mental Retardation 2:* 23-38.

Guralnick M. (1998). Effectiveness of early intervention for vulnerable children: A developmental perspective. *American Journal on Mental Retardation 102:* 319-45.

Heller, T. (1982). Social disruption and residential relocation of mentally retarded children. *American Journal of Mental Deficiency 87:* 48-55.

Hill, J. W., and Wehman, P. (1979). Employer and nonhandicapped co-worker perceptions of moderately and severely retarded workers. *Journal of Contemporary Business 8 :* 107-11.

Huxley, A., Prasher, V. P., and Hague, M. S. (2000). The Dementia Scale for Down's syndrome. *Journal of Intellectual Disability Research 44* (6), 697-98.

Jarrold, C., and Baddeley, A.D. (2001). Short-term memory in Down syndrome: Applying the working memory model. *Down Syndrome Research and Practice 17* (1): 17-23.

Jensen, P.S., and Cooper, J.R., eds. (2002). *Attention deficit hyperactivity disorder: State of science--best practices.* Kingston, NJ: Civic Research Institute.

Kahn, S., Owinowa, T., Pary, R.J. (2002). Down syndrome and major depressive disorder: A review. *Mental Health Aspects of Developmental Disabilities, 5,* 46-52.

Katerndahl, D.A., and Vande Creek, L. (1983). Hyperthyroidism and panic attacks. *Psychosomatics 24* (5): 491-496

Kessler, R.C., Chiu W.T., Demler, O., and Walters, E. (2005). Prevalence, severity and comorbidity for 12-month DSM-IV Disorders in the National Comorbidity Survey Replication. *Archives of General Psychiatry 62: 617-27.*

Krantz, P., and McClannahan, L. (1999). *Activity schedules for children with Autism: Teaching independent behavior.* Bethesda, MD: Woodbine House.

Kumin L. (2003). *Early Communication Skills for Children with Down Syndrome: A Guide for Parents and Professionals.* 2nd ed. Bethesda, MD: Woodbine House.

Landon, T.M., and Barlow, D.H. (2004). Cognitive-behavioral treatment for panic disorder: Current status. *Journal of Psychiatric Practice 10 (4):211-26.*

Lee, H. (1960). *To kill a mockingbird.* Philadelphia: J. B. Lippincott.

Levinson, D. (1978). *The Seasons of a man's life.* New York: Ballantine.

Lord, C., Risi, S., Lambrecht, L., Cook, E. H., Leventhal, B.L., DiLavore, P. C., Pickles, A., and Rutter, M. (2000).The ADOS-G (Autism Diagnostic Observation Schedule-Generic): A standard measure of social-communication deficits associated with autism spectrum disorders. *Journal of Autism and Developmental Disorders 30:*205-23.

Luchterhand, C. (1998). *Mental retardation and grief following a death loss.* Silver Spring, MD: The Arc of the United States. (Copies of the booklet can be ordered from The Arc of the United States, 1010 Wayne Ave., Ste. 650, Silver Spring, MD 20910; 301-565-3842. Or download at www.thearc.org/publications.)

Martin J. E., Rusch F. R., Lagomarcino, T., and Chadsey-Rusch, J. (1986). Comparison between workers who are non handicapped and mentally retarded: Why they lose their jobs. *Applied Research in Mental Retardation 7*: 467-474.

Martinez-Cue, C., Baamonde, C., Lumbreras, M. A., Vallina, F., Dierssen, M., and Florez, J. (1999). Murine model for Down syndrome shows reduced responsiveness to pain. *Neuroreport 10* (5):1119-22.

McGuire, D. (1999). The groove. *NADS: The Newsletter of the National Association for Down Syndrome.* November.

McGuire, D. E., and Chicoine, B. A. (2002). Life issues of adolescents and adults with Down syndrome. In *Down syndrome: Visions for the 21st century,* W. Cohen, L. Nagel, and M.E. Madnick (eds.). New York: Wiley-Liss Press.

McGuire, D., and Chicoine, B. (1996). Depressive disorders in adults with Down syndrome. *The Habilitative Mental Healthcare Newsletter 15* (1) 1996: 1-7.

McGuire, D., Chicoine, B., and Greenbaum, E. (1997). "Self talk" in adults with Down syndrome. *Disability Solutions 2* (1), July/August: 1-4.

Murphy, K. R., and Barkley, R.A. (1996*)*. The prevalence of DSM-IV symptoms of AD/HD in adult licensed drivers: Implications for clinical diagnosis. *Comprehensive Psychiatry 37: 393-401*

Myers B.A., and Pueschel, S. (1991). Psychiatric disorders in a population with Down syndrome. *Journal of Nervous & Mental Disorders 179:* 609-613.

NADS News: The newsletter of the National Association for Down Syndrome, January 2004.

Papolos, D., and Papolos, J. (1999). *The bipolar child: The definitive and reassuring guide to childhood's most misunderstood disorder.* New York: Broadway Books.

Powers, M., ed. (2000). *Children with autism: A parents' guide.* Bethesda, MD: Woodbine House.

Reid, J.R., and Wheeler, S.F. (2005). Hyperthyroidism: diagnosis and treatment. *American Family Physician 72:* 623–30

Reiss, S., Levitan, G.W., and Szyszko, J. (1982). Emotional disturbance and mental retardation: Diagnostic overshadowing. *American Journal of Mental Deficiency 86:* 567-74.

Rogers, C. (1951). Client centered therapy: Its current practice implications and theory. Boston: Houghton Mifflin.

Rosen, L. (2002). Family dynamics in the treatment of Tourette syndrome. *Exceptional Parent,* December.

Saxena, S., Brody, A.L., Schwartz, J.M., and Baxter Jr., L.R. (1998). Neuroimaging and frontal-subcortical circuitry in obsessive-compulsive disorder. *British Journal of Psychiatry (35)* (suppl): 26-37.

Schwartz, J. M., Stoessel, P.W., Baxter Jr., L.R. et al. (1996). Systematic changes in cerebral glucose metabolic rate after successful behavior modification treatment of obsessive-compulsive disorder. *Archives of General Psychiatry 53* (2): 109-13.

Seligman, M. (1998). *Learned optimism: How to change your mind and your life.* New York: Pocket Books.

Seligman, M. E. P., Klien, D.C., and Miller, W.R. (1967). Depression. In *Handbook of behavior modification,* H. Leitenberg (ed). New York: Appleton-Century Crofts.

Seligman, M. E. P. (1975). *Helplessness: On depression, development and death.* San Francisco: W.H. Freeman.

Siperstein, G.N., and Bak, J. J. (1985). Effects of social behavior on children's attitudes toward their mildly and moderately handicapped peers. *American Journal of Mental Deficiency 90:* 319-27.

Snowdon, D. (2001). *Aging with grace: What the nun study teaches us about leading longer, healthier, and more meaningful lives.* New York: Bantam Dell Publishing Group.

Sovner, R. S. (1986). Limiting factors in the use of DSM-III criteria with mentally Ill/mentally retarded persons. *Psychopharmacological Bulletin 22:* 1055-59.

Sovner, R. S., and Hurley, A.D. (1993). Commentary: Psychotoform psychopathology. *Habilitative Mental Healthcare Newsletter 12:* 112.

Vygotsky, L. (1934/62). *Thought and language.* Cambridge, MA: MIT Press.
    (L. S. Vygotsky is the Russian psychologist credited with explaining how higher thought and our inner silent dialogues emerge from childhood's private speech or self-talk.)

Yapko, M. (1997). *Breaking the patterns of depression.* New York: Doubleday.

Index

Abilify. *See* Aripiprazole
Abstract reasoning, 173. *See also* Intellectual
    disability
Acceptance
    of Down syndrome by families, 107, 133, 135,
        229
    of Down syndrome by peers, 106
    of Down syndrome by the adult with DS, 133,
        227-30, 306
    steps in, 108
Acetylcholine, 243, 246, 402
Activity Schedules for Children with Autism, 379
Addendum, medication, 402-12
Adderall, 332
AD/HD, 180, 325-32, 366, 371
Adolescence, 169-70
Adolescents with Down syndrome. *See also* School
    AD/HD in, 180
    autism spectrum disorders in, 181
    bipolar disorder in, 181
    compulsive tendencies in, 174
    conflicts with parents, 171
    delays in teenaged behavior of, 53, 175-76
    depression in, 179, 180
    drive for independence in, 172-73
    physical and hormonal changes in, 171
    sensory problems in, 181
    Tourette syndrome in, 181
Adult Down Syndrome Center
    family counseling at, 231

history of, xi-xii
    mental health assessments at, 2
    most common mental health problems seen at,
        153
    people served by, 2
Adults with Down syndrome
    and awareness of own disability, 108-12
    as a minority, 106
    as caregivers, 31, 37, 132, 229, 397
    as self-advocates, 99
    expression of feelings and, 5
    identity problems of, 35-36
    oldest, 387
    pain tolerance of, 13
    premature aging of, 182, 185
    reasons not to regard as children, 184
    rights of, to self-determination, 123, 124, 126
    special problems of highly able, 97-98
    "super stars," 127
    typical cognitive characteristics of, 53-60, 61
    typical emotional characteristics of, 50-53
Advocate Lutheran General Hospital, xii
Advocate Medical Group, xii
Affection
    lack of, outside of family home, 130
    safe expression of, 131-32
    tendency of people with DS to express, 129
Afferent cell, 241, 242
Aging, of people with DS, 182, 185, 388
Agitation, 395, 407

Aggression. *See also* Bipolar disorder
    as clue to severity of mental health disorder, 333
    case stories involving, 206, 210, 324-25, 331
    dealing with extreme, 343-46
    medication for, 381
    role of serotonin in, 244
Alcoholism, 285
Alprazolam (Xanax), 265, 284, 353, 394, 402
Alzheimer disease
    activities for people with, 395-96
    age at occurrence, 27, 386
    and changes in the brain, 386, 387, 398
    behavioral and psychological changes in, 392-95
    case stories of patients who had symptoms of, 17, 37
    conditions that may be confused with, 388
    definition of, 385-86
    duration of, 398
    incidence of, 27, 386-87
    medications for, 247, 391, 393, 394, 395
    misdiagnosis of, xi, 385
    right environment for people with, 396-98
    research into, 398-99
    role of acetylcholine in, 243, 246
    role of glutamic acid in, 242, 246
    seizures and, 390, 391, 392, 398
    symptoms of, in adults with DS, 389-90
    tests for, 388-89
    treatment of, 391-95
Ambien. *See* Zolpidem
American Association of Mental Retardation Adaptive Behavior Scales, 235
Amitriptyline (Elavil), 262, 405
Amphetamine-dextroamphetamine (Adderall), 332, 412
Anafranil. *See* Clomipramine
Anaprox. *See* Naproxen
Anger, 341, 343-46. *See also* Aggression
Anorexia nervosa, 317
Anti-cholinergic side effects, 262, 312, 406, 413
Anticonvulsants, 273, 346-47, 354-55, 392, 407
Antidepressants, 262-64, 273, 347, 353-54, 393, 404. *See also* Tricyclic antidepressants; SSRIs
Antihistamines, 406
Anti-psychotics, 266-67, 295-96, 312, 347, 355, 371, 406, 407
Anti-seizure medications. *See* Anticonvulsants
Anxiety, normal, 277
Anxiety disorders. *See also* Obsessive-compulsive disorder; Grooves; Posttraumatic stress disorder
    agoraphobia, 280-83
    Alzheimer disease and, 394-95
    as co-morbid disorder with depression, 264-65

case studies involving, 279, 282, 284, 287-90, 353
counseling for, 287-90
distinguishing from medical problems, 284-86
generalized anxiety disorder, 278-80
medications for, 286-87
misdiagnosis of, 329
panic disorder, 283-84
phobias, 79
role of GABA in, 246
role of norepinephrine in, 243, 246
role of serotonin in, 244, 246
self-injury and, 350, 353
types of, 277
Appetite. *See* Eating refusal
Aricept. *See* Donepezil
Aripiprazole (Abilify), 266, 272, 295, 296, 312, 347, 355, 371, 381, 406
Arthritis, 12, 17, 18
Arranging items. *See* Grooves
Art therapy, 237
Assessment, for suspected mental illness
    difficulties encountered during, 205
    history from adult with DS and, 206-07
    history from caregivers and, 208-09
    lack of, in hospitals, 344
    multi-pronged approach to, 206
    observations and, 209-10
    standardized tools for, 235
Assessment, mental health
    areas assessed during, 3-7
    DSM criteria and, 6, 205
    goals of, 2
    results of, 7-8
    when to have, 1
    where to obtain, 2-3
Astrocytes, 243
Atarax. *See* Hydroxyzine
Atenolol (Tenormin), 408
Ativan. *See* Lorazepam
Atlanto-axial instability. *See* Cervical subluxation
Atomoxetine (Strattera), 332, 408
Attention, 243
Attention deficit disorders. *See* AD/HD
Autism spectrum disorders
    and questions about co-morbidity with DS, 373, 374
    diagnosis of, 377-78
    differences in, in people with DS, 374-77
    eating feces and, 356
    late diagnosis of, 374, 375
    misdiagnosis of, 329
    nature of, 373
    oppositional behavior and, 338
    in adolescents with DS, 181

self-injury and, 350
sensory issues and, 26
stereotypic behavior and, 359, 376
symptoms of, 375-77
treatment of, 378-82
Bathing, prolonged, 300
Behavior. *See also* AD/HD; Aggression; Psychotic
    behavior
  adolescent, 169-82
  as communication, 95-97, 101-02, 157-60,
    239-40, 324, 329
  assessing function of, 340
  changes in, in adults, 182-85
  changes in related to pain, 14, 95
  continuum of normal vs. abnormal, 46, 62-63
  "defiant" or "oppositional," 18, 161
  developmental age and, 46-47
  disorders, 333-38
  impulsive, 325, 346
  in-home support for, 381-82
  myth of "Down syndrome," xi, 48
  "psychotoform," 310
  reasons for problems with, 324
  recording history of, 209
  sexually inappropriate, 334, 335
  standardized assessments of, 98, 234, 235
  stereotypic, 357, 358-63
  teenaged, 53
  treatment for disorders of, 339-47
Benadryl. *See* Diphenhydramine
Benzodiazepines, 253, 265, 353, 403. *See also*
    under Specific types
Benztropine (Cogentin), 402
Bilodeau, Janet, 217
Bipolar disorder, 181, 251, 269-75, 328, 338
Birth control pills, 22, 409
Bladder problems, 18, 28. *See also* Incontinence
Blood, drawing, 355
Boardmaker™, 40
Brain. *See also* Neurotransmitters
  changes in, in Alzheimer disease, 386, 398
  differences in, in people with DS, 244-45
  nerve activity in, 154, 241
Brain chemicals. *See* Neurotransmitters
Breathing difficulties, 285. *See also* Panic disorder
Buddy Walk, 135
Bupropion (Wellbutrin), 264, 286, 287, 295, 327,
    332, 354, 404
Burke, Chris, 111, 132
Buspirone (Buspar), 286, 353, 402
Caffeine, 285
Calendars, 40, 195, 196
Capone, George, 373, 375
Carbamezepine (Tegretol), 251, 273, 346, 354,
    392, 407

Caregivers. *See also* Parents
  adults with DS as, 31, 37, 132, 229, 397
  as interpreters, 86-87
  changes in, 258
  questioning authority of, 337-38
Case managers, 216
Catapres. *See* Clonidine
Celebrities, obsessions with, 303
Celexa. *See* Citalopram
Celiac disease, 21, 28, 260
Central nervous system, 241
Cervical subluxation, 11, 17, 28
Changes, preparing for. *See* Transitions
Chicoine, Brian, xi
Childhood disintegrative disorder, 375
Chloral hydrate, 402
Chlorpromazine (Thorazine), 407
Choices, making own. *See* Self-determination
Choline, 262, 391, 393, 394
Cholineacetyl transferase, 245
Cholinesterase inhibitors, 410
Citalopram (Celexa), 263, 286, 296, 404.
    See also SSRIs
Clomipramine (Anafranil), 405
Clonazepam (Klonopin), 403
Clonidine (Catapres), 402
Clozapine (Clozaril), 312
Clothing, insistence on same, 158-59
Cogentin. *See* Benztropine
Cognex. *See* Tacrine
Cognitive abilities. *See* Intellectual disability
Cohen, Bill, 373
Communication. *See also* Language; Speech
  areas of difficulty in, 86
  behavior as, 95-97, 101-02, 157-60, 239-40,
    324, 329
  nonverbal, 87, 94-95
Co-morbid disorders, 257, 264-67
Compulsions, 292, 298-302. *See also* Grooves;
    Obsessive-compulsive disorder
Concerta, 327, 332, 412
Concrete thinking, 57-58, 66-67
Conduct disorder, 333-35, 338
Consent, patient, 248-49
Contraceptives, 245, 409
Coprolalia, 364
Counseling. *See also* Counselors
  behavior-changing, 221-22
  benefits of, 211-12
  bipolar disorder and, 273
  cognitive-behavioral approach to, 223-27
  confidentiality of, 217-18
  family, 231-34, 318
  for less verbal people, 235-36
  for patients with anxiety disorders, 287-90

insight oriented, 221
involvement of caregivers in, 218
monitoring progress related to, 234-35
paying for, 214
preserving boundaries in, 216-17
self-injury and, 352
social-learning approach to, 222-23
supportive, 219-20
to help adults accept own DS, 227-30
using pictures and memory in, 236-37
Counselors
    choosing right, 218-19
    conflicts of interest and, 216
    personal qualifications of, 215
    professional qualifications of, 212-15
    signs of bias in, 238-40
Cymbalta. *See* Duloxetine
Dangling items, 359
Day programs, 185, 186
Death, of family members, 34, 73, 184, 196.
        See also Grieving
Dementia, 387. *See also* Alzheimer disease
Denial, of medical problems, 28
Dennis Principle, 41-43
Dental concerns, 12, 19-20
Depakote/Depakene. *See* Valproic acid
Dependency, 413
Depression. *See also* Bipolar disorder; Grief
        response; Stress
    Alzheimer disease and, 393
    case studies of patients with, 10, 13-14, 17, 38,
        51-52, 120, 123, 190, 233, 251, 262, 265,
        304-05, 320
    causes of, 258-61
    co-morbid conditions and, 264-67
    counseling for, 224
    diagnosis of, 257-58
    due to difficulties communicating, 96, 97
    eating refusal and, 352, 353, 354
    fear of heights and, 15
    medications for, 251
    in adolescence, 179, 180
    incidence of, 255
    medical problems and, 259-61
    overly high expectations and, 42
    pain and, 14, 259
    psychotic features and, 257
    recurrence of, 264
    returning to work with, 232
    role of dopamine in, 245
    role of norephinephrine in, 245
    role of serotonin in, 244, 245-246, 259
    symptoms of, 256-57
    treatment of, 261-64
    vision changes and, 15

Depth perception, 15, 159
Desensitization, 282-83, 290
Desipramine (Norpramin), 393
Desyrel. *See* Trazodone
Developmental age, 46-47, 143, 164
Dexedrinem 332
Dexmethylphenidate (Focalin), 332
Dextroamphetamine (Dexedrine), 332, 412
Diabetes, 12, 19, 372
*Diagnostic and Statistical Manual of Mental
        Disorders. See* DSM-IV-TR
Diazepam (Valium), 265, 286, 403
Dilantin. *See* Phenytoin
Diphenhydramine (Benadryl), 394, 406
Directions, giving appropriate, 55
Disabilities, invisible, 106
Divorce, 52, 197
Doctors' visits, fear of, 280, 282
Donepezil (Aricept), 247, 391, 399, 410
Dopamine, 243, 245
Doors, opening or closing, 298-99
Down regulation, 253
Down syndrome. *See also* Adolescents with Down
        syndrome; Adults with Down syndrome
    clinics, 2
    mouse model for, 13
    telling person with DS about, 109-12
Doxepin (Sinequan), 262, 405
Drug abuse, 285
DSM-IV-TR
    behavior disorders in, 333
    criteria for generalized anxiety disorder, 278
    criteria for depression, 256
    criteria for panic disorder, 283
    difficulties in using with adults with DS, 6, 46,
        205
Dual diagnosis. *See* Autism spectrum disorder
Duloxetine (Cymbalta), 264, 404
Dying, fears about, 84
Dysthymia, 261
Eating refusal
    diagnosis of, 316-17
    examples of, 315
    medical problems and, 316-17
    triggers for, 315
    treatment for, 317-21, 408
Efferent cell, 241, 242
Effexor. *See* Venlafaxine
Elavil. *See* Amitryptiline
Emotions
    ability to express, 5, 28, 100
    AD/HD and, 326
    changing from negative to positive, 341
    difficulties expressing, 100-03, 206
    effect of conflict on, 51-53

effect of environment on, 50-51
expressing through drawing or writing, 207, 258
grief and, 53
guilt, 72
happiness, perpetual, 49
helping people with DS express, 102-03
range of, in people with DS, 49
sensitivity and empathy, 50-51, 173, 336
using body movements to express, 361
using self-talk to vent, 140
Employment. *See also* Dennis Principle
    as source of stress, 191
    at sheltered workshops, 120-21
    case studies involving, 38, 39, 49, 51, 59, 67,
        75, 101, 117, 118, 119, 120,182, 192, 239,
        282, 287
    conflicts, 54
    dissatisfaction with, 228
    importance of choosing appropriate, 38-39,
        98-99
    keys to success in, 117
    learning skills for at school, 115
    need for ongoing support with, 120-21
    retirement from, 185-86
    social skills training for, 118-20
    too much "down time" and, 362
    training for, 118
    trying out different types of, 117-18
    volunteering as alternative to, 39
Enclaves, 120
Endorphins, 244, 350, 355, 360
Endoscopy, 317
Entertaining self, 330-31
Erickson, Milton, 302
Escitalopram (Lexapro), 263, 264, 286, 296, 353,
    404. *See also* SSRIs
Estrogen, 245
Eszopiclone (Lunesta), 266, 347, 412
Exelon. *See* Rivastigmine
Expectations
    basing on developmental age, 47
    effects of, on independence, 41
    for people with DS and Tourette syndrome, 369
    too high, 97, 98-99, 113
    too low, xii, 113
Evaluation. *See* Assessment
Family. *See also* Parents
    counseling, 231-34
    effects of bipolar disorder on, 273-74
    importance of to people with DS, 29-30, 31
    overdependence on, 33
    role of in mental health assessments, 208-09
    separation from, 175
Fantasies, 142-46, 180, 258. *See also* Reality
Feces, eating, 355-56

Flashbacks, 77. *See also* Memory
Flexibility, 166. *See also* Grooves
Fluoxetine (Prozac), 263, 286, 405. *See also* SSRIs
Fluvoxamine (Luvox), 263, 405. *See also* SSRIs
Food, aversion to, 159. *See also* Eating refusal
Free time, difficulties with, 330-331
Friedman, Andrea, 132
Friendships. *See also* Imaginary friends; Social
        interactions
    affection and, 129-32
    lack of, 228
    peer programs to foster, 125
    with other people with disabilities, 35-36, 114,
        132-36
    with typically developing peers, 35, 133
Frontal lobe, 244
Functional behavior assessment (FBA), 340.
        See also Behavior, as communication
*Functional Behavior Assessment for People with
        Autism,* 340
Gabapentin (Neurontin), 347, 354-55, 392, 407
Gait problems, 390
Galantamine (Razadyne), 247, 391, 410
Gamma amino butyric acid (GABA), 242-43
Gastrointestinal problems, 12, 20-21
Generalization, 59-60
Geodon. *See* Ziprasidone
Get Out of My Life, 170
Glutamic acid (glutamate), 242
Grieving
    assisting with process of, 200-203
    delayed, 53, 73, 198
    right time for, 199
Grooves. *See also* Obsessive-compulsive disorder
    at work, 149
    benefits of, 148, 149
    biochemical basis of, 154, 157
    caregivers' response to, 296
    case studies involving, 147, 150-51, 152, 162,
        163, 225, 289, 321
    continuum of, 62, 154-55
    definition of, 61, 148
    disadvantages of, 151 53
    encouraging development of healthy, 161-67
    examples of types, 148-49
    incidence of, 148
    in older adults with DS, 183
    maladaptive, 153-54, 165
    misinterpretation of, 338
    ordering, 150
    overlap of, with OCD, 153, 155, 156, 293-94
    related to appearance, 149
    related to personal preferences, 150-51
    relaxing, 149
    stress and, 156-57

Grudges, 79-80
Guanfacine (Tenex), 402
Guardianship, 126, 218, 249, 250
Guilt, 72
Habits, bad, 157, 165. *See also* Grooves
Haldol. *See* Haloperidol
Hallucinations. *See* Psychotic behavior
Haloperidol (Haldol), 137, 266, 312, 407
Hand flapping, 358. *See also* Stereotypic behavior
Hand biting, 359, 360. *See also* Stereotypic behavior
Hand washing, 301
Hands, keeping busy, 302, 367
Happiness, myth of perpetual, 49
Hearing impairment, 11, 15-16, 26, 56, 261
Heart disease, 285
Hebein, Chris, 109, 201
Hebein, Sheila, 109, 201
Helplessness, 259. *See also* Learned helplessness
Hoarding, 152, 299, 335
Home, fear of leaving, 282-83. *See also* Residences
Hospitalization, 344-45
Howard, Jenny, 217
Hurrying, resistance to. *See* Slowing down
Hydroxyzine (Atarax), 406
Hyperactivity. *See also* AD/HD; Bipolar disorder; Mania
    misdiagnosis of, 328-29
    thyroid problems and, 20
Hyperthyroidism. *See* Thyroid
Hypothyroidism. *See* Thyroid
Hypoxemia, 285
Ibuprofen (Motrin), 411
Imaginary friends
    case stories involving, 145, 311
    normalcy of, 47
    obsessive-compulsive disorder and, 302, 303-04
Imipramine (Tofranil), 405
Incontinence, 17, 18, 19
Independence. *See also* Guardianship; Visual supports
    conflicts over "right" amount, 126
    Dennis Principle and, 41-43
    desire for, in adolescence, 172-73, 175
    effects of expectations on, 41
    effects of memory on, 70
    fostering, 39-43, 112-13
    right level of, 121-26, 177-79, 337-38
Inderal. *See* Propranolol
Inflexibility, 152. *See also* Grooves; Routines, insistence on
Insomnia, 264
Institute on Disability and Human Development, 384

Intellectual disability. *See also* Developmental age; Memory
    characteristics of, in DS, 53-60, 61
    concrete thinking and, 57-58, 66-67
    effects of, on understanding of illness, 27
Intelligibility. *See* Speech
International Classification of Diseases, 46
Inventory of Client and Agency Planning (ICAP), 235
IQ tests, 46, 213
Isolation, 33, 120, 133, 178, 180, 228, 333
Job coaches, 119, 120
Jobs. *See* Employment
Kennedy Krieger Institute, 383
Klonopin. *See* Clonazepam
Krantz, Patricia, 379
Kumin, Libby, 56
Lamictal. *See* Lamotrigine
Lamotrigine (Lamictal), 273, 347, 407
Language skills. *See also* Speech
    abstract vs. concrete, 59
    effects of hearing loss on, 16
    effects of on mental health, 4-5, 7
    effects of processing speed on, 54
    receptive, 95
    verb tenses and, 56, 76, 336
Learned helplessness, 113, 180, 190-91
Leshin, Len, 2
Lethargy, thyroid problems and, 20
Levinson, Daniel, 143
Lexapro. *See* Escitalopram
Librium, 403
Lights, turning off or on, 298
Listening
    importance of, 190
    reflective, 93
List making, 69
Lithium, 272, 410
Loneliness. *See* Friendships; Isolation
Lorazepam (Ativan), 265, 286, 394, 403
Love. *See* Affection
Luchterhand, Charlene, 198, 200
Lunesta. *See* Eszopiclone
Lutheran General Hospital, xi
Luvox. *See* Fluvoxamine
Lying, 336
Mania, 268-69, 273, 328. *See also* Bipolar disorder
Marital counseling, 234
McClannahan, Lynn, 379
McGuire, Dennis, xi, 41
Medical problems. *See* Physical health
Medications. *See also* Addendum, medication; under names of specific medications
    choosing, 250-52
    consent form for, 414
    deciding whether to try, 248

dependency on, 413
effects of, on neurotransmitters, 241-42
for challenging behaviors, 346-47
"hiding," 249
monitoring use of, 252-54
paradoxical reactions to, 252
patient involvement in use of, 248-50, 413
professionals who prescribe, 213-14
questions to ask doctor about, 254
response to previous, 208
side effects of, 12, 22, 251, 252, 253, 262
tics and, 371
tolerance and, 253
using multiple, 252
withdrawal and, 253, 413
Medlen, Joan, 373
Meetings, involving adult with DS in, 94
Megace. *See* Megestrol
Megestrol (Megace), 319, 408
Melatonin, 244, 266, 347, 354, 394, 411
Mellaril. *See* Thioridazine
Memantine (Namenda), 247, 391, 411
Memory. *See also* Posttraumatic stress disorder
  auditory, 71
  case studies involving, 65, 67, 68-69, 73, 336
  decline of, in old age, 182
  interpretation of, 74-75
  of high-interest facts, 69
  reliving, 71-72
  repeating, 72-77, 330
  strengths in Down syndrome, 68-71
  visual, 68-69
  visual-spatial, 69-70
  weaknesses in Down syndrome, 66-68, 71
  working, 66
Menstrual problems, 22
Mental health
  definition of, x
  expressive language and, 4-5
  pain and, 13-14
  physical health and, 7, 9-10
  social health and, 3-4
Mental health assessment. *See* Assessment,
    mental health
Mental illness. *See also* Counseling; Medication;
    Specific types of mental illness
  definition of, 187-88
  difficulties expressing emotions and, 5
  difficulties expressing discomfort and, 7
  grief as a cause of, 197-201
  incidence of, 188
  stress as a cause of, 189-97
  treatment of, 211
  types of, 188
Mental retardation. *See* Intellectual disability

Metabotropic glutamate receptor 5, 245
Medadate, 332
Methylphenidate (Ritalin, Concerta), 327, 332, 412
Mice, DS model, 13
Minority, people with DS as, 106
Mirtazapine (Remeron), 264, 404
Money, difficulties with, 99, 121
Mood disorders. *See* Bipolar disorder;
    Depression; Mania
Movements, repetitive. *See* Compulsions;
    Stereotypic behavior; Tics
Movies, 80-84, 143, 165, 180, 336
Music
  repetition of, 71
  therapy, 237
Musicals, 142
Naltrexone (ReVia), 355, 411
Namenda. *See* Memantine
Naproxen (Anaprox, Naprosyn), 411
National Association for Down Syndrome
    (NADS), xi, 383
Navane. *See* Thiothixene
Neatness, excessive. *See* Grooves
Neck vertebrae, 11
Neuroleptic malignant syndrome, 413
Neurons, 241, 244
Neurontin. *See* Gabapentin
Neurotransmitters
  differences in, in people with DS, 244-45
  effects of medications on, 241-42, 253
  function of, 241
  receptor proteins of, 245
  role of in anxiety, 246
  role of in depression, 245-46, 259
  role of in mental health disorders, 242
  types of, 242-44
Noncompliance. *See* Grooves; Oppositional
    behavior; Oppositional defiant disorder
Norepinephrine (noradrenaline), 243, 245, 246,
    404, 405
Nortriptyline (Pamelor), 262, 405
Nose blowing, 301, 302
Obsessional slowness, 306-07
Obsessions, 292, 302-05. *See also* Obsessive-
    compulsive disorder
Obsessive-compulsive disorder (OCD).
    See also Grooves
  Alzheimer disease and, 392-93
  case stories of patients with, 15, 294, 296-98,
    300, 303-04, 320, 365
  chemical differences in, in OCD, 154, 293
  common compulsions and, 298-302
  common obsessions and, 302-05
  definition of, 291-92
  diagnosis of, 293-94

eating refusal and, 317
family counseling and, 232
incidence of, 292
medical problems and, 300-301
medications for, 248, 295-96
misinterpretation of, 338
over-diagnosis of, 293
overlap of, with grooves, 153, 155, 156, 293-94
psychotic features and, 295
redirection and, 294-95
symptoms of, 292
Tourette syndrome and, 371
Occupational therapists, 160, 378
Olanzapine (Zyprexa), 266, 272, 295, 312, 319, 347, 355, 371, 381, 406
Omeprazole (Prilosec), 319
Opiates, 355
Opportunity, lack of, 191-92. *See also* Expectations
Oppositional behavior, 161-62. *See also* Grooves; Oppositional defiant disorder
Oppositional defiant disorder (ODD), 336-38
Orap. *See* Pimozide
Ordering, 298-99
Osteoarthritis. *See* Arthritis
Outbursts, unprovoked, 207. *See also* Aggression; Anger; Emotions
Oxazepam (Serax), 394, 403
Oxcarbazepine (Trileptal), 354, 407
"Pace," 306-07
Pain
causes of, 13
communicating, 13-14, 324
effects of on mental health, 11, 13-14, 259
self-injury and, 350-51
serotonin and, 244
signs of, 14
"stuck grooves" and, 158
tolerance of, 13
Pamelor. *See* Nortriptyline
Panic disorder, 283-84
Paradoxical reactions, 252
Paranoia, 395
Parents of adults with DS. *See also* Family
adults with DS as caregivers for, 31, 37
aging of, 36-37, 182-84
and ability to keep children active, 124, 125
as interpreters for their children, 86-87, 236
continued caregiver role of, 32
death of, 34, 73, 184
difficulties "letting go," 177
drawbacks of living with, 33, 124
"good enough," 112, 165
marital problems of, 52, 90-91, 197, 233
Paroxetine (Paxil), 263, 264, 286, 295, 319, 320, 353, 404. *See also* SSRIs

Patterson, Bonnie, 373
Paxil. *See* Paroxetine
Peers, desire to emulate, 179. *See also* Friendships
Peripheral nervous system, 241, 243
Phenytoin (Dilantin), 392
Phobias, 279, 280-83. *See also* Anxiety disorders
Photographs. *See* Pictures
Physical health
attitude toward, 27-28
relationship of to mental health, 7, 9-10
Physical health, assessment of
Alzheimer disease and, 27
arthritis and, 18
bladder problems and, 18-19
cervical subluxation and, 17
dental problems and, 19-20
diabetes and, 19
gastrointestinal problems and, 20-21
hearing and, 15-16
medication side effects and, 22
menstrual problems and, 22
overview of areas assessed, 11-12
pain and, 13-14
seizures and, 16-17
sensory issues and, 26-27
sleep disorders and, 23-25
thyroid problems and, 20
vision and, 14-15
when diagnosing anxiety disorders, 284-86
when diagnosing eating refusal, 316-17
when to have, 10
Physical restraint, 343
Pica, 356
Pictures
as reminders of positive events, 73, 78, 80, 226
as visual supports, 60
for communicating emotions, 351
using in counseling, 236-37
using to assist with grieving, 200-201
using to prepare for upcoming events, 195, 196
Pimozide (Orap), 371, 407
PMS. *See* Premenstrual syndrome
Police, 344
Posttraumatic stress disorder (PTSD), 77-78
Premature aging, 182, 185, 388
Premenstrual syndrome (PMS), 179, 409
Pretending. *See* Fantasies
Processing speed, 53-55, 380
Propranolol (Inderal), 408
Prozac. *See* Fluoxetine
Psychiatrists, 213. *See also* Counseling
Psychologists, 213. *See also* Counseling
Psychomotor retardation, 264
Psychotic behavior
as part of depression, 266-67

misdiagnosis of, 56, 61, 81, 309, 310-11
sleep apnea and, 24, 311
Psychotic disorders (psychoses)
    diagnosis of, 310-11
    symptoms of, 309-10
    treatment of, 311-12
    types of 309
Qualified Mental Retardation Professionals, 215
Quetiapine (Seroquel), 266, 272, 295, 312, 347,
    355, 371, 381, 406
Razadyne. See Galantamine
Reality, difficulties distinguishing, 80, 84, 143,
    146, 257, 336
Recreation, 36-37, 42, 70-71, 123
Redirection of behavior, 340-42, 352
Reiss Screen for Maladaptive Behavior, 235
Relaxation techniques, 288-90, 341
Religion, 203
Remeron. See Mirtazapine
Repetition, need for. See Groove; Routine
Residences. See also Dennis Principle
    as source of stress, 191
    case studies involving, 37, 42, 51-52, 90, 91,
        122, 123, 152, 183, 337
    fear of leaving, 282-83
    independence and, 121-26
    living at home, 31-32
    living away from home, 33-35
    planning for changes in, 184, 194
    staff turnover and, 34
Residential service agencies, 124
Resistance to change. See Grooves; Oppositional
    behavior
Respect, lack of, 178, 192-93
Restoril. See Temazepam
Restraint, physical, 343
Retirement, 185-86
ReVia. See Naltrexone
Reward systems, 339
Rigidity. See Routines, insistence on
Risperdal. See Risperdone
Risperdone (Risperdal), 137, 266, 267, 272, 295,
    303, 312, 347, 355, 371, 381, 406
Ritalin, 332, 412
Rivastigmine (Exelon), 247, 391, 410
Rocking, 358, 359, 361. See also Stereotypic
    behavior
Roommates, 191, 223, 351
Routines. See also Grooves
    difficulty functioning without, 330-31
    for people with DS and autism, 378-79
    insistence on, 299-301
Rubbing stones, 290, 353, 363
Safety concerns, 40-41, 126, 130, 178.
    See also Independence

Sameness. See Groove
Scales for Independent Behavior (SIB), 235
Schedules, 40, 42, 60, 379
School
    case studies involving, 54, 59, 144, 331-32, 365
    competence in, 113-15
    needing extra time for routines at, 163-64
    postsecondary programs, 115-16
    socialization at, 125
Sedation, as side effect, 251, 262, 264, 406
Seizures, 11, 16-17, 325, 358, 390, 391, 392, 398
Selective Serotonin Reuptake Inhibiters. See SSRIs
Self-advocacy, 99, 135
Self-determination, 123, 124, 126
Self-esteem
    and acceptance of DS, 107, 227-30
    awareness and, 108-12
    benefits of, 105
    competence and, 112-29
    keys to promoting, 136
    role of love and friendship in, 129-36
    role of talents and gifts in, 127-29
Self-injury
    as communication, 349, 351-52
    case stories involving, 51, 351, 352, 353
    causes of, 350-52
    definition of, 349
    related to anxiety, 279, 287
    related to "stuck grooves," 160
    role of endorphins in, 244, 350, 355
    sleep disorders and, 354
    stereotypic behavior and, 359, 360
    Tourette syndrome and 367
    treatment of, 352-55
Self-modeling, 222
Self-redirection, 341-42, 352
Self-talk
    among older persons, 139
    case studies involving, 81, 100, 139, 144, 225,
        267, 310, 311, 342
    changing negative, 224, 225
    desirability of eliminating, 62-63
    incidence of, 61, 137, 138
    internalizing, 139
    misdiagnosis of, 61, 137
    normalcy in children, 138
    problematic, 140-42
    reasons for, 138
    related to depression, 266
    to direct behavior, 138-39, 342
    to entertain oneself, 140
    to vent emotions, 140
Seligiline (Eldepryl), 391
Sensory issues, 26-27, 158-60, 181, 333, 376-77, 378
Serax. See Oxazepam

Seroquel. *See* Quetiapine
Serotonin. *See also* SSRIs
  and connection to melatonin, 244
  in people with DS, 244
  role of in mental health, 244
  role of in anxiety, 246
  role of in depression, 245-46, 259
  role of in obsessive-compulsive disorder
  role of in producing grooves, 154
SERT, 244
Sertraline (Zoloft), 251, 263, 265, 267, 284, 286,
    295, 303, 405. *See also* SSRIs
Sexual abuse, 131, 160, 225, 226, 334
Showering, prolonged, 300
Shyness, 135
Siblings
  case stories involving, 79-80
  comparisons with, 230
  moving out of home, 193, 331
Side effects, medication. *See also* Addendum,
    medication
  agitation, 263
  anti-cholinergic, 262, 393, 394
  changes in appetite/weight, 263, 264, 319, 355
  increase of in Alzheimer disease, 392
  increased risk of suicide, 263
  of antidepressants, 262-64
  of anti-psychotics, 266, 355, 395
  of stimulants, 332
  sedation, 251, 262
Sinequan. *See* Doxepin
Sleep, levels of norepinephrine during, 243
Sleep disorders. *See also* Sedation
  Alzheimer disease and, 393-94
  apnea, 12, 23-24, 260, 284-85, 354
  effect of routines on, 25
  hypopnea, 25
  insomnia, 264
  medication and, 265-66, 347, 354
  restless, fragmented sleep, 25
Slowing down
  as avoidance tactic, 160, 164
  in retirement, 185
  obsessional slowness and, 306-07
  using video to stop, 223
  when rushed, 152
  with age, 182
Social interactions. *See also* Family; Friendships
  among institutionalized people, 3-4
  families' role in promoting, 124-25, 133-36
  importance of, 4
  obsessive, 304-05
Social skills
  importance of at work, 118-20
  in people with DS and autism, 375

Social Stories, 379
Social workers, 4, 212
Sociopaths, 334
Sonata, *See* Zalepion
Special Olympics, 133
Speech. *See also* Language; Self-talk
  as indication of competence, 97-98
  effects of donepezil on, 247
  intelligibility of, 85-86
  interpreting, 86-89
  lack of, 94-97, 235-36
  reluctance to use, 88-91
  using in a group, 91-94
SSRIs
  anxiety and, 246, 286
  depression and, 246, 262-63
  effects of, on brain, 246
  obsessive-compulsive disorder and, 295-96
  side effects of, 405
  types of, 246, 405
Staff, residential
  as counselors, 216
  turnover of, 34, 258
Stairs, 159
Stealing, 335-36
Stelazine. *See* Trifluoperazine
Stereotypic behavior, 357, 358-63
Stimulant medications, 328, 332, 366
Strattera. *See* Atomoxetine
Stress
  and maladaptive grooves, 156-57, 160
  as precipitant of mental illness, 189, 258-59, 345
  conflicts as cause of, 232-33
  hyperactivity in response to, 329
  inflexibility and, 102, 300
  stereotypic behavior and, 362
Stubbornness. *See* Grooves; Oppositional
  behavior
Suicidal gestures, 180, 352
Supervision, right level of, 164, 165. *See also*
    Independence
Swallowing
  difficulties, in Alzheimer disease, 390
  therapy, 318-19
Synapses, 241
Tacrine (Cognex), 247, 391, 410
Tactile defensiveness, 15
Talking to self. *See* Self-talk
Tantrums. *See* Anger; Aggression; Emotions
Tardive dyskinesia, 251, 266, 296, 312
Teasing, 178, 192-93
Teeth. *See* Dental concerns
Tegretol. *See* Carbamezepine
Television, 80-84, 336. *See also* Movies
Temazepam (Restoril), 403

Temperament, 153-54
Temporal lobe, 244
Tenex. *See* Guanfacine
Tenormin. *See* Atenolol
Therapy. *See* Counseling
Thioridazine (Mellaril), 266, 312, 407
Thiothixene (Navane), 287, 312, 407
Thomas Center for Down Syndrome, 383
Thorazine. *See* Chlorpromazine
Thunderstorms, 278, 280
Thyroid
  medications, 412
  underactive, 12, 20, 223, 260, 294
  overactive, 12, 20, 269, 284, 319
Tic disorders, 363. *See also* Tourette syndrome
Tics
  definition of, 363
  in Tourette syndrome, 363-65
  medications that may trigger, 371
  misinterpretation of, 338, 370
Time concepts, difficulties with, 55-57, 71-72, 76, 198, 336
To Kill a Mockingbird, 2
Tofranil. *See* Imipramine
Tolerance, medication, 253
Tourette syndrome
  case studies involving, 364, 365-66, 368, 370-71
  compared to stereotypic behavior, 367
  definition of, 363
  medications for, 370-71
  misinterpretation of, 338, 370
  responding to tics, 368-70
  symptoms of, 364-65
  treatment of, 366-68
Transitions, 195-96, 379
Trazodone (Desyrel), 264, 265, 347, 354, 404
Tricylic antidepressants, 405
Trifluoperazine (Stelazine), 407
Trileptal. *See* Oxcarbazepine
Tryptophan, 243
"Two Syndromes," xii-xiii
Upregulation, 253
Urinary tract problems, 11, 19
Valium. *See* Diazepam
Valproic acid (Depakote, Depakene), 273, 346, 354, 392, 407
Venlafaxine (Effexor), 264, 286, 296, 353, 354, 404
Verb tenses, 56, 76, 336
Videos, using to change behavior, 223. *See also* Movies
Vision impairment, 11, 14-15, 261, 355
Visual supports, 32, 55, 60. *See also* Schedules
Vitamin B6, 22
Vitamin B12, 21-22
Vitamin E, 22, 391
Volunteer work, 39, 135
Weather, anxiety about, 79, 278, 279, 281
Weight problems. *See also* Eating refusal
  celiac disease and, 28
  diabetes and, 19
  due to lack of activity, 123, 124
  overactive thyroid and, 20
  sleep apnea and, 24
  slower metabolism and, 124
Wellbutrin. *See* Bupropion
Withdrawal (medication), 253, 413
Withdrawing. *See* Depression; Isolation
Wolf, Anthony, 170
Work. *See* Employment
Workshops, sheltered, 120-21
Worry stones, 290, 353, 363
Xanax. *See* Alprazolam
Zaleplon (Sonata), 266, 347, 412
Ziprasidone (Geodon), 251, 266, 272, 295, 296, 312, 347, 355, 381, 406
Zoloft. *See* Sertraline
Zolpidem (Ambien), 266, 347, 412
Zyprexa. *See* Olanzapine

About the Authors

· · · · · · · · · · · · · · · · ·

Dennis McGuire, Ph.D., is the Director of Psychosocial Services for the Adult Down Syndrome Center of Lutheran General Hospital in suburban Chicago. **Brian Chicoine, M.D.,** is the medical director of the Adult Down Syndrome Center. Together they founded The Center in 1992 and have served nearly 3,000 adults with Down syndrome since its inception. Both authors have made numerous presentations to parent and professional audiences about their work at The Center.

Dennis McGuire received his Masters degree from the University of Chicago and his doctorate from the University of Illinois at Chicago. He has worked for more than 29 years in the fields of mental health and developmental disabilities. He lives in Oak Park, Illinois, with his wife and son.

Brian Chicoine received his medical degree from Loyola University in Chicago from the Stritch School of Medicine. He did his residency at the Lutheran General Hospital Department of Family Medicine in Park Ridge, Illinois, where he currently works. Dr. Chicoine has spent nearly 30 years working with people with intellectual disabilities in a variety of capacities. The father of three, he lives with his family in Arlington Heights, Illinois.